From the days of Hippocratic 'bedside medicine' to the advent of the CAT scanner, doctors have always relied on their senses in diagnosing and treating disease. Medical education, from the apprenticeship to the birth of the clinic and the rise of the laboratory, has sought to train the senses of students who must act subsequently like medical detectives. At the same time, debate since antiquity has pondered the relative hierarchy of the senses – from noble vision to baser touch and smell. From the rise of medical and, particularly, anatomical illustration at the Renaissance, doctors have been concerned about the relationship between image and reality.

This richly illustrated collection of essays explores many facets of these themes. They range widely over time and space and shed much new light on medical perceptions and the cultural dimensions of the healing arts.

Medicine and the five senses

Medicine and the five senses

Edited by

W. F. BYNUM AND ROY PORTER

Wellcome Institute for the History of Medicine

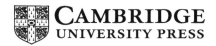

CAMBRIDGE
UNIVERSITY PRESS

PUBLISHED BY THE PRESS SYNDICATE OF THE UNIVERSITY OF CAMBRIDGE
The Pitt Building, Trumpington Street, Cambridge, United Kingdom

CAMBRIDGE UNIVERSITY PRESS
The Edinburgh Building, Cambridge CB2 2RU, UK
40 West 20th Street, New York NY 10011–4211, USA
477 Williamstown Road, Port Melbourne, VIC 3207, Australia
Ruiz de Alarcón 13, 28014 Madrid, Spain
Dock House, The Waterfront, Cape Town 8001, South Africa

http://www.cambridge.org

First published 1993
First paperback edition 2004

A catalogue record for this book is available from the British Library

Library of Congress cataloguing in publication data

Medicine and the five senses / edited by W. F. Bynum and Roy Porter.
     p.   cm.
Based on a Symposium on Medicine and the Five Senses, held at the
Wellcome Institute for the History of Medicine on 11–12 June 1987.
Includes index.
ISBN 0 521 36114 1 (hardback)
1. Medicine – History – Congresses. 2. Senses and sensation – History – Congresses.
3. Diagnosis, Physical – History – Congresses.
I. Bynum, W. F. (William F.), 1943– . II. Porter, Roy, 1946– · III. Symposium on
Medicine and the Five Senses (1987: Wellcome Institute for the History of Medicine)
[DNLM: 1. History of Medicine – congresses.   2. Sensation – congresses.
3. Sense Organs – congresses.   WL 700 M489 1987]
R1313.A2M44   1992
610′.9 – dc20   91–36282   CIP

ISBN 0 521 36114 1 hardback
ISBN 0 521 61198 9 paperback

Contents

Illustrations

Contributors

MERRILEY BORELL is a consultant working with nonprofit organizations in the San Francisco Bay Area. She is author of *The Biological Sciences in the Twentieth Century* (1989) and numerous articles on the history of nineteenth- and twentieth-century medical science. She has taught history of medicine and science at the University of California at Berkeley, the University of Edinburgh, Harvard University and, most recently, Stanford University.

GERT BRIEGER is William H. Welch Professor and Director of the Institute of the History of Medicine, the Johns Hopkins University. He has worked mainly on American medicine, public health, and surgery of the nineteenth and twentieth centuries. He is presently completing a book on the history of premedical education in America.

LAURENCE BROCKLISS is Fellow and Tutor in Modern History at Magdalen College, Oxford. He works on the social and intellectual history of early-modern France, with particular reference to problems of cultural transmission. He is the author of *French Higher Education in the Seventeenth and Eighteenth Centuries: A Cultural History* (1987) and he is the editor of the international journal *History of Universities*. At present, he is nearing the completion of a study of the early-modern French medical profession, co-authored with Colin Jones of Exeter University.

JEROME BYLEBYL is Associate Professor of the History of Medicine at the Johns Hopkins University and a co-editor of the *Bulletin of the History of Medicine*. His research has focused mainly on the history of medicine and physiology from antiquity to the seventeenth century, and he has published widely on William Harvey and the early history of clinical teaching.

W. F. BYNUM is Head of the Academic Unit at the Wellcome Institute for the History of Medicine and Professor of the History of Medicine at University College London. He has published widely on many aspects of the biomedical and life sciences since the seventeenth century and, with Roy Porter, is general editor of the Wellcome Institute Series in the History of Medicine.

SANDER GILMAN is the Goldwin Smith Professor of Humane Studies at Cornell University and Professor of the History of Psychiatry at the Cornell Medical College. During 1990–91 he served as the Visiting Historical Scholar at the National Library of Medicine, Bethesda, Maryland. A member of the Cornell faculty since 1969, he is an intellectual and literary historian and the author or editor of over twenty-seven books, the most recent being *Sexuality: An Illustrated History* (1989). He is the author of the basic study of the visual stereotyping of the mentally ill, *Seeing the Insane* (1982).

LUDMILLA JORDANOVA is Professor of History at the University of Essex. Her research interests include the relationships between the biomedical sciences and the visual arts, and the history of the family. Her publications include *Lamarck* (1984) and *Languages of Nature* (1986, editor and contributor).

MARTIN KEMP is Professor of the History and Theory of Art at the University of St Andrews and Honorary Professor of History at the Royal Scottish Academy. He is the author of *Leonardo da Vinci: The Marvellous Works of Nature and Man* (1981) and *The Science of Art: Optical Themes in Western Art from Brunelleschi to Seurat* (1991). He has edited Dr William Hunter's anatomy lectures to the Royal Academy of Arts.

SUSAN C. LAWRENCE is Assistant Professor in the Department of History and Medical Historian in the College of Medicine at The University of Iowa. Among her publications is 'Private enterprise and public interests: medical education and the Apothecaries' Act, 1780–1825', in *British Medicine in the Age of Reform* (1991). She is currently working on her book *Charitable Knowledge: Hospital Practitioners and Pupils in Eighteenth-Century London*.

MALCOLM NICOLSON is Research Fellow at the Wellcome Unit for the History of Medicine, University of Glasgow. He works on a number of topics in the history and sociology of eighteenth- and twentieth-century medicine and science. He is currently engaged with Dr David Smith in a study of the 'Glasgow School' of chemical physiology. His recent publications include 'Henry Allan Gleason and the individualistic hypothesis: the structure of a botanist's career', in *Botanical Review* (1990) and 'The social and the cognitive: resources for the sociology of scientific knowledge', in *Studies in the History and Philosophy of Science* (1991).

VIVIAN NUTTON was formerly a Fellow of Selwyn College, Cambridge. Since 1977 he has been at the Wellcome Institute for the History of Medicine as Senior Lecturer. He specializes in the history of the Graeco-Roman medical tradition and his books include *From Democedes to Harvey* (1979) and *Galen: On Prognosis* (1988). He has been joint editor, with W. F. Bynum, of *Medical History* since 1980.

RICHARD PALMER. Until his recent appointment as Librarian and Archivist of Lambeth Palace Library, Richard Palmer spent eleven years at the Wellcome Institute for the History of Medicine as a post-doctoral research fellow and subsequently as Curator of Western Manuscripts. His field of research is the history of medicine in Renaissance Italy, especially the Republic of Venice.

ROY PORTER is Reader in the Social History of Medicine at the Wellcome Institute for the History of Medicine. He is currently working on the history of hysteria. Recent books include *Mind Forg'd Manacles: Madness in England from the Restoration to the Regency* (1987), *A Social History of Madness* (1987), *In Sickness and in Health: The British Experience, 1650–1850* (1988), *Patient's Progress* (1989) – these last two co-authored with Dorothy Porter, and *Health for Sale: Quackery in England 1660–1850* (1989).

STANLEY J. REISER is the Griff T. Ross Professor of Humanities and Technology in Health Care at the University of Texas Health Science Center at Houston. His recent publications include *The Machine at the Bedside: Strategies for Using Technology in Patient Care* (1984) and *Divided Staffs, Divided Selves: A Case Approach to Mental Health Ethics* (1987).

ELIZABETH SEARS is Assistant Professor in the Department of the History of Art at the University of Michigan, Ann Arbor. She has held fellowships at the Warburg Institute, the Wellcome Institute for the History of Medicine and Magdalen College, Oxford. She is the author of *The Ages of Man: Medieval Interpretations of the Life Cycle* (1986).

Acknowledgements

This volume is the result of the Symposium on Medicine and the Five Senses held at the Wellcome Institute for the History of Medicine on 11–12 June 1987 with the generous support of the Wellcome Trustees. The editors are grateful to the authors for their forbearance during a protracted preparation of the manuscript and to William Davies and Richard Ziemacki of Cambridge University Press for their patient courtesy. Caroline Prentice provided sterling assistance with the illustrations. The secretarial and administrative assistance of Frieda Houser, Betty Kingston and, latterly, Sally Bragg has been cheerful and efficient. Chris Doubleday's work at the copy-editing stage has been outstanding.

Introduction

> So much is human genius limited, by the limits of human nature, that
> we just know what our five senses teach.
>
> Thomas Sydenham, *Works*, Vol. II, p. 182.

'Nihil est in intellectu quod non prius in sensu' runs the old Latin saying. It was a commonplace long before Sydenham reflected on the limits of our senses, or his friend the physician-philosopher John Locke (1632–1704) placed them squarely at the heart of his theory of knowledge. Even St Augustine (354–430), whose *Confessions* fretted about the dangers of the sensual world, repeated the ancient maxim that the organs of sense are 'the body's gateways to the mind'. For Augustine, sight 'is the principal sense by which knowledge is acquired', sound something to be enthralled by, smell, taste and touch created by God and thereby to be cherished. Man's highest duty and joy – the love of God – is a kind of internalized sense experience:

But what do I love when I love my God? Not material beauty or beauty of a temporal order; not the brilliance of earthly light, so welcome to our eyes; not the sweet melody of harmony and song; not the fragrance of flowers, perfumes, and spices; not manna or honey; not limbs such as the body delights to embrace. It is not these that I love when I love my God. And yet, when I love him, it is true that I love a light of a certain kind, a voice, a perfume, a food, an embrace; but they are of a kind that I love in my inner self, when my soul is bathed in light that is not bound by space; when it listens to sound that never dies away; when it breathes fragrance that is not borne away on the wind; when it tastes food that is never consumed by the eating; when it clings to an embrace from which it is not severed by fulfilment of desire. This is what I love when I love my God.[1]

If Augustine could not describe the love of God without recourse to the senses, it is little wonder that the history of a more mundane subject like medicine is rich with reflections on, and concern with, the body's gateways. As a practical activity, medicine requires its votaries to rely on their senses to come to diagnostic judgements which in turn dictate therapeutic recommendations. As members of a learned profession, doctors are forced to ponder on the relationship between sensations and reality. As speculators, observers, or as experimentalists, doctors may seek to understand just how the five senses work. As students they are taught how to use their senses and, detective-like, to interpret the clues they have picked up. As a cultural phenomenon, medicine is portrayed in a variety of ways, and through a variety of subjects, ranging from anatomical preparations to scenes of triumph effected by self-conscious and confident individuals. The history of medicine embraces ample portions of both sense and sensibility.

A volume with the title of the present one could have any of several principal themes: the history of sensory physiology; the development of physical diagnosis; the varieties and aims of medical education; medicine in its cultural manifestations. The essays touch on them all, although sensory physiology as a special subject emerges only tangentially, and that only in its classical formulations.[2] Rather, through a series of case studies, diagnosis, education, and cultural and anatomical representation predominate. Although the essays are arranged chronologically, two subsidiary themes run through several of them. The first is the traditional preoccupation with the hierarchy of the senses: which is the noblest sense and which the basest, and why? The palm was traditionally given to sight, a decision with which Denis Diderot (1713–84) agreed, as he speculated how differently a race of blind men would conceptualize the world.[3] Not for nothing are our eyes near the top of our heads, nearest to heaven and not far away from the other noble sense organ, the ears. There was less consensus over the ordering of the other senses, but St Augustine was not alone in feeling that somehow touch was the most seductive and therefore perhaps the basest. The essay of Elizabeth Sears examines some of the classical reflections on these matters, along with the iconography of the senses and their relation to the castle of the mind. Richard Palmer singles out smell – generally accorded a middle rank in the hierarchy – for closer scrutiny.

Running through many of the essays is a second preoccupation, which might be described as the nature of the castle: how do the faculties of the mind convert the raw data of the senses into something like coherence? Within the medical context, how do reason and judgement work at the bedside? In emphasizing bedside experience, the Hippocratic tradition provided an observational model for medicine which could still be invoked as a living force in early nineteenth-century Paris, when the French capital was the Mecca of the medical world.[4] Indeed, one recent reading of the whole of medical history has it as the history of tensions between empirical and rationalist traditions, between doctors who value experience and those who bow to authority and (in this particular account) reason.[5] While the essays in this volume may be more modest in their scope, and maybe even more cautious in their generalizations, several of them expose the weight of tradition and focus on the experiential within the context of the written word.

Reason can be described as the sixth sense, and even someone like Elisha Bartlett (1804–55), that ardent exponent of observational facts as the sole hope for medical progress, would have conceded that there was a mind collecting those facts.[6] Even among enthusiastic empiricists like Bartlett, however, collective experience also counted for much; tradition is inevitable and one of the functions of medical education is to induct the student into the values of one or another philosophy of medicine.

Several of the essays examine aspects of the broad themes of education, tradition and experience. Although Galen may have himself been, as Nutton argues, a medical detective, he was also an inveterate scribbler whose writings provided the touchstone of experience for thirty or forty generations of doctors. Bylebyl and Brockliss look at two episodes in the long history of Galenism. Eighteenth- and early nineteenth-century doctors may have seen the 'birth of the clinic' as the contemporary recovery of a historical ideal.[7] That ideal was Hippocratic rather than Galenic, although this may mean, as Brockliss points out, that there was more than one kind of Galenism, or at the very least, that Galenism could be commandeered into a multitude of services. As part of its bad historical press, Galenism can be seen as the bastion of those who valued reason over experience, authority over the testimony of the senses. In early seventeenth-century Paris, those who wanted to expunge the magical and the occult from medicine, who did not want to believe what they could not see, could also nestle in the wings of Galenism.

On the other hand, to teach 'Galenism' was often to teach the Word, even, ironically, in the Renaissance clinic. Bylebyl's own detective story began with historical claims made in the later age of Hippocratism, with the 'discovery' in 1808 by Giovanni Rasori that Giovanni Battista da Monte had taught clinical medicine in the mid-sixteenth century, long before French doctors in the age of Bichat and Laënnec had elevated it to the be-all and end-all of medicine.

On closer scrutiny, however, da Monte can be revealed as running a Renaissance clinic, not a proto-Napoleonic one; as using the bedside to expound the tenets of Galenism. In ways that the historical Galen would have appreciated, this did not mean a disparagement of the senses. On the contrary, da Monte urged his pupils to use their senses to 'take in those signs which are manifestly apparent, from which you will afterward perceive those things that are hidden within'.

The steps from the individual to the universal were different for da Monte and his successors three centuries later, but, as Susan Lawrence demonstrates, pedagogical rhetoric has continuity as well as change. Her examination of medical teaching and learning in London between about 1750 and 1820 rests on a systematic analysis of a tangible by-product of education – student notes.

In an age when relatively few textbooks existed, and when entrepreneurial teachers were reluctant to publish the contents of their lectures for fear that student numbers would decline, much care was often lavished on the notes, as a permanent record of the student's encounter with the subject. In 1794, French medical reformers wanted their students to 'Read little, see much, do much.'[8] Independently, London teachers were impressing upon their own students the importance of active engagement with all their senses as they learned to infer the internal diseases from the external appearances.

During the course of the nineteenth century, new methods of visualizing, including photography, and new ways of recording especially the 'graphic method', reinforced traditional reliance on sight, and, as Merriley Borell explores, placed new demands on medical education, as an increasingly powerful science lobby stressed that technology was a permanent feature of both practice and research, and that the new practical physiology could bridge the gap between science and practice, laboratory and clinic.

The meanings and the methods might change, but it is hard to escape the conclusion that creating medical detectives has long been high on the list of educational priorities. Inevitably, this centres around the bedside or consulting room, in the doctor–patient encounter. Several of the essays take aspects of physical diagnosis as their theme, with as much emphasis on the physical as on the diagnosis. Nutton, Jordanova, Nicolson and Reiser present case studies widely separated in time and space, but linked by a common diagnostic thread. Nutton reveals Galen as the rather brash and aggressive character which he undoubtedly was, but also as a shrewd Sherlock Holmes before his time, conscious of Hippocratic precedents but equally aware of his own diagnostic acumen. As a good Holmesian, he could throw all his senses into the chase, but vision remained foremost, as it was of course in the physiognomical tradition, some of whose medical reverberations are considered by Jordanova. While recognizing the subtle interactions between artistic and medical convention within physiognomy, she seeks to extend the conventional reading of physiognomy after Lavater as simply a series of footnotes to him, by contextualizing two medical theses on the subject.

Despite frequent lip-service to sight, hearing – in the form of history-taking, and of listening to the patient's complaint – had (and has) an honourable place in the doctor-patient encounter. With the publication of Laënnec's monograph on mediate auscultation in 1819, new, esoteric demands could be placed on a doctor's hearing. Nicolson's careful study of the introduction of the stethoscope and auscultation into Edinburgh medicine looks at the interplay of cultural tradition and reaction to innovation. John Harley Warner's recent work has already shown how selective the importation of medical knowledge and practice can be.[9] Nicolson in turn reinforces Warner's insight by scrutinizing the Scottish response to French innovation.

In our own century, technology has not obliterated the central cultural meaning which the stethoscope has come to have for medicine; but technology has immeasurably extended the doctor's senses and threatened, perhaps, the old-fashioned virtues of bedside diagnosis. Reiser's essay dissects two facets of this complicated story: the problems that develop when technological relations compete with and threaten to displace human relations, and the way in which the coming of the machine has placed new demands on the organization of medical institutions and created new hierarchies within the profession.

Physical diagnosis is physical, however, and its emergence as an indispensable feature of modern medicine has produced its own set of issues. In earlier times, doctors looked at tongues and felt pulses, but the doctor–patient encounter would not routinely involve anything more intimate than could be experienced in ordinary social intercourse. When seeing and touching extended to intimate areas of the body, and especially when the patient was female, new social strategies had to be adopted to desexualize a potentially charged situation. Porter's essay exposes aspects of etiquette and convention during the past couple of centuries. Even before the diagnostic ideals of the French made routine the inspection, palpation, percussion and auscultation which every medical student learns, the rise of male-midwifery had generated debate both within the medical establishment and in lay circles more generally. As Porter points out, notions of class as well as sex were at issue; although Queen Victoria had a male accoucheur, her trusted physician Sir James Reid did not know she had an umbilical hernia until after her death.

'Touching' is a loaded word, as both Porter's and Gilman's essays make clear. Gilman opens up the larger questions of the iconography and anthropology of touch, sexuality and disease, as his wide-ranging and provocative essay juxtaposes blackness and the infant Christ, the signs of the zodiac and what it means to be touched by AIDS.

Finally, the iconographic is central to the essays of Sears, Kemp and Brieger. Sears and Kemp bring to their subjects the skills and perspectives of the art historian. Through a consideration of the library of Richard of Fournival, Sears offers a reading of the senses within the classical tradition, and its assimilation by the Christians of a later age. Kemp's concern is more explicitly medical, viz. anatomical illustration from the Renaissance to the eighteenth century, as anatomists and their artists sought to depict structure 'as it really is', while at the same time exploring new media and modes of representation. Some of the high art of the period may be found in anatomical monographs and musings, as Kemp's other work on Leonardo and William Hunter has superbly demonstrated.[10]

William Hunter (1718–83) was one of the most enterprising anatomy teachers of the eighteenth century, but he was also a man of culture, a connoisseur who rubbed shoulders with literary and artistic elites (and delivered babies of royalty and the aristocracy).[11] Questions of sensibility and of artistic representation are central to Brieger's essay on two monumental canvasses which depicted two eminent surgeons in late nineteenth-century America. Thomas Eakins's *The Gross Clinic* (1875) and *The Agnew Clinic* (1889) now occupy familiar positions in the heroic iconography of modern medicine. Brieger examines both the circumstances of their composition and reception, and the ways in which 'conservative', or sensitive surgery was a product of post-Listerian surgical practice.

The essays in this volume hardly exhaust the subject. Rather, they demonstrate how inexhaustible it is; at the same time reminding us how central medical concerns can be to many varieties of historical inquiry.

1

Galen at the bedside: the methods of a medical detective

VIVIAN NUTTON

To begin a volume on the five senses in medicine with the Greeks needs no justification. The Western tradition of medical diagnosis depends very largely on principles first enunciated by them over two millennia ago, and it is only the technological revolution of this century that has brought about a substantial change in the methods of diagnosis. Although there were instruments for investigating some of the internal arrangements or malfunctions of the body even in classical antiquity – probes and, occasionally, an elaborate vaginal speculum[1] – what was taking place within the body could, in general, only be deduced from external phenomena, a situation that, in essence, remained true until the nineteenth century. Hence, an understanding of the condition of the sick patient could be gained only through a perception of the external 'happenings' – that is the direct translation of the Greek word 'symptom' – that, in some way or other, manifested themselves to the observer. How these perceptions were to be interpreted was a matter of considerable controversy among what later became known as the medical sects, but there was universal agreement on the supreme importance for diagnosis of what the doctor could perceive.[2]

But if this tradition can be traced directly back to the Greeks, it might be thought more appropriate to devote the first pages to the great Hippocrates. After all, it is in the *Epidemics* and in *Prognostic*, texts which were long presumed to have been written by the famous Coan physician himself, that one finds exemplary reports of detailed investigations of symptoms.[3] *Prognostic* contains a substantial list of symptoms that the doctor should note and which will enable him both to diagnose the past and to foretell the future course of an illness, both of which were subsumed under the same heading of prognosis.[4] *Epidemics*, by contrast, does not prescribe for the doctor what he should look for, or how he should interpret his findings, but is rather, so most Hippocratic scholars are agreed, the record of case notes collected by physicians during visits (*epidemiae*), notes presumably of what they thought most significant.[5] These notes, of which those in Books I and III are by far the most celebrated, report not only on an individual patient, his temperature, his various excretions, principally of urine and faeces, his movements, sleeplessness or the reverse, his appetite and so on; they also offer a description of the general constitution (*catastasis*) of a particular community over the course of a year, the climatic changes, and the range of diseases present. These notes are a remarkable record of observations (the work *skopein* (look) is frequently used) collected in order that the doctor may be better prepared to foretell the outcome of an illness and, in particular, of critical days, and to know whom and when to treat. It would indeed be tempting to assume, with Galen among others, that the author of *Prognostic* and that of *Epidemics* I and III was one and the same man, the great Hippocrates himself, and that it would thus be possible to see in one tract Hippocrates putting into practice the prescriptions given in another, or, because the order in which the books were written is uncertain, collecting the observations out of which was to spring a textbook on prognosis. But, alas, things are rarely so simple, and the question of the authorship of the *Epidemics* and their relationship to both *Prognostic* and Hippocrates has been hotly debated for almost half a century. To identify precept and practice as coming from the same man may here involve a dangerous circularity of argument.[6]

But there are further arguments in favour of concentrating on Galen as the model for ancient diagnosis rather than Hippocrates. In *Epidemics* I and III it is the information derived from the sense of sight that predominates almost to the exclusion of everything else. The voice of the patient is rarely remarked upon, and the sense of touch is only involved in references to tension of the hypochondrium or to tenderness of the spleen, or in rough descriptions of the heat or coldness of the patient's body.[7] Unlike the author of *Ancient Medicine*, whose discussion of bodily humours in terms of their sweetness, acridity or saltiness presupposes distinctions by taste, the writer of *Epidemics* I and III makes no use of this category in his descriptions, nor does he refer to the patient's smell.[8] This concentration on sight and, to a much lesser extent, on sound is repeated in *Prognostic*. Smell is mentioned, albeit briefly, in the sections that deal with pus, urine, faeces and vomit, but there is little attempt to go beyond the broad formulation that a very foetid smell is more indicative of a serious illness than a less pungent odour.[9] The contrast between the detailed descriptions of the *facies Hippocratica* or of the visible behaviour of the sick man and the transitory allusions to the symptoms that can be distinguished by the other senses is marked indeed. This general conclusion is modified only slightly by a consideration of other Hippocratic texts, and a more detailed reconstruction of the diagnostic methods of the Hippocratic physician would risk serious error in implying a dubious precision.[10]

There is, however, a further reason for concentrating upon Galen. Not only does he provide detailed rules and prescriptions for perceiving illness, but he is also inordinately proud of his own therapies and thus offers a substantial number of his own, generally successful, cases by which one can judge his bedside manner and his fidelity to his own precepts. In short, he sets himself forward as the very model of the modern Hippocratic physician, developing the insights of his great predecessor both practically and theoretically, and he uses his own experiences to exemplify the proper method of healing, the true 'therapeutic method'.

By Galen's day, these two words were loaded with meaning. They had been almost appropriated by a group of physicians who flourished in the first two centuries of the Christian era in the Roman Empire, especially in Italy, and who are known in English by the confusing title of Methodists.[11] It was their claim that they alone possessed the true method of healing the sick. This consisted in relating a series of observations to one of three bodily conditions: tension, or stricture; laxity; or a combination of the two. Depending on which of these three general conditions was indicated, a contrary treatment was applied accordingly. The recognition of these conditions and the consequent treatment were thus clear, simple and secure. To the Methodist, nothing was easier than relating observation to these 'causes' and thence to treatment, or than continuing this process throughout the whole length of a patient's illness. Such a method of healing, they claimed, might be taught in a mere six months, with assured success.[12]

For Galen and his fellow Hippocratics of the second century, all this was anathema. The sick man and his disease could not be neatly categorized into a trinity of conditions, and, although they too would agree that, once the cause of the disease was located, to find an appropriate remedy was not difficult, they emphasized the hazards involved in linking observation and cause. Above all, Galen, like writers on medicine before him going back to Plato, doubted the utter certainty of diagnosis.[13] Logic, geometry and scientific method might all bring certainty; but, when faced with an individual patient – or perhaps, in Galenic fashion, one should say an idiosyncratic patient – the doctor's art was necessarily uncertain, hypothetical, or, to use a Latin and a Greek word, 'conjectural and stochastic'. The doctor had to take a potshot – the meaning of στοχάζεσθαι – at the illness, and his shot might miss the target. For Galen, diagnosis – or as he would say, prognosis – was the most difficult task facing the doctor; for the peculiarities of the living human organism inevitably imposed a margin of chance, or the unexpected.[14] How wide that margin might be depended on the abilities of the physician. Only the great physician, a Hippocrates or a Galen, could disestablish chance and set in its place a true medical certainty – and, even then, he might not always succeed.

The true physician needed two things, 'reason' and experience, the two tools (*organa*), of medicine, and, of these, as Michael Frede has recently emphasized, the most important was experience.[15] This was not just the expertise of a practised surgeon, or of a physician faced with his thousandth case of malaria; nor was it book-learning, prodigious in Galen, and the assimilation of the recorded clinical experiences of the past. It involved also the proper way of approaching a practical situation, investigating the patient at the bedside, and deciding upon the nature and cause of his illness. This detective work, so typical of Galen and of the Hippocratics, required above all the full employment by the doctor of all his senses.

What Galen understood by this is clear from a long section of his commentary on the Hippocratic tract *On the Doctor's Surgery*. Whereas Hippocrates had cryptically declared that like and unlike were best discovered from what was most significant, easiest and universally recognized, Galen spent over thirty pages in explaining precisely what was meant by these terms. His conclusions were aptly summed up by a medieval Arabic author, Ali Ibn Ridwan, in his abridgement of the Galenic commentary:

For your diagnosis and the indications you observe, you should always choose things that are extremely powerful and easy to recognise, and these are what can be perceived by sight, touch, hearing, smell, taste and by the intellect. When these are properly grasped, they show the nature of the disease. Nature, in fact, has given us these faculties in order that by them we may recognise the true character of things, and the faculty of sense perception has organs that are natural to man and that can be used for testing.[16]

Two points can be made about this declaration. First, this is the only section in the genuine Galenic Corpus where Galen specifically refers to the five senses, and, like his model, Hippocrates, he adds a sixth sense, judgement, to the approved criteria.[17] Yet in the context of this passage, which Galen interprets as relating to the method of perceiving illness, he finds it somewhat tricky to explain the role of the intellect in the whole process. Secondly, Galen is here laying down a whole programme of investigation for the ideal physician, and it is worthwhile to compare his own clinical activity with the methods that he himself claimed to be following.[18]

Contrary to what might be supposed from Galen's comments in this section, the sense of smell plays only a small part in his bedside manner. It is true that the odours of urine, sputum, faeces, ulcers and a patient's breath are all mentioned at various times as important diagnostic guides, but, apart from indicating that there is something wrong, they are not sufficiently subdivided as to specify exactly what that something is.[19] Besides, to judge from other, non-medical writings, bad breath was extremely common: the purchaser of a slave had a right to return him as being unsuitable through bad breath only if he could show that this condition had some serious origin.[20] Even when bad breath is mentioned, its cause is more often ascribed to a sexual misdemeanour than to illness.[21]

Taste is involved more often than smell, especially in distinguishing between the various manifestations of sweat. The doctor should lick the sweat of a patient that has collected on his finger during the physical examination, and see whether it is sweet or salty, or variously acrid.[22] This may help to identify the disease, e.g. jaundice results in a bitter-tasting sweat, but quality is less significant than quantity and temperature.[23]

Hearing, the third of the senses, is deployed by Galen in two ways, in listening to some of the sounds within the body, and, secondly, in listening to the patient's responses. Although auscultation was employed by some of the Hippocratic writers in order to arrive at a more accurate differential diagnosis, Galen seems rarely to have used it.[24] Not that it was unknown to him, for he remarks on the different sounds coming from the abdomen of a sufferer from tympanites and one from ascites. Rumblings in the stomach might also be a indication that there was something amiss, although they could give no precise information.[25] The role of hearing is thus relatively restricted, and Galen is sorely tempted to interpret the Hippocratic passage so as to suggest that it is the patient's hearing, taste and smell, not those of the doctor, that furnish the prime indications of illness.[26] That this was the view of some other inter-preters is clear from Galen's commentary, and it was only his conviction of the value of the second type of hearing that led him to reject their explanation. In his view, the doctor's hearing (and judgement) are best utilized assessing the ways in which a patient's responses differ from the normal. In this he had a distinguished precursor in Rufus of Ephesus, whose *Medical Questions* is a remarkable manual of Hippocratic diagnosis. Almost from the start, Rufus reminds the aspiring physician that changes in a patient's voice or in his ability to respond to questioning may indicate a serious condition, especially if there are grounds for suspecting trauma.[27] Galen extends Rufus' interest in the physical causes of speech changes by looking also at possible psychological causes. A patient may refuse to answer a doctor's questions out of fear, shame or excitement.[28] Both Rufus and Galen are agreed that changes in the voice pattern may indicate some physical disorder, but their interpretation of these changes takes second place to their interpretation of the contents of the responses.

We are left with two senses, touch and sight, both of which are used more often by Galen in his practice than the other senses combined. Touch is used in three ways: in taking the pulse, taking the temperature, and in palpating the body, in particular the abdomen. This seems to have been common among all physicians in Classical Greece, and is portrayed as a typical part of the doctor's activity on a relief sculpture from the British Museum.[29] There were attempts to correlate the hardness or softness of parts of the body with the seriousness of an illness, and much of the gynaecological lore in the Hippocratic Corpus and in Soranus was formulated with the aid of palpation.[30]

Nevertheless, palpation takes second place in Galen to sphygmology. The role of the pulse in Classical medicine dates only from the fourth century B.C., when the Coan physician Praxagoras is considered to have first established a link between pulsation and disease. His more famous pupil Herophilus brought his ideas to Alexandria, extending them both by adopting a musical classification system and by devising a portable water-clock whereby to measure pulsation.[31] It is very likely also that Herophilus coined a series of distinctive names for individual pulses, e.g. the 'water-hammer', or the 'gazelle-like'.[32]

Galen was proud to continue the tradition of Praxagoras and Herophilus. Although his explanation for the pulse differs substantially from our own – he ascribed the power of pulsation to the arterial coats themselves, as they received a life-force from the heart,[33] – he seems to have regularly used it in making his diagnoses. By contrast with uroscopy, which he frequently practised, but which, as a regular and systematic procedure, seems to have been the contribution of post-Galenic physicians, sphygmology was perhaps the single most important diagnostic aid in Galen's repertoire and the technique to which he devoted most space in his theoretical expositions of medical practice.[34] Throughout his writings Galen lays down a long series of factors in the pulse that the doctor should observe: strength, frequency, speed, rhythm and so on – and prides himself on his own exquisite technique, his 'exceedingly sensitive touch'.[35] Not only does he claim to be able to detect rests at the full extent of the arterial systole and diastole, but perhaps even slighter variations within the individual movements.[36] He gives us the benefit of his great learning in a whole series of sixteen books on the pulse, which he later condensed to a double volume, to a further summary, and ultimately, to a brief diagram.[37] He tells us how to take the pulse, what different types of pulsation there are, and what causes the variations between pulses. The final four books of this large series, *On Prognosis from Pulses*, reflect two ways of using the pulse in diagnosis. One is to confirm a diagnosis reached by other means: for example, in pleurisy one expects to find one particular type of pulse, and its discovery offers necessary confirmation. The other, more spectacular, is to suggest a diagnosis that may be confirmed later by other means: for example, this type of pulse usually suggests pleurisy. Galen's pulse doctrines, which have been well expounded by C. R. S. Harris, are a monument to the great man's belief in his own powers.[38] His minute distinctions, and his careful classification of variations, may recall some of the subtleties of the bedside pulse-lore of clinicians of the nineteenth century, where one may indeed doubt how far they could, even with the most expert practice, pick out all the data they claimed to have felt.[39] One might flippantly add two more senses here: a sense of rhythm, for Herophilus and Galen often expressed their pulse doctrine in musical terms,[40] and a sense of self-delusion, for, it seems to me, at times Galen's subtle distinctions led him to find what he thought he ought to find, not what he actually could feel. But coming from a non-clinician, this verdict may be too harsh.

The second important area in diagnosis where the sense of touch predominated was that of temperature. Here it was less the fingers than the palm of the hand that mattered. Temperature, at least roughly defined, was one of the major diagnostic signs in the Hippocratic Corpus, especially in fever, when temperature changes might be correlated with the hypothetical series of days of crisis.[41] Galen hardly instructs us as to how to take a temperature, but in an anatomical tract, *De usu partium*, he discourses rapturously about the bountiful creator who has so wisely constructed the palm of the human hand to respond to the smallest of stimuli and to be able to notice the smallest of changes. Of all the body, the palm of the hand is the best-tempered, and hence can be best used as a measuring rod whereby to judge temperature. With such a natural and god-ordained instrument, the well-trained physician can easily judge degrees of heat or cold all over the body and diagnose accordingly.[42]

Finally, the sense of sight, since Hippocratic times the most important of the senses in diagnosis. As has been mentioned, the Hippocratic treatises, such as *Prognostic*, *Epidemics* and *Aphorisms*, had laid down a large number of visible symptoms that the doctor should notice on his way to forming a sound diagnosis. Some of these were immediately revealing of a cause of disease, others required correlation with a patient's normal behaviour and habits before they could be rightly assessed.[43] But, as every Hippocratic physician knew, examining the patient's body was not the sole means of gaining the necessary information; the patient could not be understood without the nature of 'the whole' – on one interpretation, without his environment.[44] This could be on the macro-scale – *Airs, waters and places* is a Hippocratic manifesto of the importance of climate and localities in health generally – or it could be on the micro-scale, the individual patient's own environment. Here anything might prove relevant. A look round the sickroom; a glance at the patient's relatives; a view of the house's relationship to the street outside; all might help to build up a picture of the disease. It is here that Galen is at his most detective, for he had a remarkably wide interest in everything around him, from the cooking practices of Egyptians to the nesting habits of birds.[45] He had a trained eye, and, as he rightly says, many of the conclusions about the course of a disease seemed remarkable to others only because they had not observed everything that he himself had seen. The practice of prognosis, he regularly declares, is not difficult; it rests on a basis of observation, and it is the duty of the physician to improve his observational powers to their full extent. Practice at observation is the key to the understanding of the sick patient.

Observation, however, was not just confined by Galen to things; he could appreciate a situation equally well, and it is in this area of a sense of situation that he claims novel expertise. He reports many cases of what might be termed stress-related disorders, in which his diagnosis is made after observation of the patient's social situation – a senator fearing the murderous intent of the blood-thirsty emperor Commodus; an orator preparing himself for a major speech; an athlete before a race; a scholar pining away after the loss of his library; a wealthy woman in love with an actor.[46] Only by attempting to observe the patient as a whole in his particular situation and environment can the doctor, like Galen, become a proper expert in diagnosis, and, like the detective, finally pinpoint the culprits.

This chapter has so far talked almost entirely in general terms, yet it would be wrong to end without some examples of Galen at the bedside, employing his senses in what is a far wider search for the causes of disease than many of his later followers could or did perform. It is perhaps in these, in one way programmatic, case histories that one gets an idea of the impression Galen must have created at the bedside, an impression that eventually gained him recognition as an imperial physician in Rome, and which may give some indication of his greatness as a clinician to go with his other achievements as an anatomist and publicist.[47]

As one example of the way in which the properly trained physician can distinguish between conflicting symptoms or select what is most significant from among a mass of varying detail, Galen tells the story of his diagnosis of a Sicilian physician.[48] This was a test case, in more senses than one, for not only was Galen's friend Glaucon eager to discover whether Galen's diagnosis was the result of medical skill or divinatory powers, but he himself had only glimpsed the patient once in the street and hence had to make his diagnosis without recourse to a knowledge of the patient's habits or constitution. A Hippocratic ideal of total knowledge of the patient and his environment had thus to be modified, and Galen was compelled to rely solely on the information he might pick up during the course of his consultation. He was fortunate enough to be passed on his way in by a servant carrying a bedpan containing a thin bloody serum like that of freshly slaughtered meat, a most reliable sign of a liver disease. Whether this was the result of inflammation or of some weakness in the liver Galen believed he could determine from taking the pulse, even though the man himself ascribed his increase in pulse rate to the effort involved in getting in and out of bed to evacuate. Galen's taking of the pulse confirmed him in his diagnosis of a liver inflammation, but he was emboldened to go further through seeing on the window-sill a small pot containing a preparation of water and honey. Since this was a standard remedy for pleurisy and since some of the symptoms of liver disease – pain in the area of the false ribs, fast and shallow breathing and an intermittent cough – were similar to those of pleurisy, Galen concluded that the patient himself thought he had pleurisy. To increase the amazement of his audience, Galen then told the patient the symptoms that he was actually experiencing, from a brief dry cough to a drawing sensation at the collar-bone, concluding with a declaration of what the physician and his attendants thought to be the cause of his condition. When his predictions were all confirmed by the patient, Galen's reputation rose still more, and he succeeded in overcoming Glaucon's scepticism about the efficacy of the medical art.

Two points require emphasis in the discussion of this case history. The first is the importance of seizing upon chance in the collection of the material on which to base a diagnosis. The meeting in the doorway with the servant and the pot on the window-sill are both ascribed by Galen to chance, yet, equally, it is precisely the well-trained and well-learned physician who can exploit these things in reaching his clinical diagnosis. Only the good physician would recognize the bloody stools, or know that they were the most reliable evidence of a liver disease. Secondly, both here and elsewhere Galen stresses the rationality of diagnosis and prognosis. Although opponents (and even supporters) might think in terms of special powers of divination, a god-directed hunch, Galen is firm in his conviction that with proper application of the senses and of a well-stocked mind, any physician can attain the degree of clinical competence he claims for himself.[49]

A similar exemplary story, but this time involving a non-medical ending, is recalled by Galen in his treatise *On prognosis*.[50] A boy under treatment suffered a baffling series of relapses, baffling because they contradicted Galen's predictions for the course of the disease. His explanation, which is not untypical of his sublime self-confidence, was that the boy himself was frustrating his physician by surreptitiously taking food. The boy's mother set herself on watch to prevent the boy from taking anything other than what had been prescribed, yet this did not stop him from suddenly developing a temperature in the night. Galen was called in, but, on taking the pulse, he declared that the lad was not suffering from any fever. His explanation was that he had been eating food hidden in the room, which he could do in safety since, when his mother went out to the bathroom, she always carefully locked the door behind her. When, after a search of the bedclothes and furnishings, a piece of bread was discovered wrapped in a scarf, Galen's hypothesis was triumphantly confirmed. In explaining the grounds for his diagnosis, Galen again rejected any miraculous powers, and his host's suggestion that simply taking the pulse had revealed the hidden food. That had shown no sign of the heat of a fever, but the racing beat had suggested to Galen that the condition had some psychological cause, the stressful fear of being caught out. By itself, the diagnosis from the pulse would not have been enough. It was only by being able to take in the whole situation that Galen was able to reach his surprising conclusion.

These two case histories were selected as exemplary by Galen himself. They reveal his skill at the bedside, his command of medical data and his wondrous powers of observation. Together they enabled Galen to practise a very optimistic form of diagnosis,[51] and to transmit his own achievements as a model for subsequent generations to imitate. The union of reason and experience, however derived, forms one side of medical practice; the other is the actual method of the doctor in making a bedside diagnosis. In this, Galen, the Hippocratics, the ancient Methodists and the humblest of practitioners were forced to rely, in the absence of more than rudimentary diagnostic aids, on the evidence of the senses, on what they could perceive. In reaching his perception of the patient and his condition, the doctor became, in his own terms at least, a medical detective. The range of possible causes might be high, but by a proper application of the senses, the truth might be established. By the appropriate use of the five senses, therapeutic conjecture might be turned into certainty, diagnosis followed by effective therapy, and, as in any good detective story, the case well and truly closed.

2

Sensory perception and its metaphors in the time of Richard of Fournival

ELIZABETH SEARS

An arresting image illustrates the prologue to Richard of Fournival's *Bestiaire d'amours* – a text composed in the second quarter of the thirteenth century – in a richly illuminated manuscript produced in 1285 (fig. 1).[1] Inside the curve of the initial T that stands at the head of the opening line, 'Toutes gens desirent par nature a savoir', a crenellated stone tower rises up pink against a patterned blue ground. Attention focuses immediately upon the tower's two arched gates, for unexpected emblems are discovered there: on one door an open eye, on the other a listening ear.

What might to a twentieth-century viewer seem a proto-surrealist fantasy proves to be a visualization of ideas current in the thirteenth century. The illuminator who situated disembodied sense organs on an architectural structure was giving pictorial form to a distinctive understanding of the body and its parts. His point of departure was a metaphor introduced in the adjacent text. Richard of Fournival, having cited at the beginning of his *Bestiaire d'amours* the opening words of Aristotle's *Metaphysics*, 'All men by nature have a desire to know',[2] had gone on to ponder the character of knowledge and memory. No single person, Richard reflected, can know everything, although everything can be known. And it is right that everyone should try to know something, so that all will be known collectively. But not everyone lives at once. No one now living could discover by his own intelligence things known from the ancients (*les anchiiens*).

This thought led Richard to the subject of memory, which he describes as a faculty of the soul (*une vertu de force d'ame*) given by God 'who so loves man that he wants to provide for his every need'.[3] An architectural metaphor seemed apt at this juncture: Richard observes that memory has two gates (*portes*), seeing and hearing. A particular path leads to each of them, namely

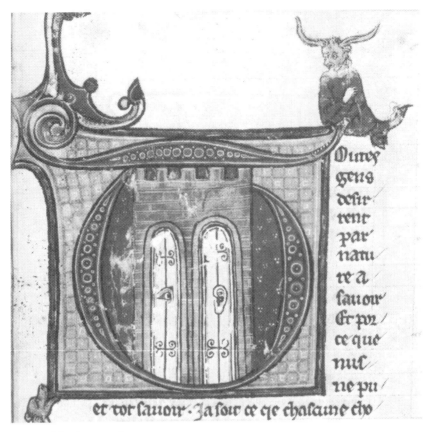

Fig. 1. The house of memory.

painture and *parole*, pictures serving the eye and words the ear. Both give access to memory's house (*a le maison de memoire*) because memory, guarding the treasures won by human intelligence, has the capacity to make the past seem as if it were present when triggered by pictures and words.[4] Richard went on to apply his learning to the immediate situation. He intends to send to his 'bele tres douce amie' an illustrated copy of his bestiary of love – one decorated with images of beasts and birds – in order that its pictures and words together will bring him to her memory, where he wishes always to reside.

When the illuminator of 1285 represented the house of memory, a task relatively few of the later illustrators of the text would undertake,[5] he did so by joining both halves of Richard's metaphor – the inorganic and organic – in a single image. It was the combination of elements, unlikely, even absurd, that ensured a proper reading of the image. Had the sense organs been omitted, the building might well have been otherwise interpreted. The miniature in a north French manuscript produced in 1277, the earliest dated copy of the *Bestiaire*

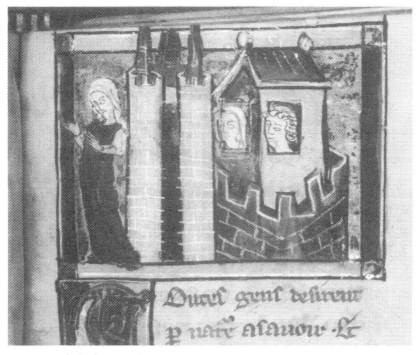

Fig. 2. Lady before castle.

d'amours to have survived, shows a lady standing beside a castle with prominent twin towers (fig. 2).[6] She can be, and has been, identified as Richard's
'amie', and the structure, by implication, as her domicile.[7] But it is possible
that the illuminator in this case, too, was intending to represent the house of
memory and its owner, Memory herself, personified as the guardian of intellectual treasures. The allegorical character of the miniature in an early fourteenth-century copy of a rhymed version of Richard's *Bestiaire* cannot fail to
be recognized (fig. 3).[8] Signs of seeing and hearing on the castle's two gates –
again an eye in profile and an ear full view[9] – establish that the gates are
sensory gates. As the status of the castle is established, the identity of the lady
standing before it is adjusted: she is seen to be an allegorical personage, the
personified Memory, holding a green branch, possibly as a token of ever-living
knowledge.[10] The viewer, compelled by the fantastic nature of the castle's
decoration to identify the image as an illustrated metaphor, is encouraged to
read further in order to gain insight into the nature of seeing and hearing.

Analogies used in explanations of natural phenomena are, of course, revealing indicators of understanding. The use of an architectural metaphor to define
the function of the eye and the ear in relation to memory is rich in implication,
as will be demonstrated in the course of this chapter. It may be suggested at
this point that Richard's figure of speech carries with it a suggestion that the

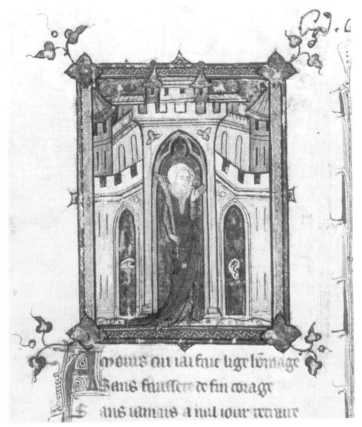

Fig. 3. Memory before the house of memory.

beneficent creator credited with having given man the faculty of memory had a role in fashioning the human body comparable to an architect's role in designing a building. It implies that the organs of sense, like the portals of a dwelling, were designed to a purpose: the eyes to see and the ears to hear, each organ constructed so as to admit a particular object – colour (*painture*) and sound (*parole*). Richard's metaphor may be said to identify, and the image to depict, the 'final cause' of the two sense organs in question, if one defines a final cause, in the way Aristotle did in the *Metaphysics*, as 'that for the sake of which a thing is'.[11]

Teleological thinking of the kind hinted at in the prologue to the *Bestiaire d'amours*, and set forth explicitly in other texts, had a long history by the thirteenth century. The urge to account for order in the natural world had led antique philosophers and, later, Christian theologians and exegetes, to define the ends for which things were created and to posit the activity of divine intelligence in their making. Organic nature was submitted to such analysis and, in this connection, the parts of the human body, including the sense organs, were found to be so constituted that they could not be more perfectly adapted to the faculties of man's soul. Final causes were introduced to explain the form, composition, position and number of the sense organs, their operation, and their relative value. So pervasive was the teleological habit of mind – as fundamental in the Middle Ages as evolutionary theory is in our own time – that its study may be considered a necessary prerequisite to any analysis of medieval speculations about sense perception.[12] In the following pages an attempt will be made to define this line of thought through the examination of texts available in Richard of Fournival's time and to use this information in the interpretation of images of the senses surviving from the thirteenth century.

Living when he did, Richard of Fournival had access to many classic expositions of organic teleology. By the second quarter of the thirteenth century it had become possible to acquire a wide range of natural philosophical works, not only long-available Latin school texts, but also recently translated works by Greek and Arabic philosophers and doctors. Richard took full advantage of the opportunities open to him and amassed a large private library, encyclopaedic in scope. In a text called the *Biblionomia*, composed probably in the 1240s, he described this library and its operation in gratifying detail.[13] Here he set forth the principles of his cataloguing system (shelf marks and shelving arrangements), and he recorded the contents of 162 of his manuscripts, volume by volume, in the order in which they appeared on the shelves. Richard made his extensive collection available to the inhabitants of his city. In the prologue to the *Biblionomia* he likened his library to a garden: here the citizens of Amiens could find many kinds of fruits, the taste of which would inspire in them a desire to be introduced into the secret chamber of philosophy.[14] The respect towards knowledge that Richard revealed in the prologue to his *Bestiaire d'amours*, founded on the idea that everything could be known and that everyone should try to know something, thus found tangible expression.

When Léopold Delisle published his edition of the *Biblionomia* in 1874 he wondered whether Richard's library ever existed, if it were not, in fact, a library of the imagination. Scholars after him, working from Richard's precise descriptions of the contents of his manuscripts, have been able to identify many surviving codexes and, thus, to establish that the library did once exist in reality. It is now known that the collection passed to Gerard d'Abbeville at Richard's death *c.* 1260, that it entered the library of the Sorbonne by bequest at Gerard's death in 1271 or 1272, and that more than forty of the manuscripts, in the succeeding centuries, have made their way to the Bibliothèque Nationale and other public libraries.[15]

Richard's collection was broadly based, but especially strong in the natural sciences and medicine. Biographical information culled from various documents has made it possible to account for his biases. Canon, deacon, and, by

1246, chancellor of the Cathedral of Notre-Dame at Amiens, Richard emerges from the sources as a man of wide-ranging accomplishment.[16] In the prologue to the *Biblionomia* he calls himself 'skilled in mathematics'; evidence of his skill in astronomical calculation is provided by a personal horoscope of his own devising which survives in several manuscripts and establishes his date of birth, 10 October 1201.[17] Son of Roger of Fournival – a physician at the court of King Philippe Auguste – Richard was himself a doctor, twice given papal dispensation to practise surgery.[18] To him is assigned an array of vernacular tracts: not only the *Bestiaire d'amours* and a rhymed version of it, but also the *Commens d'amours*, the *Consaus d'amours* and a collection of lyric verse.[19] He is also author of an alchemical tract and, possibly, of the pseudo-Ovidian *De vetula*, a poem rich in natural-historical learning, cosmological and cosmogonic.[20]

The library compiled by this erudite and multi-faceted individual provides a unique index of knowledge available in many fields in the second quarter of the thirteenth century. As such it may serve the study of the history of ideas. Since Richard's books, however disparate in terms of genre, date and place of origin, could be consulted in one place at one time, the manuscript list in the *Biblionomia* provides a control for discussions of received traditions. To read those texts Richard possessed on a given subject, especially one in the natural sciences, is to learn something about the character, range and limits of thirteenth-century thinking in that area. The task of gauging 'potential' knowledge – that which could be known – is, of course, very different in kind from that of studying 'exercised' knowledge as revealed in a work produced in the thirteenth century. As a preliminary to scanning Richard's library for information about perception it will be useful to collect statements on the subject from his *Bestiaire d'amours*. In this way it should be possible to discover what Richard, who urged everyone to know something, thought it desirable to know about the senses.

It was not Richard's immediate purpose in the *Bestiaire* to discuss the senses or sense organs. His larger aim in this novel text at once lyrical and didactic, an *ars amandi* cast in the form of a bestiary, was to describe the ever-thwarted progress of his own amorous sentiments and to define the nature of man's love and woman's love with reference to traditional animal lore.[21] Yet the theme of sense perception runs through the text as a leitmotif. Richard shows that love is awakened by the five senses, beginning with sight.[22] He himself has been captured by three of them – hearing, sight and smell; had he been taken by taste in kissing and touch in embracing, he says, he would have been put to sleep, bereft of all his five senses, and in peril of death.[23] At several points Richard indulges in learned digressions on the theme of sensory perception. Nature is presented as a force which compensates for defects in the senses by which living creatures perceive. Richard observes that no man sees as well as a deaf man, or hears as well as a blind man, or is as lecherous as one who stinks. This is because the nerves which extend from the brain to the nostrils, the palate, and the other sense organs work better when they have less to do.[24] Sight he calls the noblest sense, for from none of the others do we learn so many things, and, if deficient, it is compensated for by voice alone. Each of the senses, Richard notes, has its particular object: 'Voice serves hearing, colors sight, odors smell, and flavors taste. But many things serve touch, for with it one feels hot, cold, moist, dry, rough, smooth, and many other things.'[25] Richard compares the sensory organs of humans and animals and observes that for each sense there is one animal which surpasses all others.[26] He repeats the idea that hearing and sight are the gates of memory and he stresses that these are two of man's noblest senses.[27]

In these scattered observations Richard touched upon many issues frequently encountered in learned Latin tracts. A wider knowledge is suggested, of a kind to be gained through study in his library. Here many treatments of sense perception were to be had, located in several of the library's subdivisions. For Richard had arranged his books in considered sequence so as to reveal the very structure of knowledge. Primacy he accorded to philosophy. Tracts offering instruction in the liberal arts stood at the beginning of the first division, set out in ascending order: grammar, dialectic, rhetoric, geometry, arithmetic, music and astrology. Next came works in the physical, metaphysical, and ethical branches of philosophy. These were followed by philosophical works seen to fall outside standard categories, then works by poets, and finally secret books, kept from the public eye. The second major division was given over to the 'lucrative sciences', medicine and law. While the philosophical texts were marked by letters of diverse colours, these bore shelfmarks of silver. The third and last division comprised books on theology, their bindings inscribed in gold.

A thirteenth-century visitor to Richard's library,[28] having reached the sixth rank of the philosophical shelves – that devoted to physical and metaphysical philosophy – would have found several volumes containing tracts on the soul and the intellect. Here were shelved, side by side, works by classical writers, Arabic writers (Avicenna, Averroës, Al Farabi, Alkindi etc.), and Latin writers who had been involved in the translating enterprise in the previous century (Gundissalinus and Alfredus Anglicus). The works of Aristotle, whose fortunes were rising dramatically in Richard of Fournival's time, were given special prominence. Latin translations of his *libri naturales* were collected in the manuscript that occupied the first place on these shelves. A copy of the texts collectively entitled *De animalibus* occupied the second. The *Metaphysics* was also present, in two translations.[29]

In tracts included among Aristotle's *libri naturales* – specifically *De anima* and *De sensu et sensato* (part of the *Parva naturalia*)[30] – a good deal of basic information about sense perception could be obtained. *De anima* supplied fundamental definitions. The soul is called the cause and principle of the living body. Nature, like discerning mind, is said to do what it does for the sake of something, and that end, Aristotle claims, in animals is the soul: 'all natural bodies are instruments of the soul'.[31] In both *De anima* and *De sensu* the activities of the senses receive close treatment. Each sense in turn is defined with reference to its objects (*sensibilia*). Aristotle distinguishes between those objects special to individual senses (colours, sounds, odours, tastes, things touched) and those common to all (movement, rest, number, figure, size),[32] and he shows how the sense organs are adapted to receive particular impressions. The definition of the sense of touch is said to pose particular problems, since it is even uncertain whether this is a single or multiple sense. While each of the other senses seems to operate within one pair of contraries (sight: white and black, hearing: grave and acute, taste: bitter and sweet), touch is clearly able to discern between many (hot and cold, dry and wet, hard and soft, etc.).[33]

For Aristotle it is the possession of sensation which defines the animal, since every body possessing a soul has the power of touch. Nature gives this sense and that of taste, a particular form of touch, to all for the sake of survival. But the other three senses, those which perceive objects through a medium at a distance, are present only in creatures that have the power of movement. In *De sensu* Aristotle says of smelling, hearing and seeing that their cause is preservation (*salus*), since those possessing these senses are able to pursue their food and flee things harmful and corrupt.[34] They have an additional function in animals possessing intelligence, for through them information is collected which generates understanding in the soul. Seeing is said to be superior in this connection, but hearing, as it makes possible rational discourse, serves a greater role in developing intelligence: those blind from birth are more intelligent than those born deaf and dumb.[35]

Focused examinations of the organs of sense were to be found in the next manuscript on the shelf, a copy of Michael Scot's translation from the Arabic of Aristotle's tracts on animals.[36] In the *Historia animalium*, the first of the tracts, Aristotle had described simple and composite parts of animals and compared them to the parts of the human body, taken as standard. A reader could discover which animals have all five senses, and which perceive more acutely than man.[37] In *De partibus animalium*, the second of the tracts, Aristotle had extended the programme of the *Historia animalium* to treat the causes of nature's works.[38] Here a reader would have learned that the end is the cause of generated things, natural and man-made. If a house (*domus*) or something similar is planned, Aristotle says, first one thing is done and then another until that end is realized. It is the same in works of nature.[39] In his discussions of the sense organs in this work Aristotle demonstrates his conviction that they, like all parts of natural bodies, were formed and placed so as best to fulfil their functions. The more precise senses are located in the head – smell in the middle, sight above and hearing to the side – for good reason. The source of sensation is the heart, Aristotle claims, criticizing those who had located it in the brain. Touch and taste are directly connected with this, the hottest, organ. But it was determined that the other senses be placed near the brain, cold and wet, so that their work would not be disturbed by the heat of blood.[40] Aristotle calls attention to many niceties of design. The ears are located on opposite sides of the head so that hearing can come from all directions; the eyes are placed in front because this is the direction of movement. He identifies the functions of organs. Eyebrows and eyelids, for example, are there to provide assistance for the eyes: the brows were created to deflect fluids descending to the forehead, the lids to ward off things coming from outside, to act 'as fences preventing entry into an enclosure' (ut sepes que prohibunt introitum in ortum).[41]

Throughout De partibus animalium Aristotle was intent to demonstrate the wisdom of nature which does nothing in vain, nothing at random, nothing inadequate or superfluous. Several centuries later Galen, drawing on a more profound knowledge of human anatomy, followed the same programme. A copy of Galen's great teleological work De usu partium was to be found in Richard's library in the medical section, among a rich collection of texts recently translated from the Greek and Arabic.[42] True, a thirteenth-century reader had to make do with a Latin translation of an Arabic abridgement of the text; but even from this severely truncated work, called De iuvamento membrorum, it was possible to gain some sense of the original.[43] A comparison with Aristotle's text would have revealed contradictions in details, but harmony in fundamental assumptions. De iuvamento membrorum opens with the statement: 'The bodies of animals are instruments of their souls.'[44]

Galen begins his comprehensive description of the parts of the body with an encomium to the human hand, in it demonstrating that this instrument with its four fingers and opposed thumb, composed of flesh, nails, bones, tendons and nerves, was perfectly constructed to serve the intelligent creature.[45] Man alone among the animals, he observes, has hands, and two feet, and an elevated head.[46] When Galen analyses the structure of the head, he offers his own explanation for the fact that the sense organs are located there. For Galen the brain, not the heart, is the source of sensation, and of motion, and the hard and soft nerves, including those connected to the organs of sense.[47] He maintains that it would be wrong to think the head was made for the sake of the brain. In other animals the instruments of sensation and motion, the mouth, ears and nostrils, are located in the breast. But never are the eyes found in any but an elevated position. For they fulfil their function from on high, just as a man may climb a mast at sea or observe distances from a high place on land.[48]

The eyes thus had to be placed in the head; because soft, they could not be put on stalks, but had to be protected by brows, cheeks and nose. The brain had to be located in the head to be near the eyes, since the soft nerves which receive sense impressions are fragile. The other organs of sense, in order to be near the brain, had to be placed there too.

In a chapter on the sense organs Galen supplied further information.[49] He describes and locates the nerves along which the various kinds of sensory impressions pass, and he explains features of each organ. The ear, for example, was designed to receive waves of air which has been struck. Since the impact must make its way to the brain, the auditory nerve could not be wholly covered. Nor could it be left exposed to injury. For this reason the creator covered the nerve with a hard bone in which he put labyrinthine apertures (*foramina tortuosa*) that would reduce the force of cold and deflect hard objects.[50]

That the bodily members were fashioned to serve discernible ends neither Galen nor Aristotle doubted. This faith could be discovered in other texts in Richard's library, in descriptions of the senses even more reverent in character, if based on less sustained empirical observation. A copy of Cicero's *De natura deorum* occupied first place in the seventh rank of the philosophy shelves, that dedicated to metaphysical and ethical philosophy.[51] In this reasoned inquiry into the role of the gods in human affairs, representatives of three schools of ancient philosophy – Epicureanism, Stoicism and the Old Academy – define their respective positions. The Stoic Balbus, who energetically defends the existence of superior beings, finds the wisdom of the creator to be manifested not only in the regular and orderly movements of the heavens and in the beauties of the earth,[52] but also in the marvellous intricacies of the human body. Man – a being created to stand erect so that by gazing on the heavens he could gain knowledge of the gods – was given sense organs of consummate design.[53] 'Interpreters and messengers', set in the head as though in a citadel (*arx*), the senses are wonderfully formed and placed to fulfil their functions.[54] The eyes, acting as scouts (*speculatores*), have the highest position; the ears and nose are placed so as to receive naturally rising sounds and odours; smell, with a role to play in taste, is located near the mouth; taste is placed in that part of the mouth where nature made a path for the reception of food and drink; touch is appropriately distributed throughout the body. Nature's artistry is fully revealed in the construction of the organs. The mobile eyes are protected by fast-moving eyelids – each provided with a 'palisade of hairs' (*vallo pilorum*) – and by brows, cheeks, and a nose which acts almost like a separating wall (*murus*). The usefulness of the winding paths in the ears, organs open even in sleep, lies in the fact that they prevent objects from entering; the outer ear covers and protects the sense organ and, catching sounds, helps to make them resonate. The nostrils, always open, are narrow and moist so as to keep out harmful bodies and dust. The tongue, held in the mouth, fulfils its function while remaining protected. At the end of the passage Balbus compares the senses of man and animals and, in his enthusiasm, claims that human senses are in every case more discriminating.

Balbus makes much use of metaphor, especially architectural metaphor, in his descriptions of the sense organs. In another of Cicero's works present in Richard's library, the *Tusculanae disputationes*,[55] where the subject was the wise man and his pursuit of the good in face of adversity, further analogies were to be found. Seeking to establish that the soul is immortal, Cicero tries to establish that it is separable from the body. The sense organs do not themselves see and hear, he claims; a sleeping body does not sense. The eyes and ears are only 'windows of the soul' (*fenestrae animi*). The sense organs are but 'messengers' (*nuntii*) that bring information about colour, taste, heat, smell and sound to the soul which acts as sole judge (*iudex*).[56] A thirteenth-century reader could well be struck by patterns in the analogies employed by 'les anchiiens'. Aristotle, Galen and Cicero alike made use of similitudes to explain the working of the human body, and they frequently found their comparisons in human products and human activities – things built and actions performed (often in architectural surroundings) with a conscious end in view. Descriptive language in the same vein, even more evocative, was to be encountered in texts preserved in another section of Richard's library, texts in which teleological thinking also played a determining role.

Richard shelved apart a large group of philosophical works which stood outside the principal divisions of philosophy. Among these texts, the *libri vagi phylosophorum*, a reader would have found not only Plato's cosmological dialogue, the *Timaeus*, but also an array of platonizing Latin classics. Late antique works were juxtaposed with medieval products: authors included Macrobius, Martianus Capella and Boethius, Bernard Silvester and Alan of Lille. To read these books, shelved just before the works of poets, was to enter a world of myth and allegory, one in which philosophical truths were presented in a fabulous guise. When the wonders of the human body were extolled, it was often in cosmogonic contexts, within discussions of the creation of man and the origin of things.

In the *Timaeus*, which Richard possessed not in Cicero's but in Calcidius' fourth-century translation,[57] the creator is presented as a craftsman (*opifex*), whose end is the good. Taking as models the Forms, unchanging and eternal, he imposed reason on primeval chaos and 'persuaded' reluctant matter, controlled by its own forces of necessity, to conform to intelligent and purposive design.[58] Reason was placed in the soul, and the soul in the body of both the world and man. The creator made the World Body whole and one and all-embracing; constructed in the perfect shape of a sphere, it did not need eyes and ears, nor organs for respiration and the reception and discharge of food, nor hands and feet.[59] The immortal gods were assigned the task of creating mortal beings, and they fashioned from the four elements a frame suitable to contain the revolution of the immortal soul. They made man's head spherical, on the model of the world. But they also provided a body and four limbs in order that the head would not have to roll over the earthly terrain, and that the most divine part would be highest, supported like a citadel (*arx*). Forward motion was judged better than backward, and the front more noble than the back. The face was placed on the better side and the organs of the soul's forethought allotted to it. First made were light-giving eyes.[60]

Plato defines the operation of sight in some detail. It is a process of like meeting like: the fire within us goes forth from the eye to meet and combine with daylight, and the motions set up are then transmitted to the soul.[61] But Plato reveals that he places little value on such explanations. The lover of knowledge must pursue primary causes, the good for which the eyes were created. God gave us vision – our chief source of intellectual gains – in order that we might observe the rational and orderly revolutions of the heavens and, contemplating them, come to reproduce the movements in our own turbulent souls. Sound and hearing were similarly provided in order that, through speech and especially music, our souls might be taught harmony and rhythm.[62]

Echoes of the *Timaeus* could be recognized in a work shelved nearby, Macrobius' commentary on Cicero's *Somnium Scipionis*.[63] In this ambitious exposition of Neoplatonist doctrine, Macrobius had occasion to discuss both the macrocosm and the microcosm. Immortal souls, he claims, their proper habitation being the fixed stars and planets, are able to reside temporarily in human bodies because man walks erect and can contemplate the heavens and because he has a head in the shape of a sphere, the only shape which can contain mind.[64] In a numerological excursus, within a description of the powers and associations of the number seven, Macrobius reveals other features unique to the human form. The organization of the entire body is informed by the septenarius, justly revered.[65] Internally, there are seven black organs, seven organs for the reception and expulsion of food and air, and seven kinds of substance beneath the skin's surface. Externally, the whole body is divided into seven parts, as is each arm and each leg. Macrobius concludes, 'Since nature has located the senses and their functions in the head, the citadel [*arx*] of the body, the operations of the senses are performed through seven openings: the mouth, two eyes, two nostrils, and two ears'.[66] The body, for Macrobius as for other Platonists, is an exquisitely designed entity.

Copies of two allegorical epics composed in the recent past, Bernard Silvester's *Cosmographia* and Alan of Lille's *Anticlaudianus*, were to be found at the end of this section of Richard's library.[67] In these texts Platonic cosmology came to life. Bernard, writing in the mid-twelfth century, took as his theme the creation of the megacosmos and the microcosmos, the universe and man. At the beginning of his tale Nature, responding to the desire of Silva (primordial matter), petitions *Noys* (divine intelligence) to give form to formless matter. *Noys* agrees and fashions an ordered cosmos, teeming with life. When this end has been achieved, she determines to create man as the consummation of her labours.[68] Nature is delegated to find Urania in the heavens and Physis on earth: the three artisans together will create man, a soul and a body bound together. Urania, discovered contemplating the heavens, supplies a soul. Physis, found studying the origins, properties, and powers of natural things, shapes a body to contain it. A skilled artisan (*artifex*), she takes as her model the macrocosm. She fashions a spherical head to contain the soul, and, elevating it, makes it the body's citadel (*arx*) or capitol (*capitolium*).[69] The skull she divides into three chambers (*thalami*), each responsible for one of the functions of the soul. Speculative power is located at the front, memory at the back, and reason between; memory was not placed at the threshold (*limen*) of perception lest it be disturbed by the frequent assault of images.[70]

Bernard's descriptions of the senses, in prose and verse, contain information already familiar to readers of the texts of 'les anchiiens' or in seeming harmony with them. The 'messenger' senses, he says, are placed about the castle (*regia*) of the head to be close to the judging intellect. The soul, adapting itself to the organs it employs, perceives colours, sounds, tastes, odours, and touch.[71] In a survey of the senses extending from sight to sluggish touch (which 'serves the cause of tender love'), Bernard establishes a hierarchy among them.[72] Sight is singled out for special praise, but lower-ranked hearing is granted much. For learning itself is owed to hearing. When air shaped by the tongue enters the vestibule of the outer ear and is received into the inner chambers, Bernard says, the ear seizes its sense. If men had deaf ears, letters would perish.[73]

Shelved near Bernard's work was Alan of Lille's *Anticlaudianus*, an epic poem composed in the early 1180s which had as its theme the creation of a perfect man. Nature instigates the project, by way of compensation for earlier imperfections in her work. She appeals to the Virtues for aid and they convene at her dwelling place, a 'place of places' which has everything 'that feasts the eye, intoxicates the ear, beguiles the taste, catches the nose with its aroma, and soothes the touch'.[74] Here, in a splendid house – its walls decorated with paintings of a sequence of worthies beginning with Aristotle and the more admired Plato – Nature sets forth her plan to create a man who will be human on earth, in heaven divine. The Virtues applaud the scheme, but Prudence raises a note of caution: while it is within their capacity to fashion a mortal body, the soul must be formed by a heavenly craftsman. At Reason's urging, Prudence is chosen to travel to heaven to make their desire known to God. A special chariot is constructed by the Liberal Arts, at the command of Wisdom, and in this vehicle, drawn by five horses yoked and tamed by the charioteer Reason, Prudence journeys through the heavenly spheres. Reaching the last

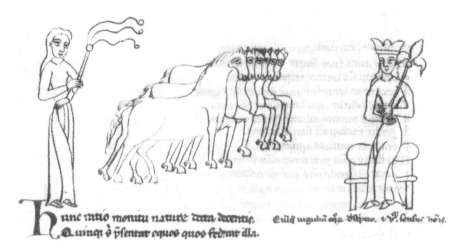

Fig. 4. Reason yokes the horses of the senses.

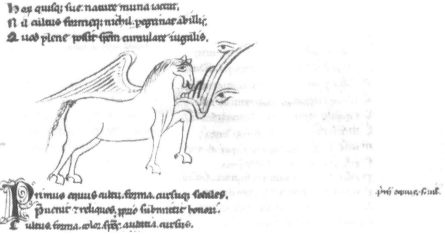

Fig. 5. The first horse: Sight.

sphere, she disembarks and, mounting the second horse, proceeds yet further, guided by Theology, and given strength by Faith. Arriving at the house of God she completes her mission and returns to earth bearing an immortal soul. Nature fashions a mortal body from the four elements and the Virtues endow the new man with their strengths. The Vices wage war upon him. With the help of Nature and the Virtues he triumphs and establishes a peaceful rule on earth.

A reader who succeeded in unveiling Alan's allegories would recognize that the five horses who carry Prudence on her celestial journey signify the five senses. Detailed accounts of the character and pedigree of each steed presented

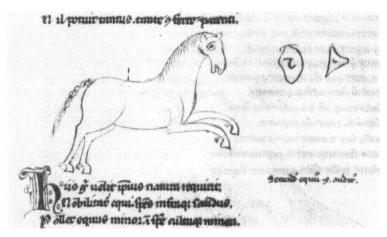

Fig. 6. The second horse: Hearing.

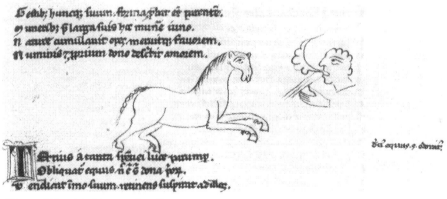

Fig. 7. The third horse: Smell.

riddles ripe for solution.[75] The first horse is the thoroughbred, sired by Pyrois, one of the Sun's horses. This steed does not walk, he flies. As fast as the air, Boreas cannot keep up with him; birds and arrows fall behind. The second horse, inferior to the first, is still greater than the others. He can travel as fast as the wind. His repeated neighs lash the air; music-making bells are suspended from his neck. The third horse, while lower in rank and less fleet than the first two, is judged to have his own beauty. Flowers adorn him, giving off perfumes. He was born to a mare impregnated by the wind of Zephyrus. The fourth horse, yet lower in rank, is not deprived of Nature's favours. A servant to the rest, he eats and drinks on their behalf. Finally, the fifth horse, so lowly he scarcely deserves comparison with the others, is seen to have no defects in form. It is the tendency of this horse, resembling the fourth, to cast his eyes to the ground.

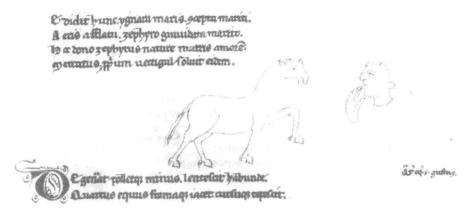

Fig. 8. The fourth horse: Taste.

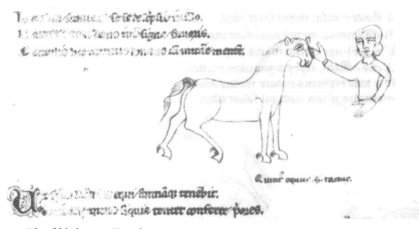

Fig. 9. The fifth horse: Touch.

Later commentators performed the task of deciphering this and others of Alan's constructions. In one thirteenth-century copy of the *Anticlaudianus*, probably of North Italian manufacture, a series of pictorial glosses was introduced to reinforce the verbal commentary. Images inserted at appropriate intervals in the text establish the identity of the five steeds (figs. 4–9).[76] The sequence begins with a scene in which Reason, brandishing a flail, tames the team of horses; the artists inadvertently granted man a sixth sense by depicting an extra equine form at the end of the row. In the next five images a single horse is represented along with a sign of sensory perception and an identifying rubric. Two disembodied eyes hover near the horse of sight, a winged animal, while the rubric (in a formula repeated five times) confirms the pictorial identification: 'primus equus scilicet visus'. Isolated ears flank the second horse.

Beside the third there appears a man's face and hand; beneath his nose a foliate flourish and a stream of air are depicted. Next to the fourth horse a man's face is again shown, but this time his hand points to his mouth. In the final image, touch is identified by means of a vignette: a half-length figure stretches out a hand to stroke the fifth horse. Like the illustrators who represented the house of memory, the artist who depicted the steeds of the senses felt obliged to render both parts of the metaphor: the horse and the sense it signified. When he depicted the organs of sense he showed no more anatomy than was essential. Eyes and ears, as on the gates of memory, appear as wholly disembodied entities;[77] nose and tongue (decorously concealed) are situated in the identifying context of the face; hands are represented on the arms of a figure in half-length.

When a reader possessed the key to Alan's allegories, he could begin to translate the veiled statements into information. The senses, he would come to understand, exist in a hierarchy, some more noble than others, though all perfectly formed in their own right. Touch, resembling taste, is the lowliest sense, and is so because it is inclined to be concerned with earthly things. If the senses are in some way like horses, it is implied, they must be strong, wilful, and potentially unruly.[78] Only when tamed do they serve a good end. The proper functions of the senses, their final causes one might say, are revealed in the storyline itself. Controlled by Reason, they carry the Mind (in a chariot crafted by the Liberal Arts) a good distance, to the limits of the visible universe. But this is not the end of the voyage. The mind has the capacity to travel further, towards the house of God. The purpose of the senses, Alan suggests, is to bring the mind to an understanding of higher things. For the twelfth-century Platonist, however, this can be accomplished only with the aid of Theology and Faith.

Richard of Fournival constructed his library on an intellectual armature which bears a relation to Alan's vision. The citizen of Amiens was to begin his intellectual journey with the liberal arts and to progress book by book, shelf by shelf, to theology. In the library's last section he would find manuscripts marked with gold. Yet Richard devotes relatively little space in the *Bibliono-mia* to his theology books. They, like the law books, receive only summary description. Richard's enthusiasm lay elsewhere, in just that knowledge which could be derived from the senses, controlled by reason. It was in the fields of natural philosophy and medicine that Richard collected most avidly. These texts he deposited with particular care and attention in his library – itself a kind of 'house of memory' where 'treasures won by human intelligence' were preserved.

Of the physical appearance of Richard's manuscripts certain things may be said. Not all the surviving codexes are contemporary with him. The older volumes he presumably purchased or inherited; those of his own time he is

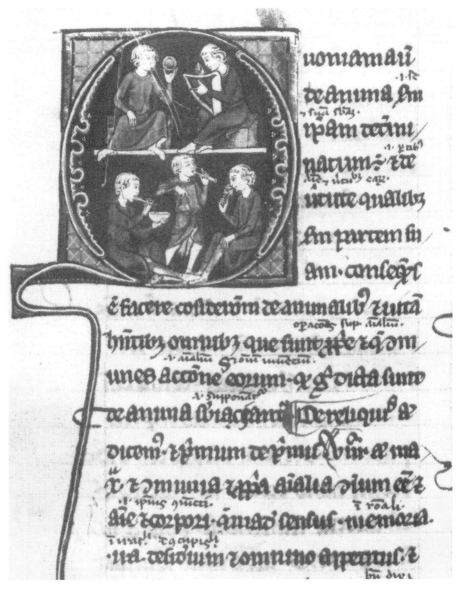

Fig. 10. The five senses.

assumed to have commissioned.[79] These volumes are characteristically unpretentious products, decorated only with red and blue filigree ornament. Whether or not Richard collected illuminated manuscripts cannot be said. Yet his insistence that the *Bestiaire d'amours* be illustrated suggests a close acquaintance with the accomplishments of contemporary illuminators.

It happens that Richard – whose *Bestiaire d'amours* would be illustrated with an image of an eye and an ear on the house of memory – possessed copies of those other texts that would, by the later thirteenth century, inspire illustrations of the senses, a pictorial theme just then coming into its own.[80] Alan of Lille's *Anticlaudianus* was one of these texts. Aristotle's *De sensu et sensato* was another. Luxury copies of the philosopher's *libri naturales* (a volume prominently placed in Richard's library) were ornamented with miniatures marking the openings of individual tracts and of books within tracts.[81] Artists responding to commissions for such manuscripts found themselves having to give concrete form to philosophical abstractions. Images created to head *De sensu* suggest the activity of sense perception in a variety of ways.

Common procedure on the part of artists was to depict individuals using objects readily recognized as stimulating specific senses. Painting being a medium which appeals only to the eye, the objects of the senses – sounds, smells, tastes, touch and even colours – had to be suggested by means of visible entities which evoked such concepts by association. In a Parisian manuscript dated *c.* 1260, the initial 'Q' of the opening words of *De sensu*, 'Quoniam autem de anima', contains a two-tiered scene showing each of five male figures actively employing a sense (fig. 10).[82] The first looks in a mirror, a device fashioned to serve the sense of sight. Next to him a figure representing touch plucks at the strings of a harp, his hands, the premier organ of touch, being given emphasis. On the bottom tier, taste, hearing and smell are represented by three figures: a man who holds a bowl and eats off a spoon, another who blows a flute and rings two bells, and a third who holds a flower to his nose. This method of representing the senses was also employed when space allowed depiction of only one or two figures.[83] In another Parisian manuscript of the third quarter of the thirteenth century a different tactic was adopted. Sense perception was represented generically. Five figures, one per sense, stand behind a table on which lie the remains of a banquet: empty bowls and fish bones signal that a sensual feast has taken place (fig. 11).[84]

In each of the miniatures sense perception is presented as pleasurable, even hedonistic activity. Aesthetically pleasing, the images are ornaments to the text. Yet viewers who brought learning to bear on their interpretation could find in the images certain information: that the senses are five, that each has a particular object, that colours, sounds, smells, tastes and touch can each be received by one and only one organ. In the most aggressively didactic of the surviving miniatures, an image at the beginning of *De sensu* in a late thirteenth-century Aristotle manuscript in Reims, the sense organs themselves become the focus of attention. The initial 'Q' encloses a representation of a bearded male head, straight on and close up (fig. 12).[85] A large bell hangs from each ear, while a red, four-petalled flower is placed below his nose. The improbability of the arrangement alerts the viewer to the fact that a specific didactic point is being made. An idea often emphasized in learned treatises is

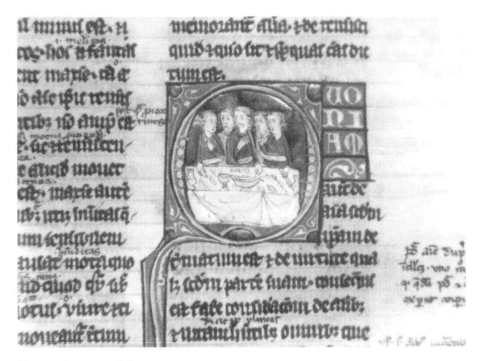

Fig. 11. Banquet of the senses.

called to mind, namely that four of the sense organs are located in the head. A viewer might notice that the eyes do not stare ahead but dart to the side, as if caught in an act of perceiving. He could supply the knowledge that the tongue is held in the mouth for its protection, and that the sense of touch is distributed throughout the body.

Just this kind of information is conveyed, even more emphatically, in an 'anatomy of the head for physicians' inserted in the mid-fourteenth century section of a natural philosophical miscellany (fig. 13).[86] In this line-drawn image, crude yet functional, the organs of sense are given emphasis: each is labelled; two nostrils are indicated even though the nose is in profile; the tongue juts out. A viewer could not but take the point that four of the sense organs are located in the head and that the locus of touch – its label arbitrarily situated in the neck – is elsewhere. If he used the diagram as intended, the viewer could trace the paths along which sensory impulses pass to the brain; he would see them collected in the first ventricle, site of common sense and fantasy, then pass to the chamber of imagination and cognitive power, and finally come to memory's place of residence.

The miniature in the Reims Aristotle has some of the same didactic aspirations as this line-drawn figure. Both offer information about the position and

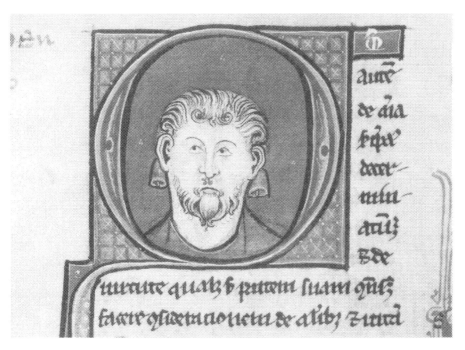

Fig. 12. The organs of sense.

operation of the organs of sense. But the illuminator, by depicting bells and a flower, also suggested that each organ has its special object and particular function. To use teleological terminology, he, like the other illuminators who provided initials for *De sensu*, represented the activities for the sake of which the sense organs were created. The miniaturists who illustrated the *Anticlaudianus* and the *Bestiaire d'amours*, literary texts, had a different task, that of giving visual form to verbal metaphors. The artist who represented the steeds of the senses gave an identity to each of the team by depicting alongside the animal one of the organs of sense. Those who represented the house of memory suggested that eyes and ears were functionally analogous to entrances in an architectural structure by placing disembodied sense organs on the gates of a castle.

Richard's metaphor, teleological in cast, would have carried with it many associations for the thirteenth-century reader. Richard and his contemporaries had access to a rich heritage of speculation about sense perception; many of the relevant texts were available in Richard's library in Amiens. Here were shelved together works of different philosophical persuasions (Aristotelian, Stoic, Platonist), of different genres and of different dates and places of origin. Linking the various discussions was the conviction that the body was created by intelligent design, and that the organs of sense were perfectly adapted to

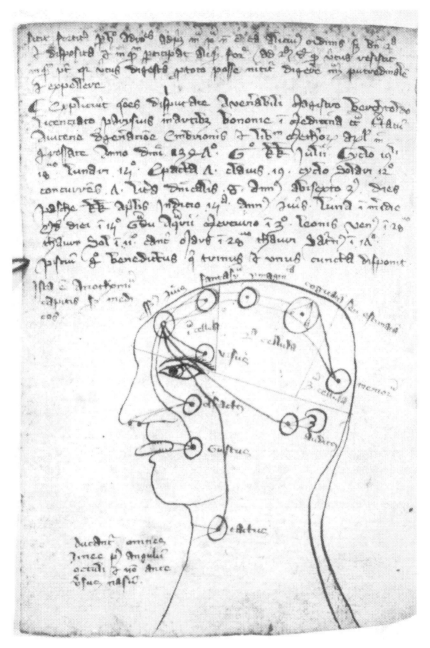

Fig. 13. 'Anatomy of the head for doctors'.

fulfil their designated functions. Metaphors of a particular cast abounded in these texts. The head was likened to a citadel or castle, the first of the three chambers of the brain to a threshold, the eyes and ears to windows, the eyelashes to fences or palisades. When Richard called the eyes and ears *portes* giving access to memory's house, he showed himself to be heir to a particular way of thinking about the body and its parts. What he conceived in words, illuminators set forth in pictures.

3

The manifest and the hidden in the Renaissance clinic

JEROME BYLEBYL

It is a commonplace to trace the beginnings of formal clinical teaching in modern Europe back to the hospital discourses of Giovanni Battista da Monte, who taught at the University of Padua from around 1540 until his death in 1551.[1] These discourses are systematic discussions of hospital patients carried out primarily for teaching purposes, and so have much in common with what would later be called 'clinical lectures'. Da Monte's students kept transcripts of these sessions, which were published during the sixteenth century together with his consultations for private patients.[2] Such discussions are rather far removed from the routine practice of medicine, but they do go beyond text-books and even retrospective case histories in representing actual encounters between individual doctors and patients. They can, therefore, provide some insights into how the exercise of the five senses – primarily by the doctor, but secondarily by the patient – might figure in these encounters. Furthermore, on such episodic visits to a hospital the one aspect of medical practice that could be taught most satisfactorily was the examination of the patient's physical person, so that it will also be relevant to try to understand the particular reasons that led da Monte to place new emphasis on this procedure.

In one of the hospital discourses, da Monte began by announcing both his didactic and his observational intentions:

In order to continue what we were discussing in the lectern with *those things that are apparent in the sick*, I shall not depart from my topic for today. Let us approach this patient, and let us suppose that he is a nobleman, since he differs in no respect from him, except by fortune.[3]

The second sentence might seem to acknowledge the interest of the patient, but alternatively or additionally it serves to establish a didactic fiction: let us

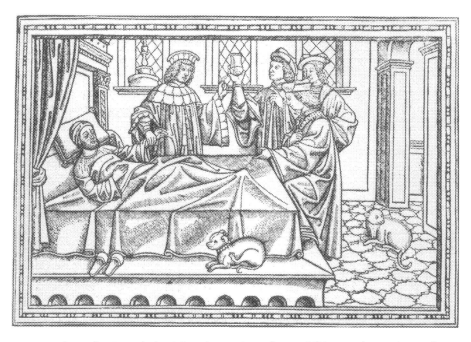

Fig. 14. Consultation of physicians in a private home. This woodcut seems to have been published for the first time on the title page of Pliny *et al.*, *Aurem opus* (Pavia, 1516) and was reprinted in several other works. It may possibly represent bedside teaching, but is more likely a consultation, since three of the four figures at the bedside appear to be taking an active part in the discussion: one takes the pulse and points to the urine glass; the second holds the urine glass and points towards it; the third gestures towards the patient.

treat this poor man as if he were someone who commands our close attention (see fig. 16).

Typically, da Monte's first visit to a hospital patient would include all the elements of practice, but on this particular day he must previously have been lecturing on the importance of the preliminary examination, because in the hospital discourse he went on to denounce doctors who do not begin by observing their patients carefully, and devoted most of the first session just to the examination.[4] He did, however, establish at the outset a therapeutic context for what he was about to do: 'We have come here to cure this man, and so it is necessary to remove whatever is against nature, and so you have the general scope of curing.'[5] In order to fulfil this general aim one must know what in particular is contrary to nature in the present patient, and it is to discover this that a careful examination is needed.

In addition, da Monte points to two other things that must be determined: what is the natural disposition of the patient, and what is the disposition of the

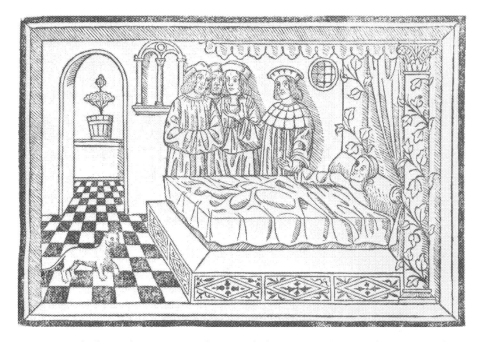

Fig. 15. Bedside teaching, or consultation of physicians. This woodcut appeared in the *Consilia Baverii* (Pavia, 1520). It was clearly based upon the scene in fig. 14, but the figures at the bedside have been modified in ways that suggest teaching rather than consultation: the one figure both takes the pulse and holds the urine glass; the other two now have their hands in their sleeves, and, like the fourth figure, appear as spectators rather than active discussants. The setting seems still to be that of a private home. (1521 edition used for figure.)

air that presently surrounds him? He was alluding to two of the central tenets of Galen's *Methodus medendi*: in devising therapy for a given patient one should take account not only of his disease, but also of such individual circumstances as his natural temperament, which must be restored, and the characteristics of the air presently impinging on him.[6] The quality of the air, said da Monte, 'is perceived by sense, so in that there is not much of art'.[7] But as regards the natural disposition of the patient under consideration he encountered a difficulty: it should be inferred from 'what is externally apparent in the colour and habit of his body, but it cannot be recognized in this patient because he has lain sick for the whole winter'.[8]

Da Monte went on to advise that, besides examining the patient, 'you should also ask either him or those who attend him about his customs and habits, what trade he exercises, whether he has anything specific to his nature, such as avoiding cheese or wine, etc'.[9] The transcript does not indicate that anything was in fact learned with regard to the latter questions, but simply continues:

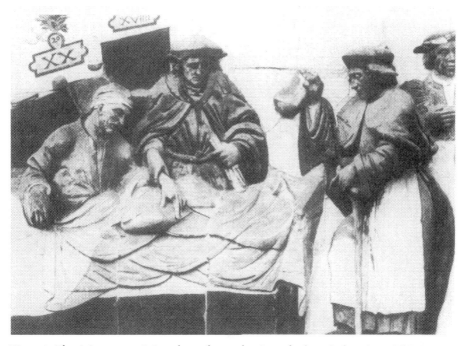

Fig. 16. Physicians examining the pulse and urine of a hospital patient. This is part of the cycle of the *Seven Works of Mercy*, executed between 1525 and 1529 by Giovanni della Robbia and others for the facade of the Ospedale del Ceppo at Pistoia. The full scene shows a second patient being treated by a surgeon. The numbered tablets over the beds clearly identify the setting as a hospital ward, although the scene has much in common with Fig. 14. In the context of the *Works of Mercy*, based upon the Last Judgement in Matthew 25, the poor sick man must be treated as if he were Christ himself. Indeed, in the preceding and following panels of the cycle, Christ is explicitly shown as one who is homeless, and as one who is in prison.

When you have learned these things, make a catalogue of them all, and then proceed in order. You will place first of all those things which are externally apparent, and so you will construct a simple description [*historia*].

Da Monte then launched a barrage at those physicians – his own teachers, in fact – whom he had seen making diagnoses without carrying out such a systematic preliminary examination. 'This is the blind pathway', he warned:

You will first declare which signs are [actually] present, those things which can also be called accidents ... then you will proceed to consider the causes of the individual accidents, and so you will proceed through the accidents in a methodical order.

Da Monte went on to outline how the patient should be examined with respect to the present preternatural disposition, that is, the disease, and here he

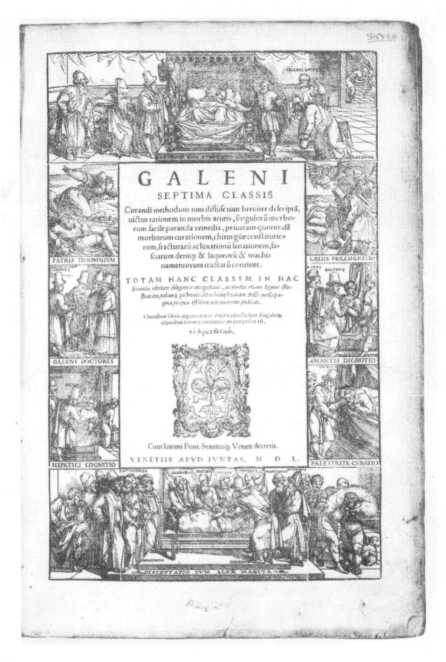

Fig. 17. Scenes from Galen's life. These woodcuts for the Giunta edition of Galen's *Omnia opera* were published first in 1541. Four of the six small scenes on the sides show Galen at the bedside; the other two (upper and middle left) show the father's dream of Asclepius, and Galen with his teachers. The large scene at the bottom shows Galen performing a vivisectional demonstration before a group of eminent Romans. The scene at the top, though not of a formal consultation, shows Galen (right) being summoned to the bedside of the emperor Antoninus, where he disagreed with the three court physicians (on the left).

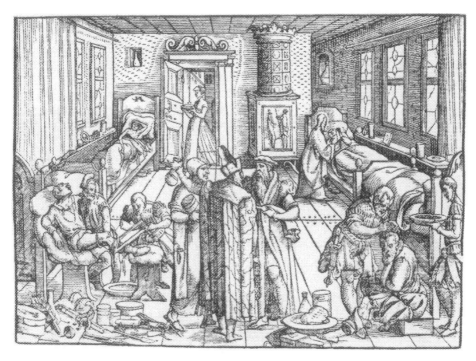

Fig. 18. Consultation in a hospital ward. The physicians in the centre of the scene appear to be engaged in animated discussion of the urine. The picture appeared in a surgical text and is probably mildly satiric: the physicians have their backs to the patients, while the surgeons minister to them, in emulation of Christ who is in the background. From Paracelsus, *Opus chyrurgicum* (Frankfurt-on-Main, 1565).

directed the students' attention primarily to the various bodily functions. These were the most important accidents in diagnosis, because by Galen's definition a disease cannot be said to exist unless the patient experiences a *functio laesa* or damaged function, and, conversely, the damaged function itself is the most reliable indicator of the underlying disease that is its cause.[10] Da Monte began his survey with the 'animal' or 'psychic' functions of voluntary movement and sensation, including the higher mental operations:

In movement there is no impediment, and the interior senses also have their powers intact, because he converses, imagines, and remembers well. The exterior senses are also good. Pain, which is a damaged function of the tactile power, appears in the head, which afflicts him more at some times, less at others.[11]

Thus da Monte was very much concerned with how the patient exercised his senses, both internal and external, although in this category the 'appearances' clearly included a good deal that he had learned, both directly and indirectly, from what the patient said. On the other hand, with regard to the

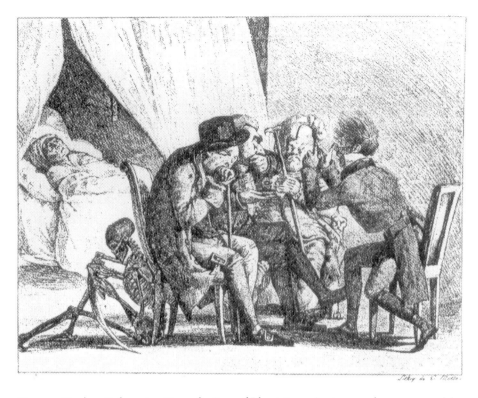

Fig. 19. Eugène Delacroix, *Consultation of Physicians*. A nineteenth-century satiric view of the traditional bedside consultation.

'vital' functions it was da Monte's own sense of touch that came into play, for under this category he carried out a minute examination of the pulse, and also determined the patient's relative hotness or coldness.[12] Finally, with regard to the 'natural' or 'nutritive' functions, da Monte declared: 'He has rugitus, he does not digest well, nor does he pass stools', things which he had evidently learned partly by hearing and partly by hearsay.[13] And although it is not mentioned on this occasion, it would not have been unusual for him to examine the abdomen by palpation as well.[14]

Examination of the excrements (in this instance only the urine) was closely related to the consideration of the nutritive functions, and here da Monte deployed a rich descriptive vocabulary: 'the urine tends towards a purple colour, there is an obscure redness, the liquor is limpid and very lucid, its substance is light ... It does not have foam, or cloudiness, or sediment at the bottom.'[15] These are all visual characteristics, although in his treatise on the excrements he also discussed how the urine should be examined with regard to smell.[16] But while he mentioned the possibility of tasting the urine, he did not expound this method in a comparably systematic way.[17]

Da Monte was an inveterate enumerator, and at the end of the examination he apparently sought to show by examples how the various sensible qualities had been taken into account: 'Accidents regarding visible qualities: the man is very pale. Regarding touch: he has much coldness. So you proceed to the other qualities in turn'.[18] The enumeration was only partial, though in one of da Monte's classroom lectures we find it in complete form:

After functions have been damaged, the sensible qualities and the objects of the senses are changed. First of all, the colours as they were according to nature are changed when the functions are damaged. Thus if someone becomes too red or too pale, you know that a red colour indicates a predominance of blood and a pale colour its privation ... Besides, the qualities which are the objects of hearing are changed, and you will perceive the sound in the intestines, and by your ears you will judge the various modes of damaged actions and functions. Also from the object of smell, for do you not judge various putridities and the parts affected by them by reason of the foetor in the putrescent humours, whether they be discharged through the bowels, the nostrils or the urine? As far as the qualities which are the objects of taste, you have the greatest indicator of the predominating humour when you perceive an acid, a bitter, a salty, an acrid, or an astringest taste, for the various humours are judged by these tastes. By touch also, from perceived heat or coldness, or from pain appearing in some part of the body, you have the greatest indicators for surveying the varieties of diseases.[19]

Thus the practitioner of humoral medicine had to be prepared to use all five of his senses in making a diagnosis, and da Monte drove home the same point in the treatise on excrements when he noted that they are unique among all the signs of disease in being accessible to all five of the senses.[20]

Both da Monte's patients and his diagnostic methods are lost to us, and therefore it would be pointless to try to arrive at an overall evaluation of how accurately he used his senses, or how well he taught his students to use theirs. But it is at least clear that he wanted the students to regard an unbiased examination of the patient ('construct a simple description') as a distinct and important entrée to diagnosis and treatment, and that his approach was systematic enough to routinely detect the absence of some symptoms as well as the presence of others. Nevertheless, da Monte was equally concerned to avoid any tinge of medical empiricism, in which practice is based solely on the external appearances. Indeed, in the particular case that we have been considering he pointed out that the external accidents would not always be considered in this way if they did not reveal 'important things', namely the internal state of the patient.[21] As he put it, a little further along, 'This way is innate to you, that we take our notion first of all from those things which are externally apparent, and from these we gather those things which are hidden.'

In the above case, da Monte began the process of interpretation at the first visit, but he had to bring the students back for a second visit to complete the diagnosis. Once again, his discussion was unusually detailed, and by the end of the second session he had not yet got around to devising an overall therapeutic strategy, much less to prescribing any specific treatment. However, a note at the end of the second discourse informs us that this marked the end of the hospital visits for that term; apparently our hypothetical nobleman was accorded a magnificent diagnosis, but no treatment.[22] The case is quite atypical in this respect, but is probably not so unrepresentative of the reasons for going specifically to a hospital to teach. In Italian medical culture of this period, a teacher such as da Monte had fairly wide leeway to take students to see his private patients,[23] and most aspects of practice could be taught more satisfactorily in that context than in the hospital. The one thing that da Monte could do better in the hospital was what he did on that first day, namely to devote as much time as he wished to teaching the students how to examine the patient.

For their part the students regarded these sessions highly enough to try to preserve records of them, although undue significance must not be attached to this fact. For the hospital discourses were preserved as part of a much larger effort by da Monte's students to publish as complete a record as possible of his teaching, with the result that we probably have more information about his public and private teaching than about that of any earlier doctor. This range of evidence provides excellent insights into his general philosophy of medical education, from which it is clear that he had very definite reasons for cultivating formal bedside teaching. But such evidence tells us very little about what others may or may not have done before him in the way of lectures on hospital cases, and hence about da Monte's priority in this regard.

Da Monte's reputation began to fade rather rapidly towards the end of the sixteenth century, so that his hospital teaching had to be rediscovered in the early nineteenth century. The immediate context was the great enthusiasm for clinical teaching that had developed by that time, with consequent interest in the early origins of the clinic. The first to call attention to da Monte's apparent priority was Giovanni Rasori, in 1808, although it remained for subsequent Italian clinician-historians to unearth the full range of evidence.[24] These efforts culminated in a monograph published by Giuseppe Cervetto in 1839, and after nearly a century and a half this is still our most detailed study of da Monte and his bedside teaching.[25]

This longevity was well deserved in some respects, but there were serious limitations on the kinds of issues that Cervetto and his predecessors felt free to explore. For they were trying to fit da Monte into a broader historiographic framework that emanated primarily from France, and whose ideology – in both senses – was that of the recently triumphant Paris clinical school.[26] In this view the clinic had come to be identified with 'the medicine of observation', and the hospital was regarded as the place where students should encounter the phenomena of disease directly and entirely, without the prejudice of any theoretical system. Such a medicine of observation was believed to have existed once before, during the time of Hippocrates, but following his death it had undergone rapid decline corresponding to the rise of the various rationalist sects. Galen had had the opportunity to revive the Hippocratic medicine of observation, but chose instead the vain pathway of subtle theorizing. This then prepared the way for the long night of medical scholasticism, when bedside observation and teaching were abandoned almost entirely. But eventually the teaching clinics served as the focus for the revival of bedside medicine, at first haltingly and imperfectly, but later with increasing authority and confidence, until in the Paris clinics the medicine of observation had been revived in all of its pellucid splendour.

It is not surprising that the Italian clinician-historians should have wished to claim for their countryman da Monte the honour of having begun this noble enterprise, but they could do so only by remaining discreetly silent concerning both the content and the context of his hospital discourses. For what da Monte had taught in the hospital was pure Galenic medicine with all of its luxuriant theorizing. And it is quite plain from the evidence that the most relevant institutional background for understanding his hospital discourses was the traditional consultation of physicians, that most ridiculed legacy of medical scholasticism, in which several doctors would gather at the patient's bedside for formal argumentation about his or her case (figs. 14, 18 and 19). Thus to call attention to what da Monte had actually taught in the hospital would only have confirmed what French historians of the clinic had already come to believe, that using a clinic to teach a theoretical system was worse than having no clinic at all. And to the countrymen of Molière, to have suggested that the consultation had given birth to the clinic might well have been to insult the legitimacy of all who taught at the bedside.[27]

Not surprisingly, therefore, the Italians chose to define da Monte's creativity in purely institutional terms. As Cervetto declared in his preface, 'It is the intention of the present work ... to provide the complete demonstration that *da Monte was the first in all of Europe, after the revival of civilization, to establish the Medical Clinic* [his emphases and capitals].'[28] However, as we have seen, one thing which our evidence cannot tell us is whether da Monte was really the first to give lectures on hospital cases. And in any event, the invention of 'The Medical Clinic', when taken out of its own intellectual and institutional context, becomes a sheer stroke of genius, something which is to be admired but not understood.

I shall try to provide a measure of intelligibility to da Monte's programme by a further examination of its relationship to his Galenism, to his more traditional classroom lectures, and to the medical consultation. On the first point my task has been made very much easier by Vivian Nutton's contribution to this volume (chapter 1) – Galen himself emphasized the importance of careful observation of the patient, hence it would indeed have been possible to mount a programme of clinical teaching based on Galenic principles. Nor was da Monte's Galenism either routine, or incidental to his hospital teaching. He was, on the contrary, a leading figure in the movement to reform medicine – and, specifically, medical practice – by the revival of authentic Galenism.[29] Before coming to Padua he had served as the editor-in-chief of the definitive Giunta edition of the works of Galen translated into Latin, and he may well have selected the scenes from Galen's life that are featured on the title page (fig. 17). In any case he would certainly have agreed with the ideal which they embody, for five of the eight scenes show Galen at the bedside, performing the feats of diagnosis, prognosis, and treatment in which he took great pride.[30] The major exception is the large scene at the bottom showing Galen performing a vivisectional experiment, but this is really of a piece with the others because a knowledge of anatomy and physiology was essential to the central feature of Galenic diagnosis, that of discovery of the 'affected part', or the internal locus of the disease.[31]

Indeed, Galen was clearly aware that an ablation procedure of the kind that he is performing in the picture – specifically the destruction of phonation by ligation of the largyngeal nerves – reproduces the essential features of his definition of disease as a preternatural condition of the body that clearly disturbs some function.[32] It would be misleading to suggest that such experiments were the sole basis of Galenic diagnosis or of da Monte's confidence in it, but the example does serve to illustrate the presumed causal relationships between bodily damage and functional damage that provided the foundation for what da Monte was attempting to teach in the hospital. In the case of the animal experiment the physician can directly perceive both the bodily damage (nerve ligation) and the resulting functional damage (loss of phonation), whereas in the human patient it is of course only the damaged function that is externally manifest, while the underlying bodily change is hidden from view. Nevertheless, Galenic physiology and pathology provided a comprehensive framework for associating specific kinds of functional damage with specific changes in the internal organs, while other external signs could further identify the humoral or other causes that affected the organ in the first place.

Thus for da Monte, as for Galen, diagnosis is a process of systematically interpreting externally manifest signs, especially disturbances of function, to answer three key questions, namely: What is the affected part? What is the nature of the affection? and, What is the cause of the affection?[33] This procedure undoubtedly involved a good deal of taxonomic reasoning, but the taxonomy in question allowed for a virtual infinity of possible species. For while Galenic medicine does admit only a limited number of general disease categories, such as distemper, obstruction or inflammation, these can in turn generate an inexhaustible variety of disease species by affecting any organ of the body, or any part of any organ, singly or in combination, and often with the involvement of two or more organs in a single pathological process.

It was because he understood this aspect of Galenic medicine with unusual clarity that da Monte took great umbrage at one of the most important parts of the traditional medical curriculum, namely the lectures on 'the practice of medicine' in which students were taught how to diagnose and treat a limited repertory of one hundred or so diseases.[34] In his own lectures on practice da Monte sought to show the futility of this approach by using the example of catarrh, which is a downward flow of humour from the brain. According to Rhazes, on whose text he was required to lecture, catarrh is just a single disease – the classic nasal catarrh caused by exposing the head to cold air – for which there is just one set of signs and one course of treatment.[35] Avicenna distinguished four species of catarrh, each with its own signs and treatment.[36] Da Monte, however, distinguished seven anatomical pathways along which the humours might flow, each resulting in a different set of symptoms and requiring a different course of treatment.[37] Furthermore, several of these pathways permitted multiple possibilities as to the ultimate locus where the humours collected, and these variations must also be taken into account in diagnosis and treatment. Nor is there any necessity that the humours follow just one of these pathways, so that, simply by taking the possible permutations of two or more, one could generate an extremely large number of species of catarrh. However, one must still go on to consider the particular qualities of the humour involved, and after that the prior cause of the flux; under each of these heads there are also multiple possibilities.

It would, therefore, have been impossible for da Monte to teach his students all the different kinds of catarrh by enumeration, or for them to learn them all by rote. Instead, he offered a methodical approach: there are certain signs that will always be present whenever a catarrh is involved; other signs will reveal the particular pathway or pathways along which the flux is occurring; others will identify the qualities of the humour involved; and others will determine the ultimate source of the humour.[38] A physician who has this knowledge does not need to try to memorize all the possible kinds of catarrh in advance of making a diagnosis, because he can (indeed, ought to) generate the diagnosis on the basis of the particular case before him.

The format of the lectures on medical practice required the teacher to conclude by telling the students how to cure the disease in question; but how could da Monte tell them how to cure an indefinitely large number of catarrhs, each requiring a potentially different course of treatment? And how could he take account of the patient's individuality, as the Galenic method of treatment required? Da Monte solved these problems by choosing a 'particular example', that is, a hypothetical case history:

Suppose a young man of twenty-five years having a hot and dry temperament, and having by nature hotness of his stomach and brain, but who on account of his age and temperament has fallen into an abuse of all of the six things non-natural.[39]

Da Monte then proceeded to specify the details of the young man's reckless way of life, as a result of which he 'began to abound in phlegmatic excrements'. From this there followed a prodigious list of symptoms, and after describing these da Monte declared:

Anyone who saw this young man would judge that he is suffering from catarrh, but to know its nature, and to choose a proper course of treatment, and to distinguish the material of the catarrh, here is the work, here is the labour.

Da Monte then carried out this task basing his approach upon the principles that he had previously outlined. His interpretation of the symptoms showed that the case was not 'simple' but 'multiple', because the phlegm must have flowed along several of the possible pathways, thus producing the great diversity of symptoms. Clearly he did not want the students to regard this case as a 'typical' catarrh; on the contrary, by choosing a very complicated example he reinforced his opposition to undue stereotyping in diagnosis.

Thus for da Monte the discussion of individual cases was not just a useful way of illustrating his lectures on practice, it was the only valid format in which to teach practice in the strict sense of the application of general rules to particular instances. And in another of his public lectures he underscored the crucial role of the senses in this regard:

The individual is known through accidents and through sensation, because sensation has particular objects, and so it is necessary to have signs and particular appearances which offer themselves to the senses, because knowledge of the nature of the body cannot be had otherwise. These [signs] are the functions and operations of each individual man, and from these we know the nature of each person. We consider the natural and the animal functions, and whatever else is apparent to the senses, and from these particulars we make universal judgements. Thus we have begun to show as under a cloud how universals are applied to particulars. The art of the physician turns on this relationship and is applied through signs.[40]

The ultimate goal of diagnosis is, then, to arrive at a rational understanding of the patient through 'universals', but it is only by the pathway of the senses that the physician can determine which of an extremely wide range of universals are relevant to understanding a particular patient and his disease.

In many of his discussions of individual cases, both in the hospital and at consultations, da Monte explicitly affirmed his commitment to rationalist medicine, as for example:

I shall not depart from the excellent custom of the ancient physicians who were unwilling to cure a disease unless they had first given exact consideration to its very essence and nature, as well as to the temperament of the body in which it occurs.[41]

By the 'very essence and nature' of a disease, da Monte understood some specific defect (*vitium*), or affection (*affectio*), or lesion (*laesio*) that inheres in some internal organ, and his discussions of individual cases were founded on the premise that it is indeed possible to arrive at an exact understanding of such hidden affections or lesions by a careful examination of the external signs and symptoms. As he put it, 'Those things which are apparent in disease usually show both the kind and the magnitude of the disease, for they follow the disease as a shadow follows its body.'[42] Or again:

When you approach a patient whom you have never seen before ... first take in those signs which are manifestly apparent, from which you will afterwards perceive those things that are hidden within, and what is the disease.[43]

But to say that certain things are manifestly apparent is not to say that they are immediately obvious, because many physicians manage to ignore them, as he warned in the continuation:

You should not do as do unskilled physicians, who only suspect that the fever is such and such ... and postulate the appropriate signs, even though many of them are not present. Beware of such things, if you wish to be physicians worthy of Hippocrates.

Hence the need for a systematic examination as a distinct prelude to diagnosis.

Another frequent motif in the hospital discourses is that of the primacy of the damaged functions among the various symptoms of disease. For example, 'Let this be your rule, that always on your first visit you should immediately see which functions are damaged. For they will indicate the disease, and they are signs which will not fail.'[44] He began the discussion of another patient by relating this concern to Galen's definition of disease:

On other occasions we have advised you that when you approach the patient, you ought first to consider the disturbed functions, for a disease is only said to exist when disturbed functions are apparent, since a disease is nothing other than a preternatural disposition that clearly disturbs the functions. Now you know that the functions are threefold, namely the animal, the vital and the natural. Therefore you should now approach this patient, and before you ask him a lot of questions, you ought to observe those things which are apparent of themselves.[45]

On both of these occasions da Monte began his survey with the animal functions, including the exercise of the senses. In the first instance he declared:

The animal functions are not damaged here, for he understands, remembers and converses rightly; all of the internal senses are healthy, therefore the physician will not consider them further. Nor are the external senses damaged: he properly sees, hears, smells, feels, tastes and carries out bodily movement, and thus exercises all of the animal functions as a healthy man does.[46]

In the second instance da Monte did find some disturbance in this regard: 'For you see that he cannot remain quiet, from which there is no doubt that he is suffering something in the senses and the animal faculty, for otherwise he would remain quiet.'[47] Da Monte conjectured that the problem might have to do with the imagination, but after determining that the patient had great fever he revised his view:

The agitation, as we have said, indicates that there is something in the animal faculty or brain. But there is no damage in the interior senses, for he reasons and imagines well, etc. The exterior senses are also healthy and it is only with respect to the sense of touch that he suffers, for he feels a great disturbance of all the members because of the bad distemper, and because of the pain he cannot remain in one position.[48]

Thus all of the internal and external senses are undamaged, so that the tactile discomfort must be a secondary consequence of the fever, or general distemper.

In fact, none of da Monte's hospital patients suffered from primary diseases of sensation, but a case of deafness in one of his private patients will illustrate how he went about the process of differential diagnosis to determine the locus and nature of the underlying disease.[49] He began by stipulating that there are five places along the auditory pathway at which the function of hearing can be disturbed: there can be a 'defect [*vitium*]', that is, intrinsic change, in either (1) the brain itself, or (2) the auditory nerve, or (3) the eardrum; or there can be an 'obstruction' in either (4) the internal, or (5) the external aural canal. Da Monte eliminated (1) on the grounds that the brain is the locus of the common sensorium, so that if it were affected the disturbance would involve all of the senses, not just hearing. He also eliminated (2), (3) and (4) on the grounds that the patient 'says that he perceives tinnitus', and to da Monte this meant that all of the organs involved in the generation and transmission of sound must be intact. This left (5) as the only possibility, and da Monte further determined that the obstruction of the external canals must be total because 'he perceives no sound from the outside, not even a very loud one'. The difficulty that no obstructions could actually be seen was dismissed on the ground that 'the passage is tortuous, and indeed sometimes worms enter the passage but can by no means be seen'. Da Monte then proceeded confidently to determine the specific nature of the unseen obstruction and the underlying pathological process that led to its formation.

Several cases of dropsy seen in the hospital also provided da Monte with opportunities to teach various facets of differential diagnosis based on Galenic principles. In discussing one of them he expounded upon the difference between general and local diseases:

It is a rule that whenever you see a patient whose whole body is affected with a bad temperament, then you will declare that the defect is in the principal organ of some faculty. For example, if no part of the body moves, you will say that the defect is in the principal of movement, that is, in the brain. But if only one part is immobile, but others mobile, then the defect is not in the principal organ. So when you see that one part suffers from a defect of concoction, as when a leg swells, but the rest of the body is in good condition, then the defect is not in the principal of the natural faculty [the liver].[50]

He then applied these rules to the patient under consideration:

In this boy there is no defect in movement, because he does move, nor are the functions of the brain damaged, because he imagines, and remembers, nor are the external senses damaged, because he sees, he hears, etc. Therefore there is no defect in the animal functions, which are in the brain. As far as the vital functions, the pulse is quite good, therefore the heat flows in from the heart [to the whole body]. The defect is in the natural faculty, which is shown by the damaged functions, for he is not nourished as he ought to be: the legs and feet are emaciated, and deprived of nutriment, but the belly is swollen ... You see that there is damage common to the whole body.[51]

'Therefore,' he concluded, 'the defect is in the liver.'

But what specifically is wrong with the liver? One possibility is a simple cold distemper, but that would produce a different set of symptoms: the liver would supply the whole body with unconcocted nutriment, and therefore all the parts would equally swell with dropsy. From the fact that most of the parts are emaciated, while the dropsy takes the form of ascites, da Monte concludes that there must be an actual obstruction preventing the flow of nutriment from the mesenteric veins through the liver, and so on to the rest of the body.[52] His prognosis is grim:

This boy will die, because he has now been ill for four years, and besides the obstruction he also suffers from hardness of the liver: the liver has become scirrhous, and I believe that it is hard like a stone, but I cannot feel it because of the swollen distension.[53]

Thus da Monte had attempted, unsuccessfully, to confirm his diagnosis by palpation.

Another dropsical patient was an elderly messenger who seemed to be in transition between general oedema, stemming from a simple cold distemper of the liver, and ascites, caused by an obstruction.[54] In another patient, a young man, da Monte found, on his first visit, the generalized dropsy that he associated with simple cold distemper,[55] but on a later visit he had to add a further complication when he got his first look at the patient's faeces and found them to be of a grey colour. Of this sign he declared:

It indicates that there is a certain obstruction in the bile duct extending to the intestine, but it is not completely blocked ... Some people conclude from grey-coloured faeces that there is an obstruction in the mesenteric veins, but that is not so if you grasp the anatomy.[56]

Da Monte expounded upon the foolishness of the latter interpretation, and then described the very different symptoms that would follow from an obstruction of the mesenteric veins.

Thus, the hospital provided da Monte with a forum in which to inculcate the particular kinds of diagnostic skills that he, as a Galenic physician, regarded as most important; but he also found another such forum ready at hand, in the tradition of consultation by a group of physicians. For this too was supposed to involve a review of the patient's signs and symptoms followed by theoretical interpretation leading to therapeutic action, and if done properly there was no reason why the strictest Galenic principles could not be followed and hence exemplified here as well. Furthermore, although such consultations were paid for by the patient, it was accepted in Italian medical culture that they might also serve a teaching function. For example, in his rules for consultation the Paduan professor Alessandro Massaria urged consultants to be moderate in argumentation and the citation of authorities, and then added, 'But I would exempt public teachers from this injunction if they conduct consultations in the presence of medical students ... for then their duty pertains not only to curing the sick, but very much to that of teaching as well.'[57] Massaria was writing in the late sixteenth century, but there was nothing new about having medical students attend consultations – da Monte reported that he had done so himself as a student.[58] Furthermore, as a famous physician he later engaged in frequent consultations, which also served a teaching function. This is implicit in the fact that the published transcripts of these consultations are known to have been based on students' notes, just as were the hospital discourses.[59] Furthermore, the transcripts show da Monte himself making occasional references to teaching, as for example when he began by addressing his fellow consultants, 'Excellent doctors, we are about to consult for the sake of this young nobleman, and we will also say much that will benefit the students, and so we will profit both of them.'[60]

Moreover, there is a good deal of evidence to suggest that this tradition of medical consultation, and its adaptation to teaching, was the matrix out of which da Monte's hospital discourses emerged (see figs. 14 and 15).[61] The latter incorporated many of the features of the consultations, but also differed from them in some important respects: the didactic intention took clear priority over the interests of the patient; da Monte conducted the hospital discourses by himself rather than in collaboration with other doctors; and the discussion of a hospital patient could be extended over repeated visits rather than being confined to just a single session.[62]

On several occasions in the hospital discourses da Monte made explicit comments about the consultations which indicate that he himself saw both similarities and differences between the two. One such occurrence was in the discourse to which I referred at the beginning of this paper, immediately following the reference to the patient as a hypothetical nobleman:

Consultations are gatherings of upright men of the sake of understanding and curing diseases, and for considering the prognostic signs of the outcome of the disease. They do not take place for the sake of boasting and ostentation. Those who only want to show off are impostors and deceivers, and nothing will succeed for them. But whatever is done without guile will lead to success . . . Therefore in every disease you ought to converse with learned men, *or with yourself*, so that having understood the nature [of the patient] or the disease, you will find the cure.[63]

Thus consultation, as a part of medical practice, is something that can be done properly or improperly, and clearly one of the aims of the hospital discourses was to teach the students how to do it the right way. And at the same time the consultation exemplifies the kind of systematic analysis that the doctor ought to carry out in every case, regardless of whether it involves formal discussions with colleagues.

But is the hospital discourse itself simply a practice consultation, or does da Monte himself see it as something distinct? A little further on, he again refers to consultations:

In my time, when I was a young man following in practice . . . [the physicians] who were then famous, a confused way of holding consultations was followed. For first they would declare the temperament of the patient, before they had even pointed out the manifest signs, and so were trying to demonstrate the known through the unknown, which is a preposterous order. And when they had considered the temperament, they would go on to name the disease. And after that they would list the symptoms of that disease as they were described by Avicenna, whether or not they were actually present in the patient. And sometimes they would declare twenty signs, but when I approached the patient I could scarcely find two of them.[64]

Here again we find da Monte, in a hospital discourse, pointing to the bad way of consulting, though now focusing on the preliminary examination of the patient.

Presumably in this respect there is also a corresponding good way of consulting, although if we look at the transcripts of da Monte's consultations we find that the one thing that he as senior consultant could not do was to conduct the initial survey of signs and symptoms; that was done by another doctor, who seems usually to have been the attending physician.[65] Da Monte then had to interpret the signs as summarized by someone else, and while he might occasionally add to the catalogue of symptoms, he might also apologize to the first doctor for doing so.[66]

Thus deference to colleagues served as a filter between da Monte and the appearances, and so also might deference to the patient. Here, for example, is the way that da Monte began at the consultation for the Venetian senator Bernardo Navagero:

Since we cannot cure the affections existing in this Magnificent Lord unless we thoroughly understand them, and because our understanding begins from *those things which are apparent*, first we will consider *the symptoms recited by him*, which ought to be diligently explained.[67]

Here the phrase 'those things which are apparent' is equated with what Senator Navagero says; contrast this with what he said in a hospital discourse: 'you should now approach this patient, and before you ask him a lot of questions, you ought to observe those things which are apparent of themselves'.[68] Thus the hospital cases offered da Monte the opportunity to examine the patient directly, without the intervention of professional colleagues, and without the need to defer to the patient's own views.

In another hospital discourse da Monte made a further comment about consultations that seems even more critical of their value for teaching. This was the instance, cited above, where he returned on a later visit to find that the patient had passed grey-coloured stools, and noted that many physicians took this to be a sign of obstructed mesenteric veins. His fuller remarks were as follows:

I frequently hear this [erroneous view] at consultations. But when I hear such things I do not contradict them, and you should also do the same, to avoid hatred and to retain favour among all ... When you hear such inept ideas, you should take great pleasure in understanding what the others do not. But if you can, always hold your silence.[69]

Here again, da Monte is using the hospital discourse to give advice on how to conduct consultations, but now in such a way as to set a considerable distance between the two. At consultations, two or more doctors necessarily took part, and the desire for good professional relations might even take precedence over speaking the truth, whereas in the hospital, by obvious implication, da Monte found no such reason to bite his tongue because he alone was conducting the session.

Finally, in one of the hospital discourses, the fourth of six pertaining to the same patient, da Monte began by pointing out the advantages of such return visits:

It makes a great difference to see the movements and changes of the disease, which take place every day, and are varied, so that often the sick person needs a sagacious cure. If you have paid attention to this boy, there have been many such alterations.[70]

Da Monte then outlined the differences between 'what we have seen on previous days' and what was to be seen 'today'. Of course, a review of the prior course of the disease was routinely provided at consultations, but the students would generally not have seen the earlier stages, and da Monte himself might even acknowledge to the attending physician that he had not seen the patient previously.[71]

Thus while the hospital discourses were probably inspired by the consultations, and clearly had many formal elements in common with them, they should not be seen solely as consultations carried out for teaching purposes on hospital patients. Indeed, if that had been their true character then da Monte would undoubtedly have asked one or more of his colleagues to join him in the hospital. He did not do so, I would suggest, because he turned to the hospital precisely to escape from the limitations that he had come to perceive in the consultation as a vehicle for teaching the practice of Galenic medicine as he understood it.

But, ironically, the very same social factors that made the hospital patients so much more available for observation and teaching also placed serious limitations on how fully da Monte could apply this particular kind of medical practice. That is, Galenic medicine is a dietetic system, in which the physician would ideally like to be able to examine the patient's whole way of life in order fully to diagnose his or her disease; and, ultimately, he would hope to make various adjustments in the way of life as an important part of therapy. Consider, for example, the case of Senator Navagero, who was suffering from vertigo:

This famous lord has many problems. He was once the consul in Dalmatia, where he became involved in affairs and litigation, and he says that he developed weakness of the brain because of the mental effort. When he returned to Venice, he followed a bad regimen, and he also gave himself over to literary studies. It is now several months since he began feeling as if he would fall to the ground, and indeed he would have fallen many times if help were not present.[72]

Here a medically sophisticated patient has provided da Monte with just the kinds of details that he would like to have for a complete aetiological diagnosis, and this is typical of the fairly circumstantial accounts of patients' lives that we often find in the consultations.[73] But when we look for such information among the hospital cases, we find only an occasional snippet – for example, that a young man got dropsy 'from sleeping on the ground', or that a boy developed scabies 'on account of poverty and gluttony'.[74] Concerning another hospital patient we learn that he went to Venice for Carnevale, and there was jostled by the crowds'.[75] And another's whole life is reduced to a stereotype: 'This man is a charlatan, a vagabond, and has lived a disorderly life, as such people are accustomed to do.'[76]

We find similar contrasts in the realm of therapeutics, where the model patient for dietetic medicine was one who had considerable discretion over how he or she lived. Thus da Monte advised a Venetian lawyer that he should seek a change of air for several months, free from all work and strong emotions, but it probably would not have occurred to him to give such a prescription to a hospital patient.[77] A more explicit reminder of social disparities is what he said of a boy in the hospital with skin eruptions: 'If he were the son of a nobleman or prince, I would have his linens changed every day so that he would not have defilement from the pustules.'[78] Also important for dietetic treatment are the attitudes that the patient will bring towards following an elaborate regimen. Thus in the case of Senator Navagero, da Monte is optimistic of a cure 'because he is a prudent man and will do whatever he is ordered for his health', but regarding a hospital patient he was more tentative: 'he seems to me to be quite a prudent man for one of his class'.[79]

There was, then, a certain hollowness to da Monte's proposal to treat the hospital patient as a supposed nobleman, and therefore a kind of paradox in his whole initiative. That is, in his zeal to teach medicine at the bedside he turned to a place where patients were indeed readily accessible for that purpose, but they were patients whose situations made them rather inappropriate to the particular kind of medicine that he wished to teach. A multiplicity of barriers – physical, social and economic – prevented him from knowing the particular circumstances that gave rise to the diseases of the hospital patients, nor could he realistically expect to be able to change those circumstances as part of the treatment. In the hospital, the patient's way of life was hidden from view, so that the scope of diagnosis was largely restricted to 'those things which are apparent in the sick', or, more precisely, in the bodies of the sick. From da Monte's point of view this aspect of medicine was important enough to warrant going to the hospital in quest of it, but I think we can see why he also continued to attach great importance to the private consultations where the patient's way of life, if not his body, was more open to examination.

4

In bad odour: smell and its significance in medicine from antiquity to the seventeenth century

RICHARD PALMER

Classical theories of smell exerted an enduring influence on medicine and on the popular understanding of disease. This chapter is concerned with the period from antiquity to the second half of the seventeenth century, when the Galenic theory of olfactory sensation began to come under attack as a result of new anatomical and physiological research. During this long period ideas were formed by the rich literature on smell inherited from antiquity. Plato in the *Timaeus*, and Aristotle in the *De anima* and *De sensu* provided ample groundwork for a debate about the nature of smell. Theophrastus and Galen also dealt with it in several works, including specialized treatises, *Concerning Odours* by Theophrastus, and *The Olfactory Organ* by Galen.[1] Medieval and Renaissance writers continued the theme in general encyclopaedias, and also in medical *consilia* and works of theory, such as the *De saporum et odorum differentiis* published in 1583 by Juan Bravo, professor of medicine at Salamanca.

Continuity rather than change in the understanding of smell was characteristic of the literature of this period. Yet the tradition was neither monolithic nor free from internal controversy. From Aristotle onwards writers noted that, amongst the five senses, smell was problematic.[2] It was easier to determine what was sound or colour than to say what was smell. It was not obvious how smell was perceived, and there was even a doubt as to which sense organ was responsible. Then again, there was the question of where smell was to be ranked in the hierarchy of the five senses. For smell had a double nature. It could be an aesthetic, even spiritual delight. But smell could equally be stench. In seventeenth-century representations of the five senses the topoi for smell ranged accordingly from the fragrant garden to the stink of vomit or the malodorous baby's bottom.[3] This chapter considers the significance for medicine of two central questions raised initially in the classical texts. First, what is the organ of smell? Second, what is the nature of smell? Finally, it examines the place of smell in the hierarchy of the senses.

In his book *The Olfactory Organ*, Galen reached a conclusion which, even he admitted, was at first surprising. The organ of smell was *not* the nose. The nose, he argued, was no more than a passage which carried smells up to the true olfactory organ, the brain itself. The same passage also carried air to cool the brain, and acted as a drainage channel for residues. Essential for the sense of smell were two olfactory projections from the front ventricles of the brain. These projections, which were clearly illustrated in the *Fabrica* of Vesalius of 1543, were of the same substance as the brain, and in effect part of it.[4] They descended to the cribriform plate separating the nasal and cerebral cavities. From the time of Galen until the research of Conrad Victor Schneider in the second half of the seventeenth century it was believed that this sieve-like plate or bone was porous.[5] Air and smells could pass through it to reach the brain. Smell, then, worked in a different way from the other senses. The nose was not equivalent to the eye in seeing, the ear in hearing, or the tongue in taste. In smell alone the brain was the primary organ of perception.

Avicenna followed these ideas closely, while noting that the olfactory projections were breast- or nipple-like, a simile repeated by writer after writer until, by the time of Ambroise Paré in the sixteenth century, 'mamillary projections' (*procez mammillaires*) could be used as a scientific term.[6] In the play *Lingua*, a comedy of the five senses published in 1607, Olfactus, the sense of smell, declared, 'I lay my head between two spongeous pillows, like fair Adonis 'twixt the paps of Venus.'[7]

Outside the medical tradition, Galen's ideas of olfactory sensation seem to have been less readily accepted. Bartholomeus Anglicus described the olfactory nipples as situated in the nose, and his account of olfaction follows the pattern of the other four senses: animal spirits pass from the brain down the nerves to the nipples, where they gather impressions to be conveyed back up to the common sense in the front ventricle of the brain. A series of illustrations of brain function popular in the fifteenth and early sixteenth centuries demonstrates the same theory. These illustrations are well known, but it has not been sufficiently stressed that they occur not so much in medical texts as in works on Aristotelian natural philosophy, or in general encyclopaedias, such as the *Margarita philosophica* of Gregorius Reisch, published in 1503.[8] They reflect the tacit assumption of Aristotle that the organ of smell lay in the nose, and as far as smell is concerned they are not representative of Galen and the medical tradition. Bartolomeo da Montagnana was more typical of fifteenth-century medicine in thinking only three theories worth consideration: that the front ventricles of the brain were the organ of smell; that perception lay in the 'olfactory breasts' attached to the ventricles, or that ventricles and breasts acted together.[9] In his opinion the 'olfactory breasts' alone were responsible, and his view was shared in the sixteenth century by Vesalius, Juan Bravo and others.[10]

The sense of smell, then, lay in the olfactory brain. But what exactly did the brain sense? When a flower was smelled, was it an immaterial quality, an image or likeness which passed from the flower to the brain, or was smell a real substance? Plato, faced with the task of associating each of the five senses with one of the four elements, found a way out by linking smells with vapour, the intermediate state between water and air. Galen followed him, though adding the idea that smells could also carry earthy or fiery qualities. Summarizing the theory, Bartholomeus Anglicus defined smell as a smoky vapour arising from the substance of a thing.[11] Once again, smell was different from the other senses. Juan Bravo noted that light and colour were immaterial qualities. Remove the object of vision, and it can no longer be seen. But remove a flower, and its perfume lingers in the air. Smells, in his view, were material.[12]

So seriously was this taken that an ancient Pythagorean tradition continued to be respected right down to the sixteenth century. Food smells, it was believed, were not merely appetising, but also nourishing. According to Pliny, an Indian people, called the *Astomi* since they had no mouths, lived wholly on the smell of wild apples. This was often discussed in medieval and Renaissance literature, and was even the subject of a woodcut by Hans Weiditz, published in 1559.[13] Marsilio Ficino, writing in 1489, likewise noted that 'Democritus . . . when he was almost dead, held on to his spirit for four days, only on the smell of warm bread, and he would have held on longer if he had wanted. He did this to please his friends.' So impressed was Ficino that he advised old people to keep out the cold by applying warm bread poultices to their stomachs – the smells would nourish them at the same time.[14] Hippocrates and Galen gave smells a particular role in nutrition, since they were absorbed directly without the need for digestion. Only Bravo expressed a doubt. Smells, he thought, could not sustain a man for long, and as for the *Astomi*, if they lived on smells, why did nature give them stomachs?[15]

This debate had a serious implication for medicine. If smells were real substances which penetrated into the brain, then their potential was great, both for causing disease and for therapy. Smells carried the qualities of the substances from which they emanated – they could be hot or cold, wet or dry.[16] Ficino noted that the cold smells of roses, violets, myrtle and camphor were beneficial to people inclined to heat, while the warm smells of lemon, mint, aloes, amber and musk were good for colder temperaments.[17] Fifteenth- and sixteenth-century *consilia* suggest that healing smells were a regular feature of the sick room, as does a seventeenth-century series of Italian engravings of the five senses, where smell is represented by an invalid in bed smelling flowers, while a perfume burner sweetens the air of the room.[18] Smells were part of

Bartolomeo da Montagnana's therapy for cold complexions of the brain, for various kinds of headache, for catarrh, for melancholy, and for nervous conditions. Anosmia – loss of the sense of smell – could itself be treated in this way, for drying smells could unblock obstructions between the olfactory nipples and the ventricles of the brain. A youth from Vicenza suffering from a cold, humid complexion of the brain with a flow of aqueous phlegm was advised by Montagnana to burn storax, mint, oregano and other dry and aromatic herbs, and to hold to his nose a pomander made from the same ingredients.[19] A similar treatment was recommended by the Paduan professor Giovanni Battista Da Monte in 1548 for a member of the Fugger family, while his therapy for the Venetian senator Bernardo Navagero, suffering from vertigo, included aromatic powders to be sprinkled on the head, and a pomander made of roses, violets, waterlilies, camphor, sandalwood and rose vinegar.[20] Bravo referred to smells used to sedate, and in pharmacy to the addition of aromatic ingredients to temper purging medicines, since good smells strengthened the mouth of the stomach.[21] Through the similarity of their nature, smells were also thought to exert a powerful effect on the spirits, the vital spirit with its seat in the heart, distributed through the arteries to vivify the whole body, and the animal spirit responsible for neurological functions, with its seat in the brain. Foetid smells, wrote Bravo, damaged and overthrew the spirits. Good smells, on the other hand, strengthened and restored them, also comforting the heart and brain.[22] Aromatic medicines accordingly had wide applications, and in general, as Avicenna advised, where several remedies brought about the same effect, the best one to use was the sweetest and most pleasant smelling.[23]

These ideas about smell were elaborated in the Renaissance by Marsilio Ficino, for whom healthy living consisted in large part in nourishing and refreshing the spirit daily with pleasant odours. Good smells prevented the compression of the spirit which spelled sadness and torpor. They also checked the excessive flightiness of the spirit, the tendency to dissipate, which rendered the body weak. For, intermediate between body and soul, the spirits had a certain mobile independence. The vital spirit, responsible for the passions, could retreat to the heart in the experience of fear, or rush from the heart outwards – the sensation of anger. Smells could be used to influence the spirits, and even to move them about the body. Fainting and even paralysis were associated with a flight of the spirit inwards, and smells were used to attract it back to the limbs.[24] Bravo noted that Paul of Aegina had recommended strong smells such as bitumen and pitch in reviving epileptics.[25] Bartholomeus Anglicus recorded that the stink of burned wool or goats' horns could recall a patient from unconsciousness (*sopor lethargicus*). He explained that in this case the spirit fled from the smell to the interior of the brain, the seat of the disease. There the spirit was better placed to digest and dissolve the substance causing the condition.[26]

In a similar way smells acted upon that curiously mobile part of the body, the womb. According to an ancient, even pre-Hippocratic, tradition, hysteria was caused by the rising up of the womb, compressing the diaphragm and other organs and causing fainting and other symptoms. The ancient therapy, popularized in the Middle Ages in the work of Trotula, and continued in the sixteenth century by Ambroise Paré, was to apply bad smells to the nose to repel the womb from above – burned wool and old shoes, asafoetida and castor – while applying sweet perfumes to the vagina to attract the womb downwards. Paré helpfully published an illustration of a fumigating device which might be used for the purpose (*un pot pour recevoir les parfums au col de la matrice*).[27] Similar therapy was recommended in the following century by John Sadler.[28] The use of bad smells in medicine was nevertheless a matter for concern. Paré was emphatic that only odours which were dry could be used in medicine. For smells emanating from dead animals, sewage and the like would infect the patient and his attendants with their putrid vapours. Here Paré was following an age-old association of putrid smells with disease. From antiquity, infections, and especially epidemic diseases, were thought to be caused by miasmatic vapours rising up from decaying and putrid matter to infect the air. The plague, according to Simon Kellwaye, writing in 1593, 'may come by some stincking doonghills, filthie and standing pooles of water and unsavery smelles'.[29]

Plato's description of smells as vapours emanating from bodies in a state of change, putrefaction, liquefaction or evaporation, was analogous to medical descriptions of the generation of disease. Galen observed that it was especially dangerous to associate with the sick whose breath was so putrid that their houses stank.[30] The stinking breath of lepers, according to Bartholomeus Anglicus, infected and corrupted the healthy.[31] Venice in 1522 ordered the compulsory hospitalization of syphilitics found begging in the town, 'with the greatest stench and infection of their neighbours' (*con grandissimo fettor et contagio delli cohabitanti et vicini*).[32] Here there was also concern that the stench of the syphilitics could bring the plague, for foetid smells produced a variety of results. Similar causes, such as the stinks raised by dredging, left in the wake of a flood, or arising from a stagnant town moat, might explain variously a diphtheria-like epidemic, a high mortality in children under ten, or the prevalence of tertian and quartan fevers.

During the Black Death of 1348 the Italian town of Pistoia regulated the depth of burials 'to avoid a foul stink' (*ad evitandem turpem fetorem*), and banned the tanning of hides within the city walls 'so that stink and putrefaction should not harm the people' (*ut fetor et putredo hominibus obesse non possit*).[33] The Venetian senate in the same crisis solemnly ordered the expulsion from the town of bad salt pork, 'which causes a great stench and in consequence putrefaction which is the corruption of the air' (*que multum*

fetorem inducunt et per consequens putredinem quod est corruptio aeris).[34]
From the Middle Ages onwards fear of epidemics motivated public health
measures governing street cleaning, sewage disposal, the free-flowing of water
courses, the zoning of industries, and hygiene in meat, fish and fruit markets. A
day in the life of the Provveditori alla Sanità, the Venetian noblemen responsible for plague control, could take them, as it did on 5 January 1501, to
inspect a rubbish tip in Campo San Stefano which was a source of local complaint. They ordered its removal, 'knowing that amongst other measures that
we can and should take to keep this city healthy, one of the most important is
to remove as far as possible all those things which give off smells and stinks
which easily produce diseases'.[35]

While magistrates strove to deodorize the air of the towns, individual
hygiene dealt with the smells of the home and of the body.[36] Juan Bravo, for
instance, advocated good-smelling clothes, changed frequently lest putrid
vapour born and confined in them should be drawn inwards through the pores
of the skin. Confinement in bad odour was especially dangerous, whether in
the home, or classically, on board ship, or in jails or hospitals, and it was
particularly feared in the privy or latrine, the smell of which, again according
to Bravo, was good for nobody.[37] Seated anxiously over the reeking vaults of
their urban privies, at the risk of a putrid fever, townspeople envied the
countryfolk who could perform their natural functions in the fields.[38]

There was, all the same, optimism that good smells overcame bad ones.
Bartholomeus Anglicus argued that if two extremes, the foetid and the aromatic, were mixed, the result was not intermediate between the two. The good
smells triumphed, for the olfactory sense delighted in the aromatic, and
rejected the foetid.[39] Aromatic fires and fumigations, scented candles, rose
water, aromatic herbs and sweet-smelling flowers, perfumed clothes and
bedding were therefore an important part of the hygiene of the home. For the
rich at least the equipment of good odour included the censer or fuming-pot,
the casting bottle for sprinkling rose water, and perhaps even the perfumed
bellows to scent the air. The traveller could also benefit. Bartolomeo da Montagnana, for instance, commended a powder, including mint, storax, incense
and aloe wood, to burn on the fire in dirty inns.[40] Medicine was allied here to
perfumery, a trade which developed rapidly from the Middle Ages onwards
with the development of distilling and the extraction of essential or volatile
oils. These were spirits, and their correspondence to the bodily spirits encouraged their use in medicine. The Middle Ages also saw the introduction of new
animal scents, such as musk, civet and amber, brought from remote parts of
the world to form the basis of myriad confections popularized through recipe
collections and books of secrets such as those of Alessio Piemontese and
Isabella Cortese.[41] During plague epidemics perfumes of all kinds were in
heavy demand. In *The Wonderful Year* (London, 1603), Thomas Dekker

noted the extraordinary inflation in the price of aromatic herbs and flowers during the plague in London: 'The price of flowers, hearbes and garlands, rose wonderfully, in so much that rosemary, which had wont to be sold for 12 pence an armefull, went now for six shillings a handfull.'[42] At the same time pomanders and sponges soaked in vinegar or perfumed water were in vogue. Tobacco smoke also joined the list of smells used to correct the air. Writing of the virtues of tobacco in 1672, John Josselyn noted that 'it ... prevents infection by scents'.[43] Pipe-smoking became, in fact, another topos for smell in representations of the five senses, for example in a seventeenth-century series by the Dutch artist Adriaen Brouwer.[44]

Smells, then, could be used in medicine in prophylaxis and therapy. They were also useful in diagnosis. At the most basic level bad smells deriving from the body or its products were symptoms of disease requiring investigation. The urine of a sick man, according to Avicenna, was never the same as that of a healthy one. Beyond this, however, lay the problem of differentiating different types of smell. Plato argued that odours could not be classified: there were in fact only two kinds, good smells and bad smells. Galen tended to agree, and he was against carrying over to smells the extensive vocabulary applied to tastes.[45] Some medieval writers were less cautious, and Reisch in 1503 referred to eleven kinds of smell, aromatic, salty, bitter, sweet and so on.[46] Avicenna described various smells of urine, such as sweet or acid, as denoting the dominance of particular humours. Foul-smelling urine might indicate ulceration in the urinary tract if it matured normally, but if not it might suggest internal putrefaction. But far more important for uroscopy were the visual signs – the nature of the sediments and above all the colour of the urine.[47]

In clinical medicine too, to judge from the *consilia* of Bartolomeo da Montagnana or Giovanni Battista da Monte, diagnosis was based primarily on visible symptoms and on those provided by touch from the pulse and temperature and from the texture of the skin. There seems to have been no suggestion at this time that some diseases had characteristic odours, an observation frequently made in the eighteenth century and later. Physicians may indeed have been reluctant to investigate too closely the bad odour of their patients. Just as Avicenna thought that in uroscopy the use of touch and taste was 'undesirable', so Gabriele Zerbi declined to sniff his patients' breath. That he admitted as much in a book on the physician and his conduct, published in 1495, suggests that Zerbi did not expect reproach.[48]

The number of the five senses was fixed by tradition, as was their order. First came sight and hearing. These senses, according to the thirteenth-century *Speculum naturale* of Vincent de Beauvais, belonged to the soul, and contributed to a higher quality of life. They were able to perceive objects at a distance, through a medium. At the lower end of the hierarchy came taste and touch, belonging to the body and contributing to mere animal existence. These senses could perceive their objects only by direct contact. Where did smell belong in the hierarchy? The sense of smell perceived objects at a distance, but only because material emanations were carried directly to the olfactory organ.[49]

On the one hand, smell was a bodily sense, less strong in men than in animals, notably the vulture, used unflatteringly to represent smell in the well-known series of the five senses by Georg Pencz, engraved at Nuremberg in the 1540s.[50] Likewise smell, in the form of perfume, was often condemned as vanity and an enticement to bodily lust. This view may be found in writings as far removed in time as the *Speculum morale* of the fourteenth century, attributed to Vincent de Beauvais, and *An Alarum for Ladyes* by Puget de la Serre, published in an English translation in 1638.[51] On the other hand, delight in sweet smells could be portrayed as an aesthetic or spiritual pleasure. As Aristotle observed, it was enjoyed as such only by man. In animals smell served merely to distinguish the edible from the poisonous, and to locate a dinner; for man it had a higher significance. Smell was therefore a contradictory sense to assess, as may be seen in the ambivalent discussion of smell in the work of Marsilio Ficino. In his commentary on Plato's *Symposium*, Ficino associated sight and hearing with the soul and with love; smell, along with taste and touch, he linked to the body, to lust and madness.[52] Yet in his medical treatise, *De vita*, Ficino made the god Mercury the spokesman for the spiritual delights not only of sight and hearing, but also of smell. Venus, in contrast, offered the transient satisfactions of taste and touch.[53] Once again, smell was ambivalent, strung uneasily between the higher and the lower senses, just as in medicine it played a contradictory role as both a source of danger and disease, and also as the bringer of health, spiritual refreshment and healing. A late thirteenth-century manuscript of the *Anticlaudianus*, by Alain de Lille, expressed the place of smell amongst the senses in a vivid series of illustrations, in which each sense was portrayed by a horse. Smell was shown as neither the winged horse of sight, nor the galloping horse of hearing. Yet neither was it the slow plodder of taste, nor at a standstill like the horse of touch. With its steady gait, the horse of smell occupied the middle place in the hierarchy of the senses.[54]

5

Seeing and believing: contrasting attitudes towards observational autonomy among French Galenists in the first half of the seventeenth century

LAURENCE BROCKLISS

In 1641 a bachelor of medicine called Roland Merlet sustained an oral thesis before the Paris faculty entitled: 'Is reason or experience the more important part of medical science?'[1] The conclusion he reached at the end of his dissertation was that judgement must be given in favour of deductive, not inductive knowledge. Admittedly, he accepted that experience had an important role to play in medicine in that observation should confirm the 'discoveries' of reason. Experience, then, was not to be dismissed as a mere 'handmaid' or 'lackey'. Nevertheless, the idea that observation could be an autonomous foundation for truth could not be entertained. Experience revealed that every manifestation of disease was a unique event: the character of a disease was always changing; the same path was never taken twice. Thus, in therapeutics in particular, the wise man, while not ignoring the experiential evidence that had been collected in favour of a remedy, would make sure that its application was strongly urged 'by the singular council of reason'.[2]

Clearly, Roland Merlet did not prescribe a high cognitive status to the evidence of sense experience. In his case, seeing was not necessarily believing. At first glance, his trite epistemological pronouncements seem scarcely worth repetition. After all, his was just the position that any Renaissance Galenist, who was a genuine adept of the Dogmatic school of medicine, could be expected to assume. Had not Hippocrates himself uttered the famous warning: 'experimentum fallax'? The significance of Merlet's epistemology, however, lies in the fact that through his father, Jean, he belonged to a coterie of Paris physicians in the first half of the seventeenth century, who rigorously honoured its rationalist prejudice in their everyday medical philosophy.[3] Most French Galenists of the period 1500–1650 merely paid lip-service to medical rationalism. In an ideal world, certainly, a physician would first identify the cause of a patient's disease and then treat it allopathically with remedies whose operation was equally understood. In reality, when confronted by diseases whose cause was as yet unknown, physicians acted empirically. The Paris group, in quite deliberate contrast, rejected this gap between epistemology and practice and promoted a holistic medical philosophy, which, it was believed, was truly in the spirit of Hippocrates, Aristotle and Galen. This group can be identified from about 1600 but it was at its most prominent in the 1630s and 1640s when led by the vituperative Gui Patin (1601–72).[4]

The purpose of this chapter is to bring to light the existence of this Paris coterie of doctrinaire Galenists for the first time, a group of singular interest because of the consequences of its medical rationalism. The chapter is divided into three parts. It begins with a brief description of the contemporary Galenic orthodoxy against which Patin and his friends reacted. It then proceeds to examine the medical philosophy of the Paris group in detail, with particular reference to its novel therapeutics. Finally, it discusses (albeit in a speculative fashion) the wider consequences of the movement to the extent it also had professional, religious and political ramifications.

French Galenism in the first half of the seventeenth century was chiefly inspired by the writings of the mid-sixteenth century Paris physician Jean Fernel (1485–1558).[5] Fernel's contribution to medicine is usually portrayed as one of synthesis; he is seen as the Renaissance pioneer who reduced the recently recaptured Graeco-Roman inheritance to a manageable textbook form and in so doing coined the words physiology and pathology.[6] In the context of this chapter, Fernel is more important as the man who addressed himself directly to the respective roles of reason and experience in medical science in a book first published in 1548 entitled *De abditis rerum causis*.[7] In this work, widely read not just in France but throughout Europe, Fernel put forward the case for observational autonomy. In his view the human body and the diseases to which it was prey could be only imperfectly understood in terms of the balance or imbalance of the Galenic humours. Very often, especially in a virulent disease, there was a hidden or occult factor which was beyond human comprehension. But if this were the case, then defects in the functioning of the human organism could not always be treated rationally. Occult diseases had to be countered by occult remedies, whose virtues could only be known by trial and error. This fact should not lead mankind to despair. Fernel began the book with a preface expressing his confidence in the achievements of the present age. The ancients were definitely not to be despised, but knowledge was cumulative.[8] He ended his work in a similar vein, with a call to arms in search for successful specifics:

Although these lie hidden, wrapped up in nature's secrets and in great obscurity, they are not to be ignored from cowardice, but carefully hunted down. They are to be discovered, not from the primary or secondary qualities of touch, not from smell, sound or colour, but from their effect and operation alone. This knowledge is confirmed and collated from long observation of their use and from the accounts of the best authors.[9]

Fernel's justification for giving due weight to the occult in his medical philosophy was empirically based, as can be seen from his treatment of the plague. According to one school of thought, the plague could be classified as a putrid fever which arose from the corruption of the air by unreasonable weather or by polluting agents such as dead bodies and privies. Fernel would have none of this. The plague was certainly transmitted through the air, but was not caused by putrefaction. If this were so, then it was impossible to explain why the disease could arrive in any season or climate and without the air being obviously corrupted. The plague, therefore, must be ultimately caused by an occult quality and should be classed as a transnatural disease. The most that Fernel would grant to his opponents was that the virulence of the scourge could be affected by different atmospheric conditions and its victims chosen among the temperamentally inclined: 'This is the reason why a pestilence does not affect and harm all regions and all men in the same way.'[10]

Fernel, however, was not simply content to distinguish between the manifest and the occult. Heavily influenced by Renaissance Platonism, he also attempted in the *De abditis rerum causis* to create a cosmology which would make sense of the existence of the occult, if not explain its mechanism. He did this through his doctrine of substantial forms which determined the essential characteristics or activity of any natural phenomenon. This form was not derived from matter, as contemporary Thomist Aristotelians argued, but directly in each instance from God, who used as his mediating agents celestial substances.[11] It was impossible, therefore, to comprehend the essence of a natural phenomenon through its qualities or temperament for it was not elementally determined. Rather, it was something quintessential, celestial, divine; it could only be known in terms of its effects. In consequence, if the cause of occult diseases and the *modus operandi* of occult drugs would always be beyond understanding, the source of their malignancy or restorative virtue was not. Fernel's theory of the occult ultimately stemmed from a nominalist theory of God which stressed the untrammelled power of the creator over His creation but at the same time the unseemliness of the Deity soiling His hands. God, the judge, could visit mankind with any disease whenever he wished, but He would always choose to act through inferior agents. An aerially contracted occult disease such as the plague would be one ultimately sent from God but mediated through a pathological seed sown in the air by the baneful influence of an adverse planetary conjunction. To thwart the effects of this visitation, mankind must search for an antidote, an *alexipharmacum*, whose therapeutic properties were the result of a specific gift from God the Father, transmitted once more through a celestial messenger.[12]

It is hard not to feel that in developing this theory of the occult, Fernel, whatever he himself believed, departed dramatically from the Graeco-Roman Dogmatic school which he claimed to represent. But the authenticity of Fernel's Galenism is here not in question.[13] Rather, what needs to be stressed is the influence that Fernel wielded over French Galenism thereafter through the promotion of his views by the two leading medical schools, Montpellier and Paris.[14] A survey of the surviving degree dissertations from the two faculties in the first half of the seventeenth century makes this abundantly clear. At Montpellier almost without exception and at Paris in the majority of instances, medical students sustained a quasi-Fernelian cosmology which emphasized the role of the occult and the heavens in medical science.[15] In the main, Fernel was explicitly or implicitly criticized only for his excesses not for his basic approach. The Paris physician had ended up claiming that virtually every transmittable disease was divinely inspired; not just the plague, but epilepsy, elephantiasis, venereal disease, even dysentery and quartan fevers. Most early seventeenth-century Fernelians were unwilling to grant the occult such a dominant sway.[16]

Unfortunately, the brevity of these student dissertations (often no longer than a single folio sheet) only permits the historian to grasp the bare essentials of early seventeenth-century Fernelianism. For a more detailed understanding of its character, it is necessary to turn to a commentary on the *De abditis rerum causis* written by the Parisian physician, Jean Riolan the elder (d. 1606).[17] Riolan's approach to the seminal text was one of critical admiration. On the one hand, he was wary of using the occult as the explanation of too many diseases. There was a perfectly respectable school of thought which derived epilepsy for one from natural causes; arguably, it was the result, not of some occult poison, but of worms or a putrid ulcer.[18] However, Riolan had no objection to the idea of occult diseases as such, even if he was much less willing, as an orthodox Thomist Aristotelian, to indulge in Fernel's Platonic rhapsodies. Thus the plague was definitely an occult disease, although one produced through the influence of the sun, not from the conjunction of the stars. Just as the sun could cause the spontaneous generation of midges and flies, so it could imprint in the air a malignant, disease-bearing quality.[19]

Like Fernel, Riolan the elder stressed the autonomous role of observation. It was well known, he told his readers, that a genuine unicorn's horn was an antidote to the poisonous bite of a scorpion or spider. Indeed, if a circle was constructed from such a horn and these creatures were placed in its midst, so powerful was the horn's virtue that they would be instantly paralysed. Some might scoff at this assertion, he went on, yet the sceptical should recall that 'almost all medicine is empirical by dint of the use of remedies proven by experience rather than reason'.[20] Unlike Fernel, however, Riolan realized that observation could be problematic. He himself drew on the early thirteenth-century philosopher Jordanus for his knowledge of the properties of *cornu monocerotis*, but he was aware that 'seeing' through the eyes of another could lead to credulity. Pliny had been completely uncritical of what he recorded in his *Natural History*. Philosophers, therefore, should be extemely careful in accepting something as true that they themselves had not observed, even if the source seemed unimpeachable. On the other hand, the solution did not lie in the individual's only believing what he himself had observed. Experience was obviously limited. How could a Frenchman verify that a crocodile was stupefied by the touch of an ibis's feather?[21] In Riolan's hands, then, Fernelianism was definitely becoming a much more sophisticated empirical philosophy.[22]

The doctrinaire Galenists of the first half of the seventeenth century took issue totally with this Fernelian inheritance. In their opinion there was no room for the occult in a truly Galenic medical philosophy. Occult diseases did not exist; nor did occult remedies. Everything that occurred in the sublunary world could be explained naturally in terms of visible qualities and temperaments. This did not mean that the rationalists claimed to possess a total understanding of the cause of disease or the *modus operandi* of a particular remedy. On the contrary, as one of their first supporters, the Paris bachelor Bonaventure Hachette, pointed out in 1598, there was much of which they were ignorant, for instance the cause of airborne diseases. Nevertheless, they refused to mask that ignorance and take refuge in the occult, repudiating any necessary connection between the obscure and the divine.[23] Nor did the rejection of Fernelianism mean that the rationalist treated Fernel himself with disrespect. To Patin, Fernel was the greatest medical practitioner France had ever known. However, as Patin explained in an undated letter of the early 1630s, Fernel's ideas were not to be taken as 'mots d'évangile'. Fernel was like Everyman, a misguided and fallible mortal:

Je l'estime le plus sçavant et le plus poly des modernes, mais comme il n'a pas tout dit, aussi n'a-t-il pas dit vray en tout ce qu'il a escript, et si le bonhomme qui est mort trop tost, à nostre grand detriment, eût vescu davantage il eût bien changé, des choses à ses œuvres . . .[24]

Unfortunately, the rationalists provide little information as to why they had come to jettison the Fernelian inheritance. None of the coterie nor any of its student supporters explicitly stated that he was led to his position by finding it impossible to square the contemporary empiricist bias in pathology and therapeutics with an Aristotelo-Galenic epistemology, which stressed the primacy of deductive reasoning based on a series of non-negotiable materialist principles. This, however, was continually implied. The Paris student J. B. Ferrand, for example, sustained a public thesis in 1628 which posed the question: 'Is the rationalist sect legitimate?' In the printed abstract of his position,

Ferrand significantly not only anticipated Merlet's view that Dogmatic medicine was based on the twin pillars of reason and experience (without developing the point), but also castigated any attempt to introduce celestial and formal explanations of disease as theoretically unsound. Arguably, only the brevity of the printed dissertation, which merely offered a series of propositions, hid the fact that in the oral debate Ferrand proceeded to justify more precisely his aversion to a recourse to the occult in terms of the divorce that was thereby encouraged between epistemology and current medical science.[25]

As it is, perhaps this reticence is not surprising. The aesthetic argument may have appealed to the initiated, but it had a limited value as a weapon for convincing the Fernelian majority. Fernel had claimed that the occult in medical science was experientially founded. The battle, then, had to be fought on the enemy's terms: it was a question of what did the evidence say. Patin himself makes this very clear. In the undated letter previously cited, he specifically rejected occult qualities on evidential grounds. Certainly, the reality of such virtues could be simply dismissed as Arabic nonsense and the credulous referred to the dogmatic authorities, Galen and Hippocrates. But Patin did not want to rely on ancient authority alone. As a Christian, he might believe in many things which could not be observationally validated.[26] In medicine, however, 'Je ne croy que ce que je voy.' Occult virtues did not exist because Patin had no personal proof that they did. What, then, was his criterion of evidential certainty? What did Patin have to see to believe? Here frustratingly Patin failed to develop his argument. Nor did he say what was wrong evidentially with Fernel's justification of the occult beyond criticizing it for being imperfect: 'ses argumens pour telles qualitez ne sont point de démonstrations mathématiques'.[27] In this particular letter, therefore, Patin blatantly dodged the issue. From other letters, on the other hand, it is clear that Patin did have an evidential criterion (albeit a crude one) for evaluating the existence of occult specifics. They could not exist because they did not work, as was proven by the ever-increasing list of their victims.[28]

Enough has been said to demonstrate the difficulties of constructing the rationalists' critique of Fernelian Galenism precisely. The problem has much to do with the sources. Not only are the printed abstracts of medical theses underdeveloped but the more substantial material consists of unrigorous exercises in propaganda, in comparison with which Patin's letters are masterpieces of compression. The rationalists have left no textbook literature, no work equivalent to the *De abditis rerum causis*. It is possible that a coherent exposition of their critique lies hidden in one of the more prolix Latin *apologia* that await perusal.[29] For the moment, however, their thought processes can be only implicitly comprehended.

Conversely, what the sources do reveal very clearly is the profound effect the rationalists' rejection of Fernelian Galenism had on their medical practice.

At the turn of the century, admittedly, the practical effect of abandoning the occult in medical science seemed minimal. The thesis of Bonaventure Hachette of 1598, already referred to, was specifically devoted to discussing epilepsy. Although rejecting completely the idea that the latter was a divine disease, Hachette none the less continued to promote exactly the same specifics (now deemed to have a manifest action) as Fernel and his followers. Epilepsy was still curable by an amulet hung round the neck, made from an elk's nail or a peony root.[30] In contrast, by 1620 Fernelians and their opponents had divided into two distinct therapeutic camps. Arguments over the reality of the occult had ceased to be academic and had come to have a practical therapeutic significance.

This was obviously the case with respect to the prescription of chemical drugs, especially the metallic remedies promoted in the second half of the sixteenth century by the followers of the anti-Galenic Swiss hermetic homeopathist, Paracelsus. Until the turn of the seventeenth century the Paris faculty had been uniformly hostile to the adoption of Paracelsian remedies, in particular antimony. Declaring the new drugs to be poisons, the faculty waged a relentless war against freelance Paracelsian physicians in the capital, culminating in the campaign against the royal doctors, Quercetanus (d. 1609) and Turquet de Mayerne (1573–1655).[31] And this was a war in which convinced Fernelians, notably Jean Riolan the elder, played a prominent part.[32] By 1610, however, the faculty had been infiltrated by a small band of neo-Paracelsian fifth columnists (albeit allopathists) who justified the use of chemically prepared *metalla* experientially. Their influence thereafter rapidly grew. By the mid-1630s the neo-Paracelsians arguably commanded a majority among the hundred or so Paris faculty physicians, for in 1638 antimony was included in the faculty's official pharmacopoeia.[33] The appearance of Paracelsian sympathizers within the faculty immediately gave the rationalists a therapeutic identity. Fernelianism became associated with supporting the chemists' *metalla*; Galenic rationalism with opposing their use.

That Fernel would one day be associated with the promotion of chemical remedies was perhaps inevitable. His attitude to experiential autonomy offered an obvious justification for the use of Paracelsian specifics, while the *De abditis rerum causis* itself hints at the need to extract the formal essence of occult remedies by chemical means.[34] As it was, the first notorious neo-Paracelsian in the faculty, Pierre Le Paulmier (Palmerius) deliberately hijacked the Fernelian inheritance for the chemical cause. In 1609 Le Paulmier published a work which attempted to square the use of metallic drugs such as *hydrargyrum, stibium* and *aurum potabile* with Galenic orthodoxy.[35] It is impossible to enter into Le Paulmier's argument in detail. Suffice it to say that he defended the use of *metalla* by articulating a cosmology strikingly similar to Fernel's, which served as the foundation for a justification for the preparation of chemical distillates. A book that purported to be an attack on Paracelsus and his disciple Libavius as poisoners rather than physicians was in fact a defence of the search for celestial essences in sublunary phenomena.[36] Not surprisingly, therefore, Fernelianism in the eyes of the rationalists became identified with the thin end of the Paracelsian wedge.[37]

The growing prominence of neo-Paracelsians in the Paris faculty not only gave the quarrel over the reality of the occult in medical science a novel therapeutic twist; it also made the quarrel increasingly bitter. In the period 1600–40 the debate was carried on in a gentlemanly fashion within the faculty schools. The bitterness that was undoubtedly there was thereby kept within bounds, only spilling out in the vituperative correspondence of Gui Patin.[38] The sole martyr on either side was Le Paulmier, ejected from the faculty for sailing too close to the Paracelsian wind. In the 1640s, however, the gunports were finally raised and both parties fired acrimonious broadsides. At the same time the conflict became complicated. The Montpellier faculty, apparently little affected in the first half of the seventeenth century by Parisian critiques of Fernel, had long since succumbed to the chemists' *metalla*.[39] Antagonized by the Paris physicians' attempt at the beginning of the decade to stop Montpellier graduates from practising in the capital, the other great medical faculty of France also entered the fray.[40] But its spokesmen muddied the waters by pretending that the Paris faculty presented a united anti-Paracelsian, conservative front. As a result, the most readable and temperate rationalist pamphlet of the period, the *Curieuses recherches* of Jean Riolan the younger (1580–1657) is in fact not an attack on his Paris opponents but a diatribe against the calumnies of the Montpellier dean, Siméon Courtaud (d. 1665).[41]

Given that the struggle between Fernelians and rationalists thus tended to degenerate into a quarrel over restrictive practices (i.e. the Paris physicians' corporate rights), it is easy to miss in the literature of the 1640s that the debate had a significant philosophical dimension.[42] Given, too, that the discussion predominantly focused on the issue of the use of *metalla*, it is equally easy to miss the fact that the rationalists of the Patin era did not just reject Paracelsian remedies but also many traditional drugs. At the same time as they outlawed *metalla* as poisons, they outlawed a variety of other specifics as vain, useless and superstitious. These were all drugs judged by the Fernelians to be occult, but acceptable to the first generation of rationalists, like Hachette, on the grounds that the remedies did indeed have a manifest cause if one that was still obscure. Presumably, as the first objection to using these empirical cures (now significantly called by the rationalists 'occult') comes from 1610, the change of heart was directly inspired by the nascent Paracelsian challenge. The only way to counter the neo-Paracelsian recourse to an experiential justification for their chemical drugs was to drop purely experientially justified remedies from the pharmacopoeia altogether.[43]

Admittedly, there was little attempt to downgrade the general antidotes, theriac and mithridate, whose peculiar therapeutic power supposedly came from the mixture of a variety of otherwise anodyne ingredients such as viper's blood.[44] The rationalists' target was primarily the age-old specific remedies whose occult virtues could supposedly combat the virulent effect of the most fearful diseases. Typical of the scorn poured upon these age-old specifics was the attack launched by the bachelor René Moreau (d. 1656) in 1617. In discussing the treatment of the plague, he dismissed all the traditional remedies out of hand. Gone was the *lapidus bezoardicus*; gone too the *bolus armenia*. Nor would victims escape the scourge by devouring the palpitating heart of a turtle.[45] In fact, the only traditional occult antidote for the plague Moreau failed to mention was the much vaunted unicorn's horn whose properties had been trumpeted by Riolan the elder. The *cornu monocerotis*, however, was not allowed to escape the axe. If Moreau neglected to administer the *coup de grâce*, it did not escape the ire of Gui Patin.[46]

The most interesting feature of this onslaught on traditional specifics was the attack on the use of charms. Fernel and his followers had always insisted that there was an important distinction between the deployment of charms and the deployment of *magia*. Ritualistic incantations, hanging parchment inscribed with hieroglyphics around the neck, wearing lucky jewellery – none of these things could naturally protect or cure. Charms, on the other hand, where a natural substance endowed with a specific celestial virtue was placed next to the body, were therapeutically sound, acting much like a magnet in drawing malign qualities.[47] The rationalists, in contrast, treated this distinction as invidious, seeing charms as no different from *magia*. This was made abundantly clear in a thesis sustained by Louis Robillart in 1615. Discussing remedies for epilepsy, he specifically lumped together as unsound 'amulets, written texts, graphics, characters, [and] three songs whispered three times'. Charms made from peony root and rings of elk's nail were to be henceforth confined to the medical dustbin.[48]

What rationalists were doing, in short, for the first time in France was making a strict division between popular and academic medicine.[49] By outlawing the experientially derived, they were dividing medical science from folklore. Their aim was to create a purified and simplified therapeutics, where the emphasis would be on phlebotomy. As a result, their opponents labelled them bloodsuckers.[50] In fact, this was totally unfair. Patin and his friends certainly bled their patients frequently. When the Paris physician, Cousinot the younger (d. 1646), was attacked by a violent rheumatism in 1633, he was bled on the orders of his father and his father-in-law, Charles Bouvard, fifty-four times in eight months.[51] Nevertheless, the rationalists did not reject the use of Galenic simples *tout court*. Their treatment, as Riolan the younger emphasized, combined phlebotomy with mild, locally gathered drugs and a sensible diet:

Ils se servent de la saignée reiterée selon la grandeur de la maladie & les forces du malade . . . Ils ont aussi diminué la quantité des remedes en diverses façons, qui incommodoient & estouffoient les malades, & se sont contentez de peu, bien choisis, & de grande vertu.[52]

In addition, as both Riolan and Patin stressed, the rationalists took full account of the role that climate, patterns of consumption and lifestyle must play in developing a specifically Parisian therapeutics. Parisians were bled profusely because, citing the contemporary Poitevin physician Citoys (d. 1652), 'depuis le 45. degré iusqu'à 49. ou 50. les habitants sont à leur aise, oisifs, grands carnassiers, abondans en sang'.[53]

Undoubtedly, the development of a simplified, more 'scientific' pharmacopoeia was the one consequence of the rejection of the Fernelian medical orthodoxy which the rationalists of the second generation would have unanimously recognized and welcomed. There were other consequences of the movement, however, that not all may have so readily intended or acknowledged.

In the first place, lying behind the move for a purified therapeutics was an implicit criticism of contemporary medical ethics. In a Fernelian world there was little room for hygiene, self-help, or leaving nature to cure herself. The Fernelians were interventionists. Indeed, they had to be, for according to Le Paulmier the world was growing older, nature was decaying, and mankind was becoming increasingly unhealthy. Modern medicine, then, had to be different from the ancients' variety.[54] But if this were the case, Fernelian medicine placed a premium on the learned physician-magus and his equally subtle assistant, the apothecary. The physician was not just an essential presence when sick; he was needed daily to ward off the evils that might suddenly beset the fragile human frame. The apothecary similarly would be as frequently patronized as the *marchand-épicier* to whom he had been originally joined. It was a contemporary medical world, moreover, where the temptation to exploit the gullible client must have been great. Molière's Purgon and Fleurant were not just plucked out of the sky.[55] Even the Fernelians themselves recognized that the difficulty of obtaining the exotic ingredients of some of their drugs could encourage the use of low-grade substitutes; finding a supplier of genuine unicorn's horn was no easy business.[56]

The rationalists, in contrast, offered mankind the chance of controlling his medical destiny and turning his relations with the medical profession into an occasional event. They did this by placing a novel emphasis on hygiene. Unlike the Fernelians, they stressed that man could determine his health to a large extent by cultivating a life of moderation, especially moderation in diet. As good Aristotelians they were not ascetics,[57] but they did condemn a life of indulgence. Thereby they provided an alternative non-medical solution to the problem of self-preservation and released contemporaries from the Fernelian tyranny of charms and amulets. The most important figure in this development was René Moreau (already encountered), who gave evidence of his commitment to the cause in 1625 with the publication of an edition of the *Schola salernitana*.[58] Moreau, furthermore, strenuously supported the idea of public, not simply private hygiene. He had his predecessors in the first generation of rationalists, physicians such as Nicolas Ellain (d. 1621), who suggested sanitary measures that could be taken by the city authorities in time of plague.[59] Moreau, however, seems to have been the first, in a memorandum of 1630, to advocate that these expedients should not just be temporary but be codified into a permanent body of law. Essentially, he sought the creation of a civic refuse service, the incarceration of mendicants, an inspectorate of the sales of perishable goods, and *maisons de convalescence* where the sick could recuperate away from the general public.[60]

At the same time, by emphasizing the efficacy and sole legitimacy of cheap, simple remedies occasionally used, the rationalists offered the chance of scientific medicine to a far larger section of the population than was usually its beneficiaries. The physicians' consultancy fee would still have to be paid, but only infrequently, while the apothecary's bill in particular would be henceforth greatly reduced. Indeed, the rationalists went out of their way to popularize their purified therapeutics in print so that the literate could make up their own drugs and bypass the apothecary altogether. It was the rationalist movement which produced the most successful self-help manual in seventeenth-century France, the *Médecin charitable* of the Paris doctor, Philbert Guybert (or Guibert, d. 1633). This was a work initially published in 1623. Interestingly, the edition of 1632 apparently included a treatise by Patin on the conservation of health.[61]

The rationalist movement, then, was implicitly one that aimed to improve the health of the population at large at the expense of the wealth of the medical profession. Perhaps the majority of its supporters failed to grasp this, but Patin certainly did not. In his 'Préceptes particuliers d'un médecin à son fils' (date unknown) he positively revelled in portraying the good physician as a man of frugal means sacrificing wealth for the good of the poor.[62] In his letters, moreover, Patin took particular delight in anticipating the bankruptcy of the greedy apothecary. Under the old dispensation, he declared in 1649, patients, expecting to be prescribed a clutch of remedies, called in the apothecary first to save the physician's bill. Today, in contrast, now that 'une medecine facile et familiere' had delivered the people from the hands of these 'cuisiniers arabesques', the proper order of things had been restored. The physician was called first and the apothecary was starved of clients. As a result, the Paris apothecaries had difficulty in gaining apprentices: 'Leur métier est si sec que personne n'a envie de s'en meler'.[63]

Of course, Patin was over-optimistic. The rationalists had not, nor ever did, capture control of the therapeutic *espace* in mid-seventeenth century France. *Le malade imaginaire* could not have been written had they done so. They should perhaps better be seen as the Jansenists of the Parisian medical profession, the minority guardians of its conscience. Jansenism was a mid-seventeenth century religious movement which drew its inspiration from the austere predestinarian theology of St Augustine. Its aim was to destroy the dominant doctrinal humanism and moral laxism of the French Church associated with the Society of Jesus. To the extent both Jansenists and medical rationalists looked for a reformation of manners and a purification of doctrine, the two movements were analogous.[64] Indeed, some rationalists may have been Jansenists in reality. Certainly Patin was close to the movement, evincing a bitter hatred of Jesuits and decadent monks.[65]

If many rationalists were Jansenists, then this immediately put them on the wrong side of contemporary Catholic orthodoxy. From its appearance Jansenism was seen as a covert Protestant heresy, and in 1653 the Jansenist Bible, the *Augustinus* of Jansen, Bishop of Ypres (hence the movement's name) was outlawed by the Pope. Thereafter the movement was repeatedly hounded by Louis XIV.[66] Even if the link between the Jansenists and medical rationalists was tenuous, however, the Parisian physicians may have been viewed with suspicion by the ecclesiastical establishment because of their attitude to demonic possession. If the first only partly understood consequence of rejecting the Fernelian inheritance was that Galenic rationalists undermined contemporary medical ethics, the second was that they challenged the witch-craze.[67]

Jean Fernel in his *De abditis rerum causis* had evinced a firm belief in the power of Satan in the world. Understandably, Fernel's cosmology entertained the idea of a hierarchy of angels and devils juxtaposed between God and man, and under the head of transnatural diseases he specifically included maladies conjured by evil men and contracted through demonic agency. The difference between these and normal diseases was the fact that they were apparent not real, for demons only had the power to produce the symptoms not the disease itself. Such diseases, as a result, could not be treated in the usual manner but had to be spirited away by a counter-magic in the hands of the Church or a white witch. Fernel, moreover, did not claim to be speaking simply on a theoretical plane. He had himself seen a boy demonically possessed, unnaturally speaking foreign tongues, and he had witnessed the healing power of the Church in several possession cases. 'I have seen', he related, victims freed from the spirit's control by 'curses, prayers, holy words, vows and fasting', victims who still today 'live healthily and in their right mind'.[68]

By and large the Fernelians of the late sixteenth and the first half of the seventeenth centuries shared this belief in the presence of malign supernatural forces. Witness the case of the expatriate Scot, George Scharpius (d. 1638), later professor of medicine at Bologna. In 1617 Scharpius presented a thesis at Montpellier attributing cures by fascination, incantation or the application to a wound of a dry piece of lint to the invisible power of devils. Twenty years later another Montpellier graduate, Pierre Cognard, emphasized, like Fernel, that the linguistic feats of madmen and melancholics stemmed from demonic possession.[69] Only Jean Riolan the elder, a staunch Aristotelian, had serious doubts. In his commentary on the *De abditis rerum causis*, Riolan identified demonic possession as a Platonic myth and seriously questioned the existence of demons *tout court*, let alone their power in the world. The Aristotelians, he maintained, insisted that demonic possession could be naturally explained as the result of an atrabilious humour. In Riolan's opinion, this was a reasonable view and he cited the case of a boy from Spoleto who spoke German while suffering from worms. If in the end Riolan gave his consent to the reality of demonology, he did so grudgingly: 'I would find on the side of the Peripatetics, were not the Platonic position more consistent with the Christian religion. I prefer to err with the Church than to judge rightly with the philosophers'.[70]

Riolan's suspicions, however, would have been shared by the majority of the rationalists, even of the first generation. Consider the role of one of their number, Michel Marescot (d. 1606), in the examination of the supposed demoniac, Marthe Brossier in 1599. Marthe was a young peasant woman who claimed to have been possessed by a devil from whom she derived the gift of tongues and divination. Brought to Paris, the bishop handed her over to be examined by a group of physicians and theologians, one of whom was the rationalist, Marescot. By careful questioning the latter succeeded in destroying Brossier's credibility before her judges. As a result, Marthe was condemned as a fraud, much to the horror of many prominent Catholics in the capital, notably her Capuchin sponsors. Marescot, however, was undismayed by the storm he had raised. He stuck to his guns and subsequently published an account of his findings, admittedly at royal behest because Marthe was being used by Catholic ultras to stir up anti-Huguenot propaganda.[71]

Understandably, no rationalist had the temerity to deny publicly the existence of witchcraft or demonic possession *per se*. Gui Patin, on the other hand, was quite ready to do so in the privacy of his correspondence. In a letter of 1643, Patin refused to believe that either the infamous case of the 'Devils of Loudun' (1634) or a contemporary possession case at Louviers in the Spanish Netherlands was genuine evidence of Satan's power in the world. Demonic possession, he suspected, did not exist. The best book to read on the subject was that by Johannes Wierus; the worst the *Disquisitiones magicae* of the Jesuit Del Rio (very much a bestseller). In fact, according to Patin, the idea of demonic activity in the world was a fabrication of the regular orders out to increase their power. There were no possession cases (so he claimed) in England, the United Provinces and [northern] Germany, whence monks had been banished.[72] This point was made even more forcibly in a letter of 1660 where Patin dismissed Del Rio's book as 'fables loyolatiques', and where the arch-sceptic Naudé was praised as the 'puritan du péripatétisme'. In Patin's opinion, the devil was a bugaboo, 'une vilaine bête noire, qui n'a point de blanc en œil, de la laideur duquel se servent les moines à faire peur au monde'.[73]

Patin's objections to the existence of demonic possession also had a political foundation. In the letter of 1643, he emphasized that the trial of Urbain Grandier as the sorcerer who had sent the devils into the Ursulines of Loudun was a cynical political manoeuvre. It was one of the many 'fourberies' of the late Cardinal Richelieu, who had wanted Grandier out of the way as a known opponent of the Cardinal's ministry.[74] This reading of the event was scarcely surprising given Patin's political beliefs. The Paris physician hated both Richelieu and Mazarin as agents of despotism, and welcomed the Fronde as a means of restoring the rule of law and a more representative political regime.[75] Whether other rationalists of the second generation felt equally hostile towards the rule of the cardinals is impossible to say. Certainly Riolan the younger was out of the country in the 1630s and early 1640s in the entourage of the exiled queen-mother, Marie de Médicis, but some sources say he was acting not just as her *médecin* but as Richelieu's spy.[76] Whatever the truth of the matter, there can be little doubt that if Patin's political antipathies had been known at court, then the coterie as a whole would have been immediately under suspicion and their medical rationalism deemed a political front.[77]

As it was, the rationalists had little influence at court, for the royal family and the cardinals, Richelieu in particular, were enthusiastic supporters of post-Fernelian therapeutics. The archetypal court physician, as Patin continually reminded his correspondents, was a neo-Paracelsian, usually a graduate of Montpellier, who purged his elevated clients with alarming regularity and with the most violent drugs.[78] Even the odd Paris-trained physician who did find favour at court and was given the Patin seal of approval was in reality tainted with the Paracelsian brush. Take the case of Charles Bouvard, Louis XIII's *premier médecin*. To Patin, Bouvard was a 'diamond' of the faculty, one of the group of heroes who had helped to deliver mankind from 'la tyrannie de ces cuisiniers arabesques'. If Bouvard in his old age had faults (he had become venal and pious), then this was the inevitable result of exposure to courtly corruption.[79] But Bouvard was not quite the rationalist saint whom Patin describes. In rejecting the chemists' *metalla* the rationalists also waged war on the contemporary enthusiasm for 'taking the waters'. The natural consumption of minerals was just as dangerous as imbibing Paracelsian potions.[80] Yet on this issue Bouvard clearly broke ranks with his colleagues. It was the *premier médecin* who had first encouraged the queen, Anne of Austria (and doubtless Richelieu, too) to make a regular pilgrimage to the fountain at Forges in the 1630s.[81]

Indeed, the very fact that the court supported the neo-Paracelsians may have made the rationalists politically suspect anyway. In an era of absolutism all opposition was political; hence the treatment meted out by Louis XIV to the Jansenists; their professions of loyalty counted for nothing when measured against the scandal of their religious deviance.[82] And, as has already been suggested, the rationalists were medical Jansenists. Moreover, in the 1640s, politics and medicine were closely entwined. As was earlier noted, the Paris faculty in this decade was attempting to stop Montpellier graduates illegally practising in the capital. The faculty's *bête noire* was the neo-Paracelsian court physician, Théophraste Renaudot. The latter had established a *bureau des pauvres* (a sort of government pawnshop) in the capital in 1629, which quickly became a people's dispensary where Renaudot and other Montpellier graduates gave free medical treatment. Renaudot, however, was not just a medical interloper. He also ran the *Gazette*, the official government newspaper. He was Richelieu's *créature*. No wonder, then, if opposition to chemical *metalla* might be thought by the government to have a political dimension. No wonder, too, that rationalist-backed attempts to get Renaudot and his Montpellier friends banned from practising in the capital were unsuccessful until after Richelieu's death in 1642.[83]

The failure of the court, and almost certainly by extension the elite in general, to embrace medical rationalism had significant consequences for the movement's progress. Thereby it was guaranteed to generate limited support among the medical fraternity. The rationalists were condemned to being a sect. Indeed, the absence of court patronage arguably played an important part in the movement's rapid demise after 1660. In 1666 the Paris Parlement legitimized the use of antimony. By that date purportedly only ten of the hundred or so members of the Paris faculty were against the drug, an indication of the rationalists' crumbling influence.[84] There were to be only two generations. When Patin died in 1672 the movement died with him. Thereafter the Paris faculty became the scene of different struggles as the Fernelian majority was faced with new and more dangerous opponents: Harveians, iatrochemists, and eventually iatromechanists. In the fight against these later foes the traditionalists were far less successful. By 1700 Paris Aristotelo-Galenism in any manifestation was moribund.[85]

This chapter has exposed the existence of two distinctive ways of regarding observational evidence among French Galenists in the first half of the seventeenth century. On the one side, the majority, whatever their ideal epistemology, accepted the autonomy of observational experience: seeing was believing. On the other side, an important coterie of Paris physicians refused to compromise with their epistemology and constructed a medical philosophy where seeing was only believing if the observation could be understood.

At first glance the majority view appears to be the more worthy of exploration. After all, the ability to accept the evidence of your senses regardless of the damage this may do to your inherited cosmology is surely the *sine qua non* for the development of the seventeenth-century experimental philosophy. The barrenness of epistemological purity, moreover, is only too apparent in the anatomical conservatism of Jean Riolan the younger. In the early decades of the seventeenth century, Riolan *fils* was the most important anatomist in Europe, the first to provide an adequate textbook map of the human body.[86] He is remembered today, however, as the man who refused to accept the reality of the circulation of the blood. Although willing to alter details of Galenic physiology, he was ultimately unable to reject the fundamental concept of the venal blood as the source of nutrition and the arterial blood as the source of the vital spirit. As a result, whatever the experimental evidence for the passage of the blood from the minor veins to the vena cava, Riolan always insisted that the movement was in the opposite direction. What Harvey and others saw, Riolan could not believe.[87]

On deeper acquaintance, on the other hand, the rationalists seem by far the more modern. With their disdainful attitude towards folk medicine, their willingness to open medical knowledge to all, their suspicion of demonic possession and their dedication to regime, they have the characteristics of the Enlightenment physician *avant la lettre*. Indeed, they seem to be the perfect illustration of Charles Schmitts's belief that Renaissance Aristotelianism (in this case Aristotelo-Galenism) could be a dynamic and original philosophical force.[88] Patin and his friends were not the slaves of a dying divinity but the standard-bearers of an iconoclastic cult.

For this reason, then, Galenic rationalism deserves studying in detail, especially the linkage between its epistemology and its novel therapeutics. Unfortunately, as this chapter has shown, a rigorous analysis is very difficult given the sources, and at present only an interim report is possible. Further work needs to be done. The most obvious strategy is to widen the scope of the enquiry. So far the phenomenon has been treated as if it were a specifically Parisian one. But this is most unlikely.[89] Galenic rationalism was presumably an international movement and its devotees in other faculties and countries may well have left more malleable material.[90]

6

'The mark of truth': looking and learning in some anatomical illustrations from the Renaissance and eighteenth century

MARTIN KEMP

No one looking at the landmarks in the history of modern anatomy, during the years following Vesalius's *Fabrica* of 1543, can doubt that illustration played a crucial role in conveying anatomical information on a widespread basis through the medium of printing. Indeed, it has been claimed that the Vesalian revolution in anatomy was predicated upon the new modes of visual represention in the Renaissance – that the revolutionary procedures for the systematic imitation of real forms from specific viewpoints were themselves ultimately responsible for developing new modes of looking amongst investigators and for breaking the mould of scholastic commentaries, which were dominantly shaped by verbal formulae.[1] The two anatomists who mark the chronological limits of this study, Leonardo da Vinci and William Hunter, both agreed that accurate representation of forms could be viewed as a 'universal language' of the eye which transcended the confusion of tongues and verbal categories. At its simplest, this idea relies upon the kind of assumption expressed by Hunter's statement that 'Representation in the imitative Arts is a Substitute for reality'.[2]

However, I think that it can be demonstrated at the outset with no difficulty that the new technique of naturalistic representation forged in the Renaissance could – even accepting the basis of Hunter's formulation – serve a far less unequivocal function than its partisans have suggested. The pictorial skill of naturalism in the Renaissance could serve as a distinctly double-edged sword.[3] An example from botanical illustration will show what I mean. The roots of the legendary and potent mandragora were supposed to assume the form of a homunculus. Abraham Bosse, the great seventeenth-century French engraver and teacher of perspective at the Academy, provided a splendidly convincing illustration of a female mandragora (fig. 20), using his skills to convince the

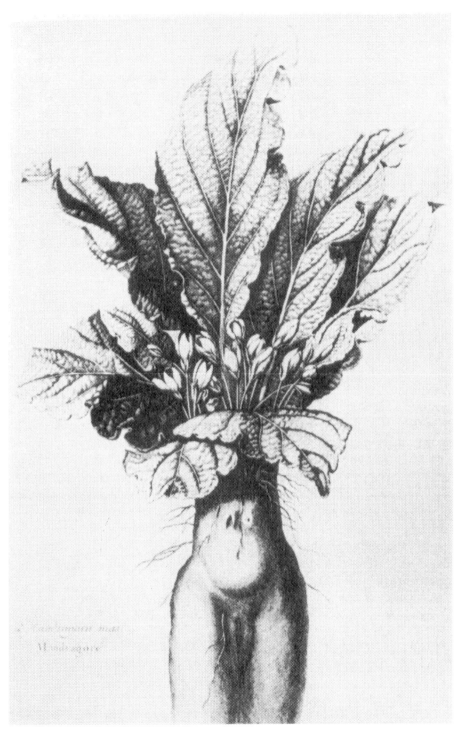

Fig. 20. Abraham Bosse (after Nicolas Robert?) 'Mandragora'. From N. Roberts, *Plantes* (Paris, 1701).

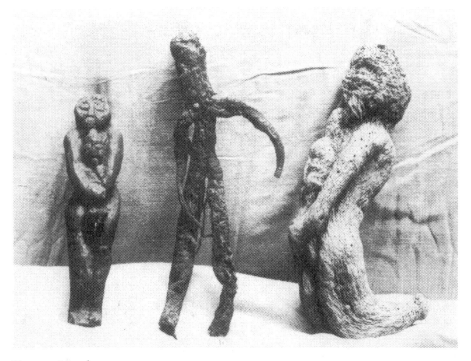

Fig. 21. Mandragora roots.

spectator that it is depicted (as they say) 'from life'. We know of course, as
Jacopo Ligozzi had shown some years earlier, that mandragora roots do not
look precisely like the human figure – though actual roots (fig. 21), with or
without the assistance of a human sculptor, suggest that the visual evidence is
more slippery than the straight denial indicates.

Hunter was himself well aware, through his wide-ranging studies in the
history of anatomical and other scientific illustration, that apparently convincing depictions could be entirely misleading. Having praised the 'art of
drawing' as exhibiting forms in a language 'so plain that the unlearned as well
as the learned understand it at first sight', he declares all the more strongly that
'impositions and misrepresentations are more unpardonable in this way: for in
as much as they have more credit, they do more mischief', since they are all
'presumed to be taken from life'.[4]

It will also be worth noting at the outset, using a Hunterian example, that
the kind of display used in naturalistic illustration relies heavily upon knowing
how to read a series of conventions. The representation of a moose commissioned by Hunter from George Stubbs (fig. 22) was intended to be a precise,
functional tool of morphological description.[5] Indeed, Hunter took it with him
three years later to compare with another specimen. On the ground, Stubbs

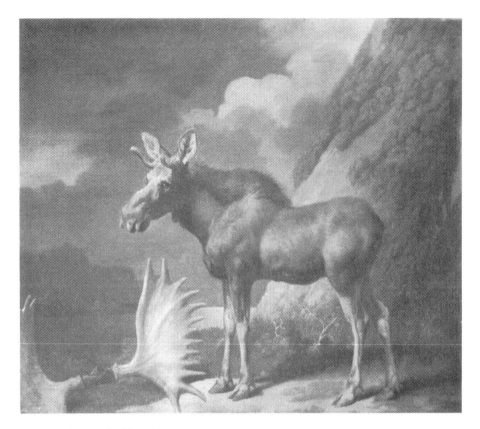

Fig. 22. George Stubbs, *Moose*.

illustrated for reference the horns of a mature animal, much as a botanical illustrator might show an open flower or seed beside the main image of a plant. However, this device, probably considered as unambiguous by Hunter and Stubbs, was (and is) open to misinterpretation. Recently one author described the animal as 'looking rather gloomily at its fallen antlers'.[6]

These two major problems – the potential of illustrations to mislead on account of their apparent naturalistic authority and the need to know how to read the conventions – become entangled with an intricate series of other considerations when we turn specifically to anatomical illustration. I think it will be worth enumerating some of them (in no particular order), even if only a few can be directly tackled in this chapter.

(1) Should the illustrator depict a particular, individual example, or aspire to show the typical or exemplary model?

(2) Should the representation only show what can actually be seen at a specific stage of dissection from a particular viewpoint or

attempt to depict the forms as synthetic demonstrations (e.g. by showing the whole vascular system in isolation)?

(3)   Should all redundant visual information be suppressed? At its most simple this raises the question as to whether the legs, for example, should be shown in a dissection of the abdomen. More profoundly, it concerns the depiction of apparently 'irrelevant' naturalistic detail, such as surface blotches on an organ or accidental damage.

(4)   Should the illustrations aim at a comprehensive visual description or act in a more limited way as points of reference or demonstrations in the service of the text?

(5)   How are the illustrations and text to be organized and what division of labour is appropriate for the visual and written material?

(6)   What medium is to be used for the illustrations and how far does the nature of the medium (its strengths and limitations) affect the information conveyed?

(7)   Are diagrammatic demonstrations to be permitted, using openly schematic forms of representation?

This far from exhaustive list of relatively technical, visual problems also needs to be viewed in the context of the historical-social frameworks from which the illustrations originated. This will involve not only an assessment of the intellectual stance of the author of the text, but also such questions as patronage (the patronage received by the author and the author's patronage of illustrators), the intended and actual production of the text, the intended and actual audience, and a series of broad values in society relating to the roles of books, medicine, observational science and so on. This is nothing short of a plea for a revised agenda for the history of anatomical illustration. Although there are now encouraging signs in some of the specialized areas of research, the standard histories remain largely untouched by the range of historical questions which are now widely practised in other fields of visual history.

In this chapter, I can only provide highly selective examples of possible approaches to the role of illustration. I have chosen to concentrate on two main areas which complement each other: the Renaissance, in which the problems and potentialities receive their earliest rehearsal; and the eighteenth century, particularly in Britain, when the analysis of the issues in the period itself reaches a point of some sophistication. In the Renaissance I will be looking at Leonardo, Berengario, Vesalius and Valverde, while in the later period I will be concentrating on the regal picture books of anatomy by Cheselden, Albinus and Hunter.

Leonardo, our first case study, serves well to establish the visual terms of reference, in that almost all the illustrative possibilities are explored in some shape or form; but in other respects he is quite atypical, in as much as his work was never brought to a publishable point of resolution.[7] It remained in his notebooks as a series of magnificent fragments, and he had not, therefore, to confront the practicalities of producing a finished text in which all the technical questions we have posed were answered in terms of an actual book, produced by a publisher for a specific audience. Indeed, one of the problems of all Leonardo's scientific work is that its intended audience is far from clear. Sometimes he seems to be indulging in a scholastic debate with known authorities, at others to be developing an entirely new form of exposition for a knowledgeable readership (as Vesalius was to do), but it is never entirely clear what kind of work he was planning in terms of actual book production. The nearest he comes to confronting the practical problems is his expression of hope that the question of cost will not dictate the production of his illustrations in an unsuitable medium.[8] The extraordinary inventiveness and unlimited ambition of Leonardo's illustrations only became possible in a context in which practical considerations remained in the background.

Broadly speaking, the anatomical illustrator has to consider two main variables: the state of anatomization of the subject; and the particular view of the form to be illustrated. All later anatomists, following the lead of Vesalius, recognized the need to economize in the face of the virtually infinite series of representations if each stage was to be depicted from various points of view.[9] Leonardo's schemes show his extreme reluctance to compromise the completeness of visual survey by compounding the variables within an economical set of views. For the muscles and bones of the foot, for example, his system appears to require at least forty-four separate drawings.

His boundless ability to invent new systems of representation only made his difficulties worse. There is hardly a later technique he did not envisage: representations of dissected forms (with or without an indication of the outlines of the undissected shape) (fig. 23); a variety of sectioning techniques (fig. 24); the use of 'transparent' organs to show underlying structures; wire diagrams to represent the spatial relationship of muscles within a limb; systems in isolation as three-dimensional 'trees'; cavities illustrated by wax injections; components demonstrated in exploded diagrams; cinematographic views of a form from successive viewpoints (fig. 25); and a range of diagrammatic techniques to illustrate the mechanical principles in operation.[10]

Early in his career, he seems to have assumed that drawings could themselves communicate all he had seen and all he wished to say, not only on questions of form but also on matters of function and cause. The fact that he was his own draughtsman, using drawing as a way of visualizing thought and conducting 'visual experiments' encouraged him to assume that the spectator could, as it were, read his thoughts through the visual representation. In his later work, after about 1510, he developed a sharper understanding of the

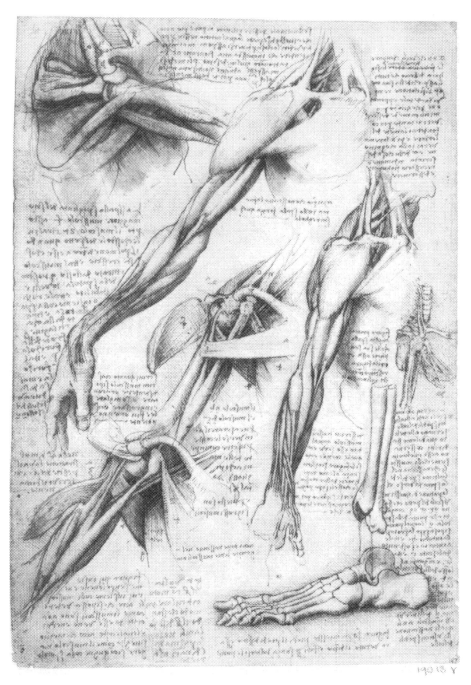

Fig. 23. Leonardo da Vinci, *Demonstrations of the Muscles of the Human Shoulder*.

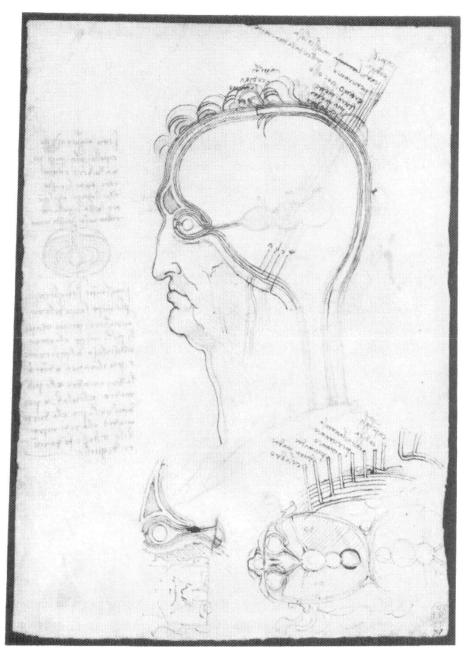

Fig. 24. Leonardo da Vinci, *Vertical and Horizontal Sections of the Human Head, Showing the Eyes and Ventricles.*

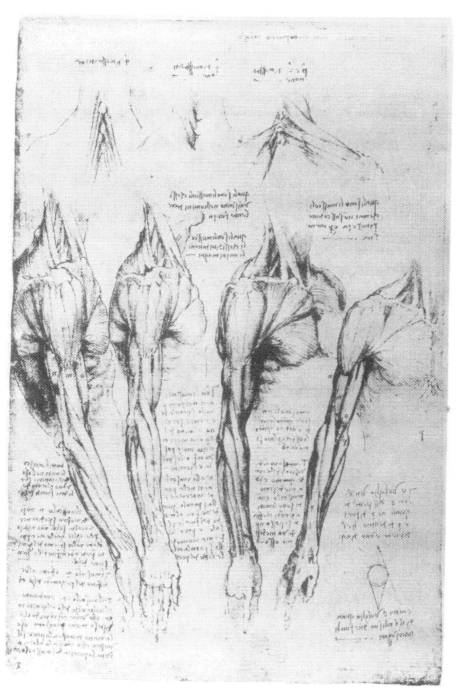

Fig. 25. Leonardo da Vinci, *Four Sequential Views of a Human Shoulder (from a Series of Eight)*.

relative competence of words and images in anatomical exposition. As his contacts with the Galenic tradition encouraged him to explain functionally every detail of created form, so he became aware that illustrations reigned supreme for description, while the text remained best adapted to explaining how something worked.[11]

'You who claim to demonstrate in words the shape of man from every aspect ... dismiss such an idea, because the more minutely you describe, the more you will lead the reader away from the thing described'. Whereas 'if you wish to demonstrate in words to the ears, speak of substantial and natural things and do not meddle with things appertaining to the eye ... Therefore it is necessary both to illustrate and to write'.[12] This practical assessment of the roles of illustration and text was not, however, accompanied by a realistic acknowledgement of the *amount* of illustration required to give a complete visual account of all forms in terms of their mutual shapes, proportions and spatial dispositions. His ultimate commitment to totality of visual representation as the sovereign end of science presented him with an unattainable goal.

In many respects, Berengario's devotion to *anatomia sensibilis* is comparable to Leonardo's stance, and it is tempting to see his pioneering use of naturalistic illustration as a profound expression of his method of sensory scrutiny.[13] It is true that someone less committed to direct looking at anatomical material is unlikely to have pioneered the use of illustration, but when we look at the nature and role of the illustrations in his text, their use seems to be more limited and pragmatic than his method might lead us to hope. The true illustrations to his text were, like those envisaged by Mundinus (upon whom he wrote a commentary), the actual forms of the body seen 'in the flesh'. His comments on the illustration of the spinal column (fig. 26) show his awareness of the limitations of the somewhat schematic wood-art technique of his illustrator: 'note, however, reader, that this figure does not exhibit a true likeness of the vertebrae, except in their number ... their actual form is better seen in dried vertebrae in the cemeteries'.[14] Even the notable series of pre-Vesalian muscle-men (fig. 27) have clearly defined functions. They guide the physicians into routes between the muscles, and they 'also assist painters in delineating the members'.[15] Similarly, his illustrations of blood vessels in the arm are dedicated to procedures adopted by physicians. There is no suggestion in the way that he uses each illustration that it is to be regarded as a true *demonstratio* serving the end of *determinatio*.[16] Only the first-hand material can perform that function.

Part of the problem for Berengario was obviously the relative failure of the somewhat schematic woodcuts to act as an adequate 'substitute for reality' (to use Hunter's phrase). It was this problem that Vesalius worked so spectacu-

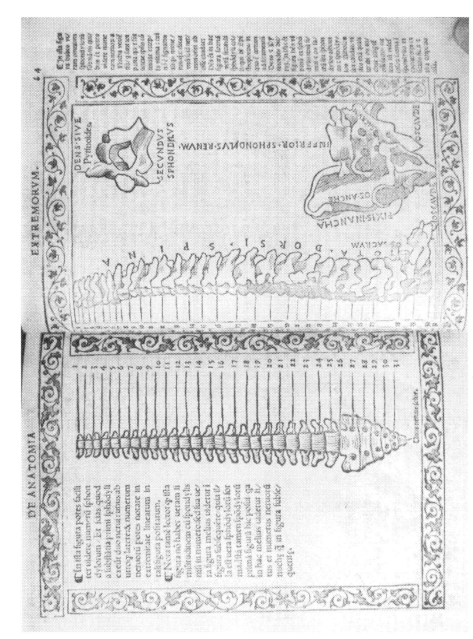

Fig. 26. Berengario da Carpi, Demonstrations of the spinal column. From *Isagogae breves* (Bologna, 1522).

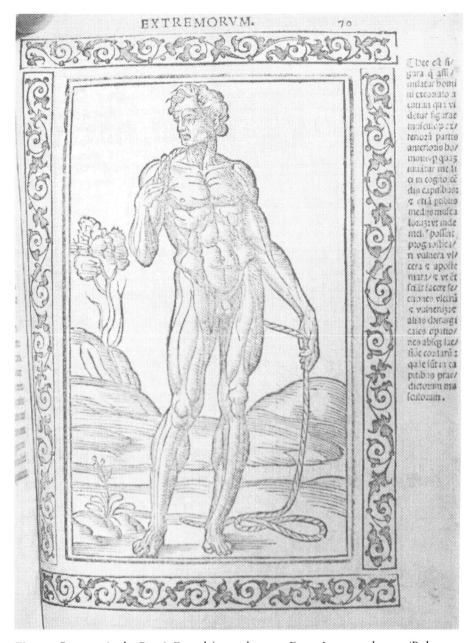

Fig. 27. Berengario da Carpi, Ecorché muscle-man. From *Isagogae breves* (Bologna, 1522).

sophistication with which Vesalius mastered all our technical questions is one of those great episodes within cultural history in which the full complexity of form and content in a new conception achieves virtually instant maturity. In art, Masaccio's *Trinity* and Leonardo's *Last Supper* stand in much the same position. The range of techniques – 'dissection' drawings, solid sections, systems in isolation (fig. 28), separate and united forms, varied viewpoints and a series of diagrammatic conventions – is little less than Leonardo's but they are exploited with an amazingly secure feeling for which technique is appropriate at each place in relation to the text.[17] The annotations to the plates convey a remarkable sense of the self-consciousness with which he orchestrates the various kinds of demonstration and conducts an unprecedentedly direct dialogue with the spectator. Typical in tone is his comment that 'the fact we have stripped the skin entirely from the right thigh and only partially from the left will, I imagine, confuse no one' (fig. 29).[18] I have argued elsewhere that in the series of muscle-men he has orchestrated the states of dissection, poses of the figures and points of view with astonishing skill, balancing the conflicting requirements of completeness and economy in an exemplary manner.[19] To achieve this series, which departs from a simple progressive depiction of a 'single' dissection, he must have exercised a direct and meticulous control over his illustrator – whom I still take to be Jan van Kalkar. The orchestration of variables in his *Epitome* of the *Fabrica* is if anything even more skilled, since the smaller number of illustrations presents even greater problems. The arrangement of the *Epitome* was, to use Vesalius's own description, 'selected from various possibilities with respect to typography and methods of illustration'.[20]

The correspondence with his publisher Johannes Oporinus, indicates that his concern with the editorial and technical aspects of the production of his books was no less meticulous and knowing. He wrote twice to Oporinus explaining how the illustrations in the *Fabrica* were to be keyed to the text through his system of marginal references, and he regularly took care in his annotations to explain to the reader why a particular illustration appears where it does rather than in a more obvious place in the sequence. He made particular efforts to ensure that Oporinus should understand the quality of printing required to do justice to the illustrations: 'Special care should be employed on the impression of the plates which are not to be printed like ordinary textbooks with line engravings.'[21] The inking of the woodblocks, quality of the paper and evenness of printing pressure could all have detrimental effects on the close shading lines, and Vesalius enclosed a 'proof struck off by the engraver as an exemplar'. The printer should 'take care of what I consider to be artistic and so pleasing in these pictures, that the density of lines which produce gradation in the shadows is tastefully rendered'.[22] He was fully aware that his 'pictures' were translations of the seen object via the particular

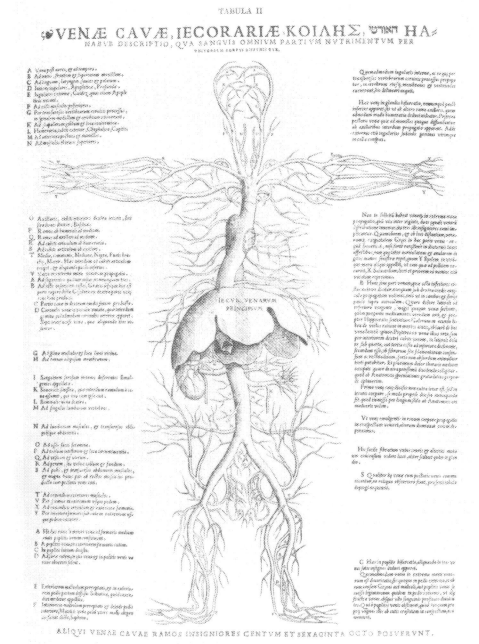

Fig. 28. Andreas Vesalius, A delineation of the entire vena cava freed from all parts. From *De humani corporis fabrica* (Basle, 1543).

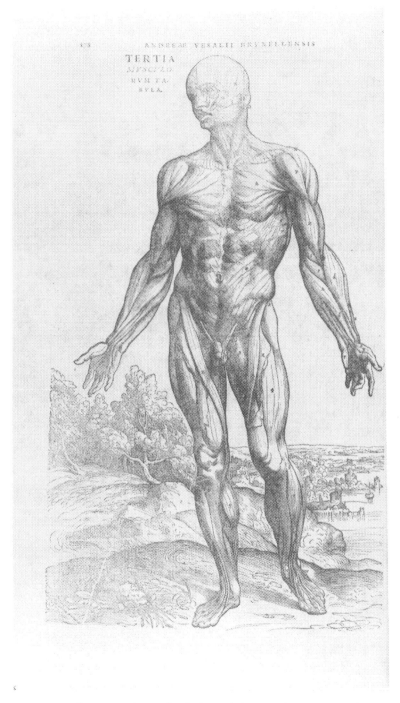

Fig. 29. Andreas Vesalius, Third plate of the muscles. From *De humani corporis fabrica* (Basle, 1543).

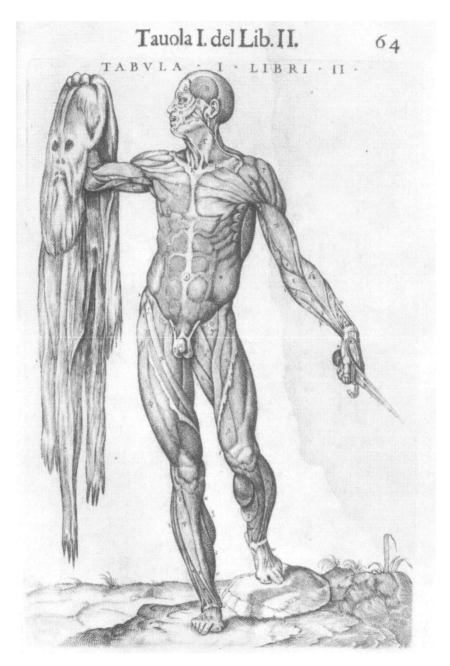

Tauola I. del Lib. II.   64

TABVLA · I · LIBRI · II ·

Fig. 30. J. Valverde de Amusco, Ecorché muscle-man holding his skin. From
Anatomia del corpo humano (Rome, 1560).

conventions of the woodcut and was keen that the pictorial skills of his graphic artists should be realized as fully as possible within the limits of the medium.

We perhaps tend to lose sight of how severe were these limits. The necessary use of line for cross-hatched shadows as well as for contour provides a source of potential confusion, and leaves little room for the differentiation of texture between muscle, bone, brain etc. Ultimately we need to be ready to accept the conventions of the woodcut if we are not to think that muscles are in part covered with a criss-cross of black fibres.

This problem of linear convention was one of the aspects of illustration in which the Spanish anatomist Valverde showed his sensitivity and inventiveness – demonstrating qualities in his work which have been all too frequently denied. His decision to have his plates cut in copper engraving resulted in little advantage in the examples transcribed directly from Vesalius, but in his own original illustrations he was able to take advantage of the finer detail possible in copper plates. He explains, with reference to his famous image of the *écorché* figure holding his own flayed skin (fig. 30) that 'in this shading I demonstrate the course of the fibres of the flesh, according to their particular orientations in each muscle'.[23] The lines within each muscle are, therefore, descriptive of linear details as seen, rather than conventional hatching lines. His choice of copper, however, causes difficulties in organization and production, since the illustrations cannot be printed with the text in the manner possible with woodcuts: 'Because my illustrations are engraved on copper, it is not possible to mingle them with the text without great confusion. I have placed all the figures which pertain to each chapter at the end of each.'[24] The system of marginal reference in the sets of figures becomes horrendously complex. One typical reference to the illustrations on an individual feature reads: 'h. li. ii. t. xvi. fi. xi. c. fi. xii. xiii. d.'.[25]

The sharp concern of Vesalius and Valverde for the visual *quality* of the illustrations does not only reflect their desire for visual lucidity but also their consciousness that their proposed publications were to take their places within the genre of fine books with magnificent illustrations. The *Fabrica* belongs with a series of great printed picture books, including the botanical books by Brunfels and Fuchs, in which printed publications came to assume their own kind of visual magnificence, having at first been the poor relations of illuminated manuscripts.[26] The *Fabrica* was in every sense – from intellectual to economic – a prestige publication for author and printer. We should also not forget that such publications arose in many instances within a context of private patronage, much like illuminated manuscripts. In Vesalius's case one of the targets of the *Fabrica* was the patronage of Charles V, to whom the first edition was dedicated. This target, as we know, was successfully struck.

In such contexts the language of style becomes very important. The

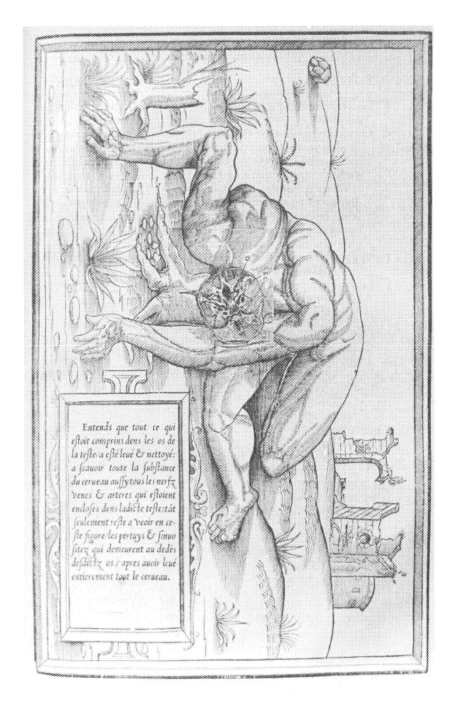

Fig. 31. Charles Estienne, Anatomical figure demonstrating the base of the interior of the skull. From *La dissection des parties du corps humain* (Paris, 1546).

picturesque backgrounds of the disarmingly energetic muscle-men in the *Fabrica*, the elegant nudes in the *Epitome*, the School of Fontainebleau adornments around the carefully posed figures in Estienne's *La dissection des parties du corps humain* (fig. 31), and Valverde's conscious use of canonical poses from works of art are not so much 'arty' irrelevances as clear signs of the intellectual and social contexts in which the authors judged their works could flourish.[27] This will be no less true when we turn to the eighteenth-century picture books.

In many ways the illustrations in an eighteenth-century book like Hunter's *Gravid Uterus*, with their uncompromising 'flesh-and-blood' quality, suggest that we are entering a very different world. However, on deeper examination, the elements of continuity are remarkable. To some extent this is deliberate, in that the Age of Enlightenment was ready to boast its Renaissance pedigree. But the continuity more profoundly arises from shared intellectual and social assumptions.

Even the debate about the necessity and value of anatomical illustration was far from dead. When Alexander Monro published the first edition of his *The Anatomy of the Humane Bones* in 1726 he provided no illustrations. His book, like that of Mundinus or even Berengario, was intended to be read with the actual objects before the eyes. His text shows that one of his dominant concerns was the naming, classifying and ordering of parts, relying upon the system of taxonomy that has so depressed the spirits of successive generations of medical students. I have chosen a passage virtually at random:

On the surface of a great many of the bones there are cavities or depressions. If these be deep, with large brows, authors name them *cotylae*. If they be superficial, they obtain the designation of *glenae*, or *glenoid*. These general classes are again divided into several special of which *pits*, are small roundish channels sunk perpendicularly into the bone. *Furrows* are long narrow canals, found in the surface ...[28]

Similar definitions follow for *niches* or *notches*, *sinuosities*, *fossae*, *sinuses*, *foramina*, *canals* and plain *holes*.

It was not that Monro *primus* was unsympathetic to illustration, but that the purpose of his text seemed not to demand it. As he said himself in later editions:

I am still of opinion, that figures of the bones would at any rate have been unnecessary in a book that is intended to be illustrated and explained by the originals themselves; but would be much more so now, when my late ingenious friend Dr Cheselden, Dr Albinus and Mr Sue have published such elegant ones.[29]

Illustrations in anatomical books were, therefore, still not inevitable, and the production of a regal picture book like Cheselden's was a major exercise predicated upon particular perceptions of function, style, production, patronage etc. The appearance and the circumstances behind the production of

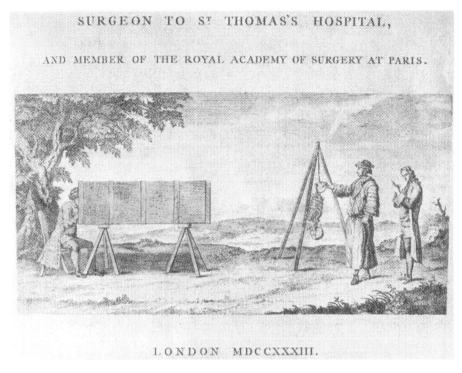

SURGEON TO Sᵀ THOMAS'S HOSPITAL,

AND MEMBER OF THE ROYAL ACADEMY OF SURGERY AT PARIS.

LONDON MDCCXXXIII.

Fig. 32. William Cheselden, The camera obscura in use for anatomical drawing. From *Osteographia or the Anatomy of the Bones* (London, 1733).

Cheselden's splendid folio, the *Osteographia or the Anatomy of the Bones*, published in 1733, displays these issues in an entirely transparent manner. The title page begins with a roll-call of Cheselden's honours: 'Surgeon to His Majesty, F. R. S., Surgeon to St. Thomas's Hospital, and member of the Royal Academy of Surgery at Paris' (fig. 32). An engraving of Galen discovering the skeleton of a robber in a rocky valley declares his intellectual pedigree, while opposite the dedication to the Queen is a magnificent engraving of her arms above a pedestal on which is a low relief of philosophers practising astronomy, geometry, arithmetic, geography and anatomy (fig. 33), activities which are flourishing 'under her MAJESTY's protection'. The system of subscription established by Cheselden to ensure the economic viability of his project was not unusual for fine books in eighteenth-century Britain. He offered subscribers a pre-publication rate of four guineas 'with a promise that none should be sold afterwards for less than six' and a guarantee that 'the plates shall be destroyed' after the printing of 300 sets of plates for the English edition and a further 100 for a Latin or French printing, in order that 'the price of the book may never sink in the possession of the subscribers'.[30] This scheme (unsuccessful

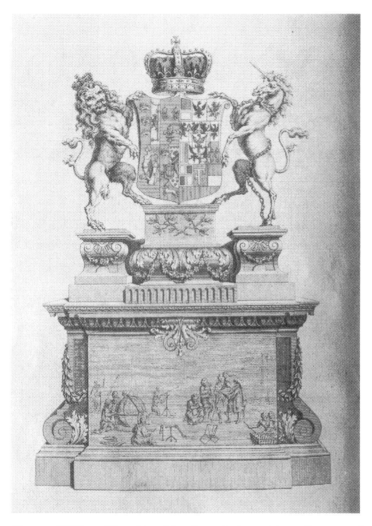

Fig. 33. William Cheselden, The Queen's Arms. From *Osteographia or the Anatomy of the Bones* (London, 1733).

as it happens) hardly gives the impression that Cheselden was providing a student's handbook.

The visual magnificence was not, of course, only a question of status and economics. It also expressed, no less directly, what was to become characteristic of the eighteenth-century picture books, namely the belief in the need for illustrations to portray a direct, uncompromising and (as far as possible) unmediated image of a form as it actually could be seen in all its reality. Like Leonardo and Hunter, Cheselden defined the descriptive superiority of visual depiction: 'I thought it was useless to make a long description, one view of

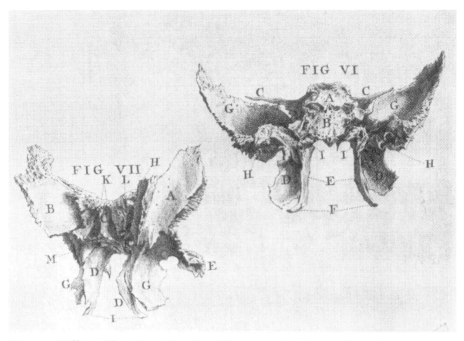

Fig. 34. William Cheselden, Os sphenoides, engraving by Vandergucht. From *Osteographia or the Anatomy of the Bones* (London, 1733), pl. VIII, figs. 6 and 7.

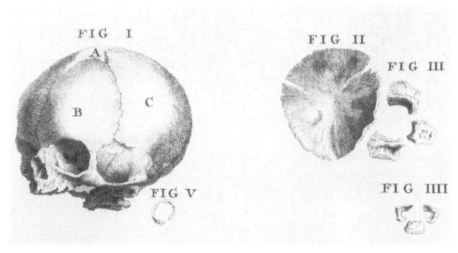

Fig. 35. William Cheselden, Skull, engraving by Shindvoet. From *Osteographia or the Anatomy of the Bones* (London, 1733), pl. XXXI, fig. 1.

such prints showing more than the fullest description can possibly do.'[31] In the text he intends to concentrate on accounts of 'mechanical contrivances' rather than shapes.

His demand for veridical representations led, as it did with Albinus and Hunter, to a rigorous analysis of how to mitigate the mediating effects of the artists' eyes and hands. Cheselden, as is well known and as is represented visually on his title page, turned to the camera obscura to achieve his ends. He tried at first to achieve objectivity by 'measuring every part as exactly as he could', but

soon found it impossible this way ... Upon which I contrived (what I had long before meditated) a convenient camera obscura to draw in, with which we corrected some of the few designs already made, throwing away others which we had before approved of, and finished the rest with more accuracy and less labour, drawing in this way in a few minutes more than could be done without in many hours, I may say in days.[32]

His artists, Vandergucht and Shindvoet, he tells us, 'knew too well the difficulties of representing irregular lines, perspective and proportion, to despise such assistance'.[33]

Cheselden did not doubt, however, that the translation of the camera obscura images drawn with 'black-lead pencil on the rough side of glass' into the engraved plates involved complex questions of mediation. He recognized the different capabilities of the engravers' styles. Vandergucht's 'open and free style' (fig. 34) was particularly good at 'expressing the different textures', while Shindvoet's 'neat and expressive' manner (fig. 35) was more limited in its pictorial range. He also paid attention to the potential of the media of engraving, mixing different techniques in one plate (fig. 36). 'The expressing of the smoothness of the ends of the bones by engraving only with single lines, while the other parts were all etched, was also my contriving.' The sense of sheen imported by the uniform parallel hatching lines of the burin technique does indeed work well against the more delicate, fuzzy and softer effects of the lines etched by acid.

Cheselden also faced the problem of any author of an anatomical text who was relying upon illustrations drawn by others to give a precise rendition of what he wanted the reader to see. There is a strong impression that Vesalius, Cheselden, Albinus and Hunter maintained a powerful presence at the draughtsmen's and engravers' elbows, making sure that the artists' hands were obedient to the anatomists' eyes. Cheselden indicates that 'where particular parts needed to be more distinctly expressed on account of the anatomy, there I always directed'. This problem of remote control was removed when the anatomist was also the artist, as in the instances of Leonardo and Stubbs.

Albinus went so far as to explain that his artist, Jan Vandelaar, had worked almost exclusively for him for ten years and that Vandelaar 'was instructed,

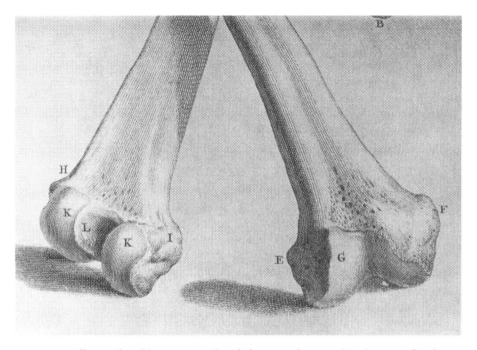

Fig. 36. William Cheselden, Femur, detail showing the mixed technique of etching and line engraving. From *Osteographia or the Anatomy of the Bones* (London, 1733), pl. XXVII, figs. 1 and 2.

directed, and entirely ruled by me, as if he was a tool in my hands, and I made the figures myself'.[34] Like Cheselden, he looked to the tradition of artists' devices for the precise imitation of nature in order to find a way of circumventing the subjectivity of the artists' eyes and hands.

He heard that the engraver was able to portray the full human figure well enough, as he had been schooled, but 'the further he proceeded amongst the internal, the figure of his parts growing more and more imperfect, was of less assistance to him'.[35] The results 'were quite different from these which I had planned in my own mind'. Albinus was not content to leave to the artist the drawing of the unfamiliar forms in correct proportion and shape 'for fear of a mistake, as he could not demonstrate to me that he was sure of doing it right'. Albinus therefore hit on the idea of adapting the artist's 'window' or 'veil' to control the demonstration. The system he used was an adaptation of a famous device, well known in the Renaissance and associated particularly with Albrecht Dürer.[36]

He placed a squared grid of strings four feet from the subject (A), and a second grid a further four feet away (B) (fig. 37). Since this second grid was smaller by 10 per cent, the grids would perfectly coincide when the artist was

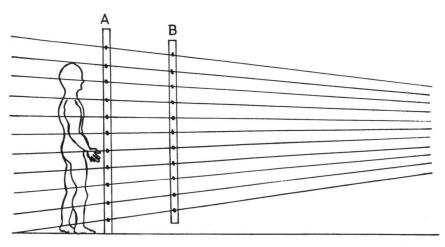

Fig. 37. Reconstructed plan of the system of grids used by Albinus for his *Tabulae*. (A) grid of ten squares placed close to the subject; (B) second grid, smaller by one tenth, placed four feet from the first. The original viewpoint is to the right at a distance of forty feet from the first grid.

stationed at a fixed eye-point forty feet away from the figure. The overall disposition and proportions of the figure were laid in from the distant viewpoint, while the details were added on closer inspection, the artist aligning the points of 'decussation' of the two grids at each point to ensure that each detail was observed in the correct part of the larger visual field. This laborious technique, on Albinus's own confession, 'occasioned an incredible deal of trouble to the engraver'.[37]

Albinus's careful description of his method and illustrative intentions is perhaps the most self-conscious and openly acknowledged account of such procedures since the annotations in Vesalius's *Fabrica*. His explanation serves to show 'by what means he [the reader] will be rendered more capable to judge' the illustrations. 'Thereby he may more easily understand what is to be avoided and what is to be observed, in a work of this nature.'[38]

His welcome openness with the reader also extends to other aspects of his procedures, visual and intellectual. His remarkable, beautiful and apparently irrelevant backgrounds (fig. 38) performed an optical function, as he tells us: 'By the shading of those ornaments . . . the light and shades of the figures might be preserved, and heightened, and the figures themselves raised or rounded.'[39] The anatomical tables should ideally be seen from a 'proper distance', with the viewer's hand 'placed before the eye in the manner of a spy-glass, so that the surrounding light may not hinder the viewing of them distinctly'.[40] The mid-tone backgrounds and shielding of external light were thus designed to reduce the ambient glare which hampers our seeing the full nuances of tonal

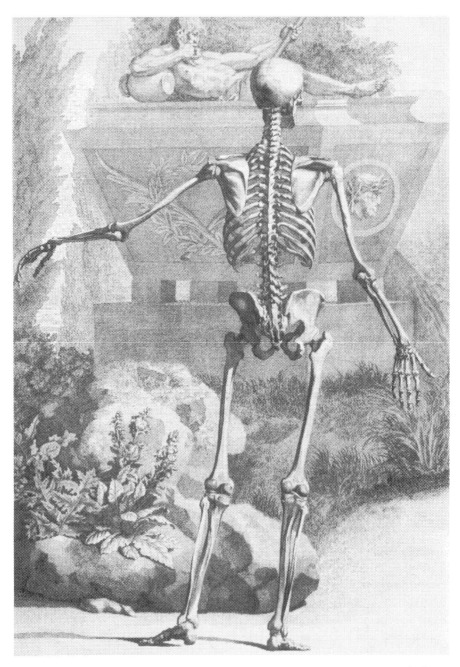

Fig. 38. Bernard Siegfried Albinus, Second plate of the skeleton. From *Tabulae sceleti et musculorum corporis humani* (Basle, 1747).

gradation in the engraved figures. This concern is typical of his almost obsessive care with the visual effect of his illustrations. This care also extended to a double-printing technique to cope with the reversal of the images, and involved research to mitigate the problems of the dampened paper stretching during printing. His very early exploration of the potential of the newly invented technique of colour printing in three of his other publications is also characteristic of his desire to push techniques of printed representation to the limits of illusion.[41]

His attention to *what* was portrayed was no less sustained than his concerns with *how* the visual effects were to be achieved. His desire for lucidity and control led him to favour a classical synthesis of 'normal' anatomies rather than an unmediated portrayal of all the accidents of a single specimen. In investigating the muscles, 'I had a great number of scattered observations. I began to digest them ... making choice chiefly of those which I found most frequently, and which I thought answered most of the intention of nature.'[42] Where the bodies used by the engraver 'manifestly and remarkably differed from what I had more frequently observed in others, these things were supplied from other bodies'. The result of Albinus's concerted efforts of visual and intellectual control is to give clear depictions of features that 'can very hardly, and others not at all, be exposed so plain in bodies themselves'.[43]

Albinus was sensitive to the charge that his attention to visual precision and magnificence had become excessive and that all his efforts were 'needless and unnecessary' in practical terms. His answer was that the 'greatness and dignity' of his subject and his illustrations went hand in hand.[44] He saw his illustrations as constructing the architecture of the body on the skeleton (fig. 39) just 'as architects, having laid a certain foundation, upon it build the edifice'.[45] The illustrator's duty was to neglect nothing that could bring his plates closer to a perfectly proportioned vision of the divine architecture of the human body – depicted according to the most sophisticated pictorial techniques that had been developed within academic art.

The pictorialism of Albinus did not pass unchallenged. Pieter Camper, in Holland, was the sternest critic, not only disparaging the ornamental backgrounds but also objecting to the whole basis of Albinus's attempt to exploit a consistent one-viewpoint perspective.[46] Camper argued that the non-diminishing perspective system of orthogonal projection – showing the figure as if seen from an infinitely distant viewpoint – would avoid the distortions of standard pictorial perspective for technical depictions of the human body.

The other eighteenth-century challenge to Albinus's style of illustration came from those who rejected any attempt to synthesize information from various dissections in a single plate. The extreme visual refinement of Albinus's plates was undoubtedly accompanied by a measure of synthetic idealization which made them remote from the 'flesh-and-blood' reality of the

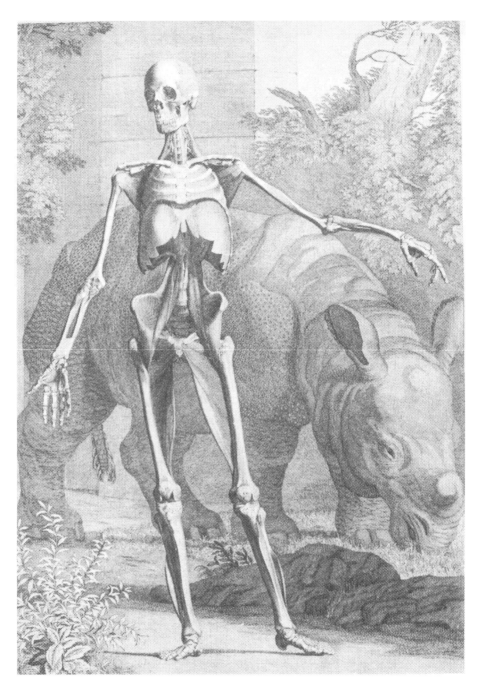

Fig. 39. Bernard Siegfried Albinus, Fourth plate of the muscles. From *Tabulae sceleti et musculorum corporis humani* (Basle, 1747).

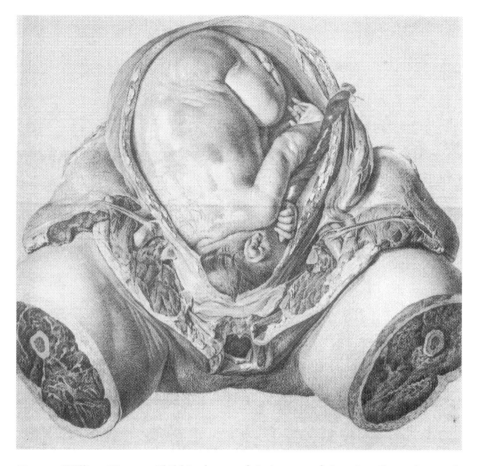

Fig. 40. William Hunter, Child in the womb in its natural situation. From *Anatomia uteri humani gravidi* (Birmingham, 1774), pl. VI.

forms. Muscles and bones tend to look as if they are uniformly made from a waxy-surfaced plastic, in contrast to the differentiated textures of Cheselden's bones. The extreme advocates of the 'flesh-and-blood' school of illustration were to be found in Britain amongst Cheselden's successors. None was more prominent than William Hunter (fig. 40).

William Hunter himself provided a neat analysis of the two main modes of illustration: 'One is a simple portrait in which the object is represented exactly as it is seen; the other is a representation of the object under such circumstances as were not actually seen, but conceived in the imagination.'[47] The character of the first kind, 'which shows the object or gives perception', is that it is 'somewhat indistinct or defective in some parts', yet exhibits the 'elegance and harmony of natural objects'. The second kind, which 'only describes or gives an idea of it ... may exhibit in one view, what could only be seen in

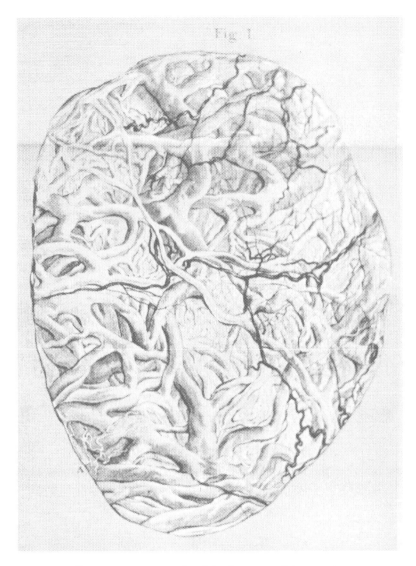

Fig. 41. William Hunter, Outside of the forepart of the womb. From *Anatomia uteri humani gravidi* (Birmingham, 1774), pl. x, fig. 1.

several objects', and tends to show the 'hardness of a geometrical diagram'. Hunter unequivocally favoured the first kind of depiction, using the artist to depict what could actually be seen in a particular specimen at a given moment. In the notes to one plate in his *Gravid Uterus* he typically records that 'the deeper seated veins could not be distinctly seen through the dried substance of the womb, and are therefore represented with the same obscurity and confusion which appeared in the object itself' (fig. 41).[48]

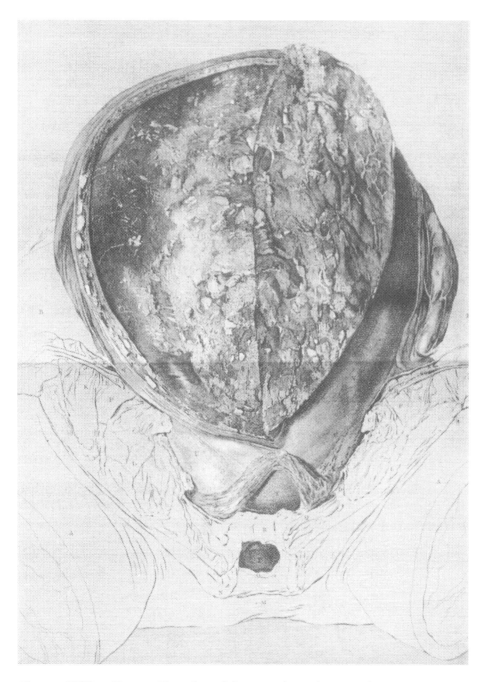

Fig. 42. William Hunter, First view of the opened womb. From *Anatomia uteri humani gravidi* (Birmingham, 1774), pl. v.

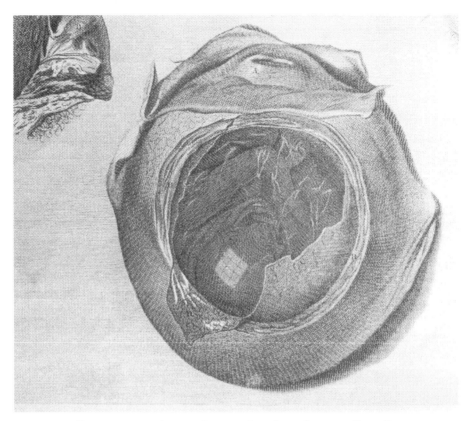

Fig. 43. William Hunter, The womb opened to show the secundines. From *Anatomia uteri humani gravidi* (Birmingham, 1774), pl. XXVI, fig. 4.

To achieve the unvarnished reality he requires that the 'work be conducted by an anatomist who will not allow the artist to paint by memory or imagination, but only from immediate observation'.[49] Effects of artistic suggestiveness or sleight-of-hand are to be strictly avoided. While the 'slight manner of producing an effect, without labour, is very agreeable in a painting' – we may recall he owned a Rembrandt oil sketch – the anatomical illustrator must aim at utter fidelity of detail.[50] Each blotch, irregularity, pockmark or blemish, however minor, must be faithfully recorded (fig. 42), regardless of its significance for the task of demonstration in hand. The sheer size of Hunter's book is justified in that the details should be displayed literally as 'large as life'. In one instance, the observation of 'accidents' is taken so far as to record the reflection of a twelve-pane window on the moist membrane over the foetus's head (fig. 43).

The plates in his *Gravid Uterus*, and other less grand books using this manner of illustration (such as John Hunter's *The Natural History of the*

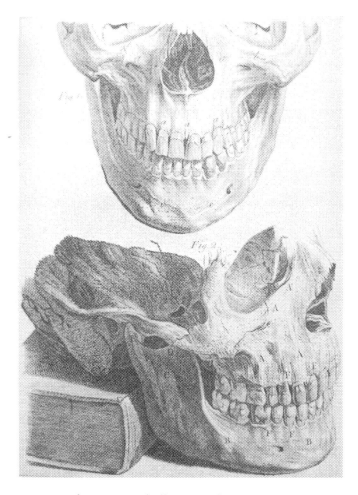

Fig. 44. John Hunter, Skull. From *The Natural History of the Human Teeth* (London, 1771).

Human Teeth) show that the 'warts-and-all' style developed almost to the point of mannerism.[51] Jacob van Rymsdyk was the greatest master of this style, in which the graphic technique is devoted to the emphatic description of surface 'accidents' of form, texture and colour (fig. 44).[52] The language of surface realism spoken by the illustrations signalled the intellectual commitment of the anatomist to an uncompromising empiricism which shows everything 'exactly as it is'.

The choice was also, in a sense, an aesthetic one. Hunter's lectures to the Royal Academy of Arts, no less than the preface to the *Gravid Uterus*, show that the highest pleasure to be evoked by a work of art arose when the effects

were most truly equivalent to those of Nature herself. The more real the
effects, the more the work 'makes stronger impressions on the mind' – a statement from the *Gravid Uterus*, but one which fits equally well in his Academy
lectures.[53]

The unadorned realism of Hunter's great book, far from being aimed at an
audience of students and general members of the midwifery profession, was no
less regal in purpose than Cheselden's production. Its sheer size, which makes
it mightily inconvenient to use, and its presentation make it clear that it is
consciously planned as a super-prestige publication. The Latin title accurately
conveys its flavour: 'Anatomia Uteri Humani Gravidi tabulis illustrate auctore
Gulielmo Hunter / Serenissimae Reginae Charlottae Medico Extraordinario /
in Academia regali anatomiae professore / et societatum, regiae et antiquariae
socio.' The work carried a prominent dedication to the King, commencing
'This work had no other claim to the honour with which it is distinguished by
YOUR MAJESTY . . . '. Like Cheselden's volume, it was financed by subscription.
In answer to the charge that 'a great part of the expense might have been
spared and the work thereby rendered of more general use', Hunter counters
that any sacrifice in visual quality and size would have vitiated its commitment
to total naturalism.[54]

Hunter's devotion to the use of the 'universal language' of drawing, which
'gives an immediate comprehension of what it represents', is less simplistic
than might at first sight appear.[55] He well knew that the same visual feature
could be interpreted in quite different ways. His involvement with forensic
science in his paper 'On the uncertainty of the signs of murder in the case of
bastard children' centred upon the difficulties of reading apparently obvious
signs, such as a swollen and strongly coloured head, as evidence of foul play: 'I
have often seen common and natural appearances . . . mistaken for marks of a
violent death'.[56] (It may be added that this paper shows Hunter in a more
humane light – with a sensitive appreciation of the plight of unmarried
mothers – than generally emerges from his writings.)

Although Hunter, as a highly intelligent man, knew that interpretation of
'signs' could err widely, he did not lose his faith that the foundation of knowledge must consist in striving for an untainted looking at the raw material. The
role of the illustrator is to capture the innocent, Lockian 'perception' rather
than the recording of the 'idea' after the interference of interpretation and
memory. He was aware that the artists' 'unselected' portrayal of what is seen
could result in the inclusion of features that are, strictly speaking, redundant in
fulfilling the purpose of the illustration. For example, on the first plate he
writes rather lamely that the prominently displayed 'thighs and *pudenda*
require no explanation'.[57]

The illustrations were also demonstrably translated into a graphic code
(fig. 45), involving dots, dashes, cross-hatching, wavy lines, etc. This code is

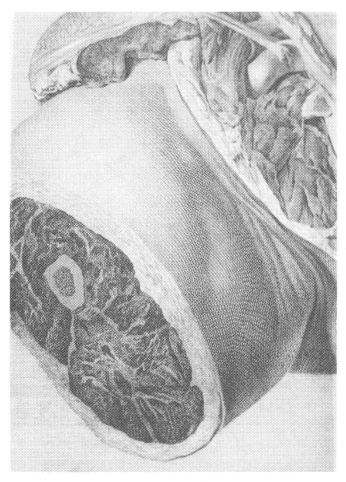

Fig. 45. William Hunter, Detail of plate VI from *Anatomia uteri humani gravidi* showing the engraving trechnique.

highly sophisticated in optical effect but does ultimately rely upon the specta-tor's collusion with the conventions. Cheselden, as we have seen, was well aware of the relative merits of different techniques of engraving, and one of the corollaries of the 'flesh-and-blood' style was that anatomists became increasingly conscious of the conventions of printing. C. N. Jenty, in trans-lating drawings by Rymsdyk into prints for his *Uteri praegnantis mulieris* of 1761, preferred the visual subtleties of the relatively new medium of mezzotint (fig. 46) as 'being the best means to Imitate Nature when coloured', notwith-standing the generally softer and less precise detail in mezzotint.[58] Anatomists during the eighteenth century were discovering that there was no single manner of printing that could simultaneously encompass all the variables of

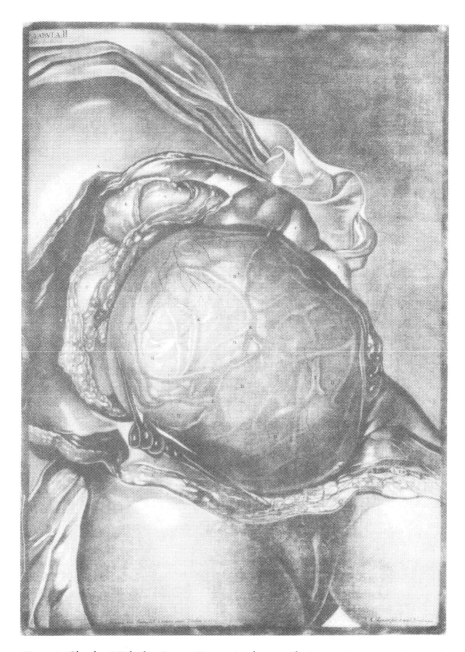

Fig. 46. Charles Nicholas Jenty, Foetus in the womb. From *Demonstratio uteri praegnantis mulieris* (Nuremberg, 1761).

the visual process in the scrutiny of anatomical form. However, there remains something heroic in the unyielding devotion to the 'real' object, and to illustrations which carried what Hunter called 'the mark of truth'.[59]

What I hope this anthology of case studies will have suggested is that we are not so much dealing with a single 'mark of truth' in anatomical illustrations, but with complex varieties of 'truths' which carry the 'marks' or imprints of a wide range of factors – intellectual, visual and social. The patterns made by the marks are not susceptible to tidy generalization, and different kinds of marks may assume greater or lesser prominence in different cases. But all of them must enter consideration in a rounded historical investigation. I am convinced that no system of anatomical representation can be properly understood without giving due weight to the questions 'how' and 'why', as well as the more traditional 'what'.

7

The art and science of seeing in medicine: physiognomy 1780–1820

Ludmilla Jordanova

The sense of sight is central to medical theory and medical practice. Practitioners are looking when they are taught anatomy, when they examine patients, when they diagnose illness, when they operate and when they perform post-mortems. Like artists, they learn that the ability to make fine visual discriminations is an essential skill. It is easy to characterize medicine in these general terms, which also serve to highlight its kinship with art. But both art and medicine have long sought to systematize, to organize, to theorize their own practices. Physiognomy has been one of the most important ways in which this has been done in medicine, and its history reveals much more than the art–medicine kinship; it shows that thinking visually made practitioners aware of methodological, theological and linguistic issues. In analysing physiognomic accounts from the late eighteenth and early nineteenth centuries, we shall find that they discuss modes of inference, knowledge of the soul, natural languages, and the book of nature and its author.

I want to examine two little-known physiognomic texts, that are not 'great' works, but which provide a sense of workaday physiognomy by medical people in the period. Unfortunately, we know very little about the context that gave rise to them, or in which they were used. This is partly because of the paucity of biographical information on their authors, who were not 'notable' in any conventional way. But it is also because the institutional setting of physiognomy in art academies and medical institutions has not yet been studied. In the absense of good historical studies, two points must be kept in mind: physiognomy was a practice as well as a system, even if at this point we can approach its formal aspects more easily, and, given this situation, the

Much of the material for this essay is drawn from my 'Physiognomy in the eighteenth century: a case study in the relationships between art and medicine' (University of Essex, M. A. dissertation, 1986).

highest priority must be accorded to laying out what it entailed at specific historical periods.

It must be admitted that, important as physiognomy certainly was in medical practice, it is extraordinarily difficult to recover this aspect historically. One reason is that we are reliant upon practitioners' descriptions of what the relevant visual signs for any particular condition were, and of how they responded to these. Few of the physiognomic texts I have seen were illustrated, and, in the absence of cheap colour reproductions, physiognomists were bound to place great store by verbal accounts. Furthermore, they were perpetually transforming their visual experience into verbal form, while those who read their treatises were doing the reverse. The slippage here is enormous, and it bears directly on the relationship between words and images. It is hard to know how physiognomy actually worked in medical practice – the necessary evidence is simply non-existent – all we can say is how some practitioners *thought* it functioned. In explaining physiognomy, late eighteenth and early nineteenth-century medical writers frequently looked to art, and also to literature, as a special kind of exemplification, and they employed particular metaphors through which to convey their ideas. It is therefore necessary to understand physiognomy in the context of art, language and literature.

Physiognomy must also be placed in its historical context. The period chosen for this chapter marks the end of an era. By the mid-nineteenth century, physiognomy was part of a larger enterprise that recorded social and racial types. Together, popularized Lavaterian ideas, phrenological theories and nineteenth-century physiognomy led to the use of photography, they entered the psychiatric hospital and responded directly to the prevailing interest in crowds, cities and dangerous classes.[1] Earlier physiognomic writings exhibited none of these traits. They negotiated on the one hand the unstable boundary between magic and physiognomy and on the other the relationship between God and nature. Accordingly, the work of Charles Bell was the culmination of a physiognomic tradition, which was closely linked with the arts and with natural theology rather than with the construction of social typologies.

The period 1780 to 1820 was thus a transitional one. We can see this clearly in a paper read to the Manchester Literary and Philosophical Society in 1790 by its Vice-President, Thomas Cooper.[2] In his lengthy article on the history of physiognomy Cooper repeatedly bemoaned the 'disgraceful' relationship between physiognomy and the divinatory sciences, which he treated as a source of contamination. Cooper wished to accord physiognomy the status of 'science', and this entailed separating it from its occult legacy. He used this shameful legacy to explain its neglect in his own time. Although his judgement as to its importance in the late eighteenth century was, I believe, faulty, his approach is exceptionally revealing. Like many writers sympathetic to the subject, Cooper used its ancient lineage as a form of legitimation and in order to emphasize his point that it had gained its reprehensible partners only in the sixteenth century. The link with divination was, for Cooper, purely fortuitous; the true kinship of physiognomy was with 'the science of man'. Cooper acknowledged that there were heated debates about what physiognomy actually is, which extended to the etymology of the world itself – does its second part derive from 'to know', from 'a mark', or from 'an index'? We can infer from Cooper's paper that physiognomy was an unstable term, and that by the 1790s, any association with the occult was especially unwelcome.

What then was physiognomy? There can be no single answer to the question. Rees's *Cyclopaedia* of 1819 defined it as 'the art of knowing the humour, temperament or disposition of a person, from observation of the lines of his face, and the character of its members or features; or of designating the powers and dispositions of the mind by a peculiar combination of the features'. Dictionaries sometimes distinguished between physiognomics – 'such signs as are taken from the countenance to judge of the state ... of the body and mind' – which is linked to medicine, and physiognomy – 'the art of judging of a person's nature, fortune, or disorders, by the lineaments of the face'.[3] In its pre-nineteenth century form, there were several important aspects to it which should be mentioned here. First, it generally spoke about knowledge of the soul of other human beings; the face acting as the mirror of or window onto it. Although there was no consensus as to exactly what this knowledge entailed, it implied that the subjectivity of the individual was involved. Second, this knowledge was understood as having a moral status; it was a special form of natural knowledge because it seemed to touch the vital core of what it meant to be human, to be social and to be created by God. Third, physiognomy inevitably embodied assumptions about the relationship between mind and body, with the latter acting as the key to the former, although the language used to express this idea was strikingly diverse. Physiognomical discourse easily accommodated different ways of thinking about the mind–body relationship. Physiognomy was thus both a subject area and a mode of inference.

If physiognomy seems confusing, even incoherent to us, it is because it was simultaneously doing a number of different things. In order to see more clearly what procedures were involved, it is necessary to distinguish between three distinct levels of operation. First, and most concretely, physiognomy operated as a technique, a vehicle for description. For example, long-standing medical and artistic traditions that focused on the temperaments involved a physiognomic approach in that a whole range of internal qualities were assumed to follow from the presence of visible external ones. Endless cataloguing of the latter was possible as was the correlation of different characteristics. Many physiognomic treatises positively revelled in their empirical detail, containing potentially infinite lists of the amazing variety of forms found in human bodies. The second level was that of action and practice. Physiognomy was a form of classification of visual signs, which allowed people to make discriminations between, for example, different illnesses or moods. It followed from these diagnostic and taxonomic procedures that prognosis and treatment were informed by physiognomic knowledge. Physiognomy, in a nutshell, helped people know what to do.

There was a third, more abstract dimension to physiognomy, which made it no less than a moral science, a science of man, as writers of this period often called it. This interpretative level arose out of two related qualities central to the physiognomic enterprise – its preoccupation with the human soul and the status of the visual signs it used as a language either of nature or of God, but either way as a universal text. Here physiognomy represented a form of knowledge, a paradigm of science. All three of these levels are present in most texts of the period. Indeed, the more significant ones knowingly spanned an exceedingly wide range of intellectual issues. None the less it is useful to distinguish them in order to understand the different kinds of conceptual work a field like physiognomy undertook and to explain its relationships with other domains, such as philosophy, literature, art and social theory.

If we examine late eighteenth and early nineteenth-century writings for their *content*, it is immediately apparent that there was remarkably little unity about the core beliefs of physiognomy. Did it apply to people *and* animals? Could plants and stones have physiognomies? What counted as a visual sign? Could transient emotions be used as well as permanent traits? What then was the role of habit?[4] It would therefore be mistaken to seek specific beliefs in the hope of finding in them the core of the subject, for this was, rather, methodological. Physiognomy was a form of inference. The human body gave rise to signifiers, which systematically led to the signified – this process was discussed in terms of the soul, mental state, essential qualities or character. Sometimes, the extrapolation was taken further than the particular object in view and moved on to nature as a whole or to God as the sources of signification. The inferential procedures passed from the full complexity of the observed world to the most abstract and metaphysical dimensions, allowing physiognomy to ally itself simultaneously to natural history (description), to medicine (practice) and to theories of language, art and authorship (interpretation).

In order to see these levels at work, we need to examine some specific physiognomic texts. I have chosen two medical dissertations, the first American, the second French, for detailed discussion. There are many other physiognomic writings like them in the period, so a comparison between them makes it possible to establish the leading themes that concerned medical physiognomists.

In 1807, Richard Brown submitted a dissertation for the Doctor of Medicine degree to the University of Pennsylvania. It was on 'the Truth of Physiognomy, and its Application to Medicine'.[5] Over the course of some eighty pages Brown discussed the nature and the scope of physiognomic knowledge, the special status of 'man', literature as a source for physiognomy, its role in everyday life, possible objections to the field, its status as a language, beauty, and, finally, the application of physiognomy to medicine, principally through a theory of the temperaments. In a wide-ranging essay, Brown devoted less than thirty pages specifically to medicine. This reveals, I would argue, that whereas his strictly medical material was well known, relatively conventional and even common-sensical, the epistemological status of physiognomy and the rationale behind its procedures required careful exposition.

It was, in fact, with the kind of knowledge that physiognomy aspires to that Brown began. Having defined it as no less than 'the knowledge of nature', he narrowed it down to the following: 'a knowledge of the connection that exists between the external or visible appearances, and the internal or invisible quali-ties of the works of nature'.[6] For Brown, physiognomy therefore had two aspects – its subject matter (i.e. nature) and its method (i.e. inference from appearances). In explaining the nature of the enterprise, Brown made two additional key points. Those who study physiognomy have 'to decypher and comprehend ... certain lines or marks', that is 'external signs'. To speak of decyphering is to evoke the act of decoding, the effort of interpretation and the concealed nature of the meaning that is sought. Yet, in the very same breath, Brown asserted that the ability to interpret facial expression was neither exclusive to human beings nor dependent on a sophisticated intellect: 'For where is the child of nine months old, that cannot discriminate between a smile and a frown?' – an argument that applied with equal force to spaniels![7] There was indeed a tension between the urge to present physiognomy as a science demanding intellectual application and the wish to support its truthful-ness by appealing to its taken-for-granted, common sense, even innate char-acter. This tension goes to the heart of physiognomy.

Brown took an assertive line when it came to arguing for the larger sig-nificance of the physiognomic enterprise. For him it could be extended legiti-mately to the whole of nature – clouds, the earth, plants and, naturally, all animals. Here 'adaptation' was the key idea, although it was not a term Brown used: 'They [animals] are all perfectly calculated by their forms structures and dispositions for the particular modes of life they are severally destined to pursue',[8] The natural theological undertow here – note the verbs 'calculated' and 'destined' – is a point to which I shall return. While Brown was happy both to show that physiognomy could be generally applied to nature and that the necessary skills were found in other animals, there was, none the less, a special place reserved for human beings in his scheme of things: 'but it is in the person, the deportment and the countenance of Man, that the fullest and brightest constellation of Physiognomical characters exists. It is here that the irresistible eloquence of signs breaks forth, and at once overwhelms us with conviction'.[9] In effect, Brown continued, physiognomy provides a *window* on the mind.

It was at this point in his dissertation that Brown appealed to authority in support of his arguments. These authorities are literary, not medical, and include writers such as Homer, Virgil, Tasso, Shakespeare and Pope. Aware perhaps that this heroic lineage might cause surprise, he asserted that poets are 'universally acknowledged to be, next to painters and sculptors, the more correct observers of the human exterior' – art was in effect being given the status of science. This impression is reinforced when Brown stated that he had used poetry to demonstrate 'the existence of a natural and necessary connection and correspondence, between the general aspect of man, and the particular qualities and attributes of his mind'.[10] Brown followed this assertion of universal physiognomic relationships with a renewed appeal to our intuitive understanding of such matters – and it is at this point, in the context of a general defence of physiognomy, that Brown explicitly raised the question of language: 'Let us, then', he implored, 'listen to the universal language of mankind, as far as it reaches our ears, and we will find in it, abundant evidence of an universal belief in the truth of Physiognomy'. He was thus able to show that 'the universal language of men' is not only rooted in nature but is the vehicle for all social relationships by virtue of which it becomes at once a moral and an aesthetic language – appearance reveals good and bad characters through beauty and ugliness.[11] There was one more level to be added to Brown's analysis of physiognomy – its providential dimension. For him the passions and their related expressions revealed 'the wisdom and goodness of Providence'. There was a divine benevolence at work here, making the face a 'kind monitor' and 'faithful index' of the mind, where index means a sign, token or indication of something, once again implying the need for interpretative labour.[12]

Only at this point did Brown turn to medical physiognomy. Not content with claiming its prognostic value, he asserted its usefulness for prevention – an assertion never further explored in the course of a fairly conventional discussion of the temperaments, indebted to Hippocrates, Galen, Cullen, Erasmus Darwin and Benjamin Rush. Brown himself focused on three temperaments – sanguineous, bilious and lymphatic, for each of which he offered a cameo sketch thoroughly in keeping with late eighteenth and early nineteenth-century traditions in environmental medicine. In the last ten pages Brown focused on specific parts of the body such as eyes, tongue, teeth and voice. The section on medicine returned to the issue of language to point out, for example, that to practitioners ignorant of physiognomy, the human 'exterior speaks not a word, or … speaks a language which is not understood'.[13]

This particular treatise on the centrality of looking in medicine contained no illustrations, presented physiognomy as a language to be either read or listened to, and drew authority from poetry. Brown described his own project as the demonstration of 'the existence of a natural and necessary connexion and correspondence between the visible exterior, and the invisible interior of man, both in health and disease'.[14] Such a statement suggests a world-view informed by natural theology, by a concern to read the book of nature and by the drive to decipher the physical world – to all of these physiognomy, as theory and as practice, was pivotal.

It will be useful to compare Brown's dissertation with one presented to the Paris faculty of medicine in the year 10 (1801/2), written by a follower of Bichat, Francois Cabuchet: 'An essay on facial expression in health and sickness'.[15] Both the differences and the similarities between these two texts are instructive. Again, a rather small proportion – roughly a third – of Cabuchet's work was devoted to strictly medical matters. His starting point, however, was somewhat different – a part of the body rather than a specific kind of knowledge. Cabuchet began by asserting that the face is the mirror of the soul – a commonplace in physiognomic writings, but a metaphor of notable complexity. Where Brown found windows, indexes and monitors, Cabuchet found mirrors, veils and pictures. Having established the value of the face in diagnosis and prognosis by drawing on the authority of Pinel, Hippocrates and Stahl, among others, he stated that the nature of his project was distinctive in that he 'has tried to draw a picture [of the face] in health and sickness, and to support this with recent physiological knowledge'.[16] The last phrase is to be understood as referring specifically to Bichat.

The main body of the dissertation was divided into three parts: on anatomy, and on facial expression in its normal and pathological forms, respectively. In the first part, Cabuchet displayed his familiarity with the comparative anatomy tradition in physiognomy, not mentioned at all by Brown, which had been preoccupied with lines, angles and brain size, and is often associated with Camper.[17] But very quickly he too began to use language as a guiding theme – for example, in claiming that gestures and facial expressions together constitute the 'language of feeling'. Like Brown, Cabuchet took for granted a broadly environmentalist approach in discussing such questions as facial variations with age, temperament, habit, sex and climate. For him these variations were as much aesthetic as medical. While conceding that beauty was largely a matter of habit, he none the less defined it in terms, such as exact proportion, which are more absolute than relative. Integral to his whole way of thinking about variations in appearance was the theory of temperaments. Like Brown, he focused on three: lymphatic, bilious and melancholic.

It was at this point in his dissertation that Cabuchet introduced another kind of evidence – paintings by great masters. Here a painting by Raphael was held to 'present the perfect expression of the traits of each temperament'.[18] Where Brown used literature as the correct depiction of nature, Cabuchet used art. Two points should be noted in this connection. First, Cabuchet's whole vocabulary was more visually orientated than Brown's. So it was not just that he went to art where Brown went to literature, but that his style of thinking was more pictorial. Second, he none the less wanted to find languages in facial movements. He stated in the second part of his dissertation, which concerned facial expression in the state of health, that there are two different sets of movements in the face, one of the passions, the other of the intelligence. These were for him two kinds of language.

What produced this drive to find languages of nature?[19] Languages have two aspects that may have made the *idea* of language especially appealing: they are systems with consistent, coherent relationships between defined parts, and they contain elements understood as having meaning. Both of these features were central to physiognomy, which could not function without the existence of systematic relationships between visual signs and which would have been devoid of interest if these signs were meaningless. However, there is another aspect to the idea of language which was equally attractive to physiognomists, who saw themselves as readers of nature. Languages imply the existence of writers as well as of readers.[20] Authors of physiognomic works were just as concerned with God and nature as authors, as they were with the practical value of the signs themselves.

There is an interesting internal dynamic in Cabuchet's writing between visual and verbal forms. When looking at the passions and their expression he used the vocabulary and ideas of a well-established tradition, often associated with LeBrun, to whom he explicitly referred. He took his pictorial examples from Poussin, Raphael, Michelangelo and Rubens, among others, under the guidance of the painter Pierre-Paul Prud'hon (1758–1823). When he mentioned paintings he treated them as data and as legitimately claiming truth status. Art was, by this token, a branch of medical science. Furthermore, his metaphors were often visual in character. At the same time, he presented expressions and gestures as languages, even calling the eye 'the language of intelligence'.[21]

The pictorial examples were in the second section of Cabuchet's treatise, which also rehearsed many well-known ideas about human variety, using terms such as habit, climate and national difference. Only in the third part did he come to the implications of his approach for medical practice, and there, significantly, he focused mainly on colouring rather than passing expressions or fixed facial features. The illnesses he described were therefore classified in terms of the colour changes they produced. This was supplemented by a very brief discussion of illnesses affecting the muscles of the face. There are no pictures accompanying the text.

A number of important points emerge from a reading of these two early nineteenth-century treatises on physiognomy. First, their similarities included: a broadly environmentalist view of health and disease, an interest in language, a belief in the general validity of moving from visible signs to invisible qualities, and broad claims about the medical value of physiognomy supported by rather thin clinical material.[22] These same features are found in many contemporary works. Second, the major differences between them were as follows: Brown took physiognomy as a paradigm of science and placed that science within a providentialist framework, while Cabuchet located it within anatomical and physiological traditions, and made no mention of God. There can be a physiognomy of everything for Brown, but not, by implication, for Cabuchet. Brown relied upon literary metaphors, Cabuchet on artistic ones, while the former used the idea of language more extensively than the latter. These differences help us to focus more sharply on the controversial areas in physiognomy of the period. Third, a comparison of these works points up some general issues: the difficulty of writing about the clinical application of physiognomy; the way in which it touched on a wide range of intellectual, moral and aesthetic matters; the tensions between its everyday, commonsense aspects and the project of developing a systematic science; and, finally, the lack of unanimity on such basic questions as what counts as a sign. Were signs traits produced by habit, expressions, or permanent, fixed features like bones or body proportions?

By its very nature then, physiognomy operated at a number of distinct, if interwoven levels. In studying it we can see that it was important for many medical practitioners to consider their own visual practices in the context, not just of the theories they espoused, but of their entire world-views and *also* how very hard it was for them to conceptualize those practices. The foregoing remarks suggest that it may be fruitful to pose our historical questions about physiognomy in the following terms: for what kind of epistemological, metaphysical and aesthetic concerns was physiognomy the appropriate vehicle? In other words, what did physiognomy mediate? In the final part of this chapter I shall consider the intertwining of theological and aesthetic interests at work in physiognomy through a brief discussion of Sir Charles Bell (1774–1842). In his writings, which came out of both his artistic and his medical practice, a number of the issues so far raised can be seen with clarity.

In the work of Charles Bell we find a deft blending of anatomy and physiology, art and theology; a marriage of attention to empirical detail with the most abstract theoretical concerns. For Bell it was not only possible to read nature, an operation that entailed bringing art and medicine together, but there was almost an obligation upon the devout to do so. He was particularly preoccupied with the idea of natural languages. His *Essays on the Anatomy of Expression in Painting* of 1806 is a classic example of the use of this idea. 'Anatomy', he asserted at the beginning of the book, stands related to the arts of design, as the grammar of that language in which they address us. The expressions, attitudes, and movements of the human figure, are the characters of this language; which is adapted to convey the effect of historical narration, as well as to show the working of human passion, and give the most striking and lively indications of intellectual power and energy.[23]

In arguing for the value of anatomical knowledge to artists, he returned to the theme of language:

Suppose that a young artist is about to sketch a figure of a limb, feeble indeed will his execution be, if without knowledge he endeavours merely to copy what is placed before him. In thus transcribing, as it were, a language which he does not understand, how many must be his errors and inaccuracies.[24]

This same sentiment was expressed by Brown. Continuing the theme of language, Bell described facial muscles as 'instruments of that universal language which has been called instinctive'.[25]

For Bell this use of language was part of a larger framework, a providentialist one. He made many points conventionally asserted by physiognomists, such as that the face is an index of the mind – but only in human beings. He therefore could not agree with Brown or with the French medical physiognomist Jean-Joseph Suë that anything in nature could have a physiognomy.[26] Two characteristics of Bell's writings are of particular interest: first, he was himself an artist, a fact that perhaps explains why he could appreciate that words and images were *not* strictly equivalent. For example, he spoke of using drawings 'in order to express what [he] despaired of making intelligible by the use of language merely'.[27] Second, in this book Bell was concerned to address the artistic community and made no attempt to codify clinical practice. I do not think that a biographical explanation of this would be satisfactory. It is better understood, I submit, in terms of the capacity of physiognomy to act as a systematic framework for the study of nature – deemed by Bell an artistic as well as a scientific enterprise. This point is borne out by the fact that physiognomic treatises of the period, however much they described, codified and classified visible traits, either stressed the soul, the book of nature and/or God, or treated the subject as being no less than the science of man. When late eighteenth and early nineteenth-century medical people looked, they saw far more than patients and diseases; they perceived a natural and/or divine universal order and they invested that order with aesthetic value.

We can see how this was the case for Bell by turning to his 1833 Bridgewater Treatise: *The Hand, its Mechanism and Vital Endowments as Evincing Design*. The hand had long been recognized as an expressive organ. Bell acknowledged the importance of the hand as an instrument of expression, invoking 'the great painters' as evidence of its 'eloquence'. This expressive capacity derived from its participation in a muscular and nervous system, the ultimate workings of which remained inaccessible to the human mind. In the last analysis, bodily expression had to be seen in terms of God's design: 'it is important to learn with what extraordinary contrivance, and with what a perfection of workmanship, the bodily apparatus is placed between that internal faculty which impels us to use it, and the exterior world'.[28] Bell concluded the treatise with a telling comparison between the eye and the hand. Both display 'convincing proofs of design'; he continued, 'the sense of vision depends on the hand', and there is a 'strict . . . analogy . . . between these two organs'.[29] By bringing the eye and the hand together, Bell could unite the different strands of his thesis. Consider, for example, his remarks on the upward direction of the eyes in prayer:

The posture, and the expression of reverence, have been universally the same in every period of life, in all stages of society, and in every clime . . . Independently altogether of the will, the eyes are rolled upwards during mental agony, and whilst strong emotions of reverence and piety prevail upon the mind. This is a natural sign, stamped upon the human countenance, and as peculiar to man, as any thing which distinguishes him from the brute.[30]

Evidently for Bell, all this talk of language is far more than a metaphor. The world *is* a language, composed of signs, designed by God. Accordingly, 'man' occupied a doubly privileged position in this universe, since his body exhibited signs unique to him, and he, uniquely, was able to interpret them. However, God's natural, universal language is not completely transparent to the human mind; we must work through that 'bodily apparatus', that is through anatomy and physiology. Once again physiognomy is linked with the labour of interpretation and understanding. Furthermore, there is an *active* force behind the 'bodily apparatus', that is, the soul or its equivalent. Bell debarred us from offering a genuinely causal account of mind–body interaction, for this would be to venture into God's territory, but failing that, the language of expression permitted human beings to speak about mind–body relationships without making false claims.

In this chapter I have suggested that in the case of physiognomy, the relationship between medicine and the sense of vision was highly complex and historically specific. Practitioners recognized the importance of visual discriminations, yet they could not theorize fully and consistently what making them entailed. This was partly because the human body generated so many different signs in distinct categories that the taxonomic challenge was quite daunting. But, more interestingly, it was also because they were, by and large, deeply committed to the idea of nature in general, and the human body in particular, as a text, to be read. This idea in turn was appealing for a number of reasons, one of which was that it could be used to construct an author, a designer, who held the world together. There was thus a continual and elaborate interplay in many physiognomic writings of this period between images and words.

Medical writers were drawn to both art and literature as authoritative sources. Yet when they deployed such sources, they treated them as simply more or less accurate reflections of nature. None the less, the relationships between medicine and these domains were exceedingly intricate. This was especially true when there were medically trained people, like Bell and Suë, who sought to or actually did instruct artists, and who wanted to make medical science aesthetically authoritative. If paintings or literary works are treated as data about nature, then those who produce natural knowledge can legitimately become arbiters of matters aesthetic. It has not been possible to examine here the social and institutional settings which made these intellectual relationships possible. Rather, I have argued that the intellectual project embodied in late eighteenth and early nineteenth-century physiognomy both allied medicine with other fields at the theoretical level, and enabled medical practitioners to use the surfeit of visual bodily signs to move from the visible to the invisible, from nature to God, from the face to the temperament, character or soul. Underpinning this project was no direct, simple relationship between medicine and one of the five senses. In fact, thinking about sight in medicine became the occasion for epistemological and metaphysical reflection.

8

The introduction of percussion and stethoscopy to early nineteenth-century Edinburgh

MALCOLM NICOLSON

The late eighteenth and early nineteenth centuries saw the development of several methods of physical diagnosis, and with them a remarkable enhancement of the role played by the physician's senses within the clinical encounter.[1] The introduction of thoracic percussion and auscultation expanded the diagnostic potential of the ear. At the same time, visual and manual examination of the patient's body became both more routine and more comprehensive, thus increasing the clinical scope of vision and touch. Visual information was also accorded a new significance as increased importance was given to correlating the results of clinical examination of the living patient with the evidence obtained by post-mortem dissection. New uses for the senses in the clinic and the autopsy room provided the empirical foundation of the anatomico-clinical method, which was to transform the nineteenth century's approach to disease.[2] This chapter seeks to illuminate an episode within this historic expansion of the role of the senses in medicine by investigating the introduction of percussion and stethoscopy to clinical practice and teaching in Edinburgh's Medical School and Royal Infirmary.

Historians have advanced two somewhat different interpretations of the reception of mediate auscultation in Britain. Some authors, most notably Edward Bluth and Stanley Reiser, have argued that the introduction of stethoscopy was a slow and difficult process, bedevilled and obstructed by a tenacious, conservative opposition.[3] Indeed, to certain commentators, Charles Newman for one, the introduction of physical methods of diagnosis counts as one of the classic battles between the forces of progress and the forces of

During the period of preparation of this chapter, I have been supported by the Wellcome Trust, to whom I wish to record my gratitude.

reaction in the history of British medicine.[4] However, other scholars have conceived of the same events in less adversarial terms. While acknowledging the occurrence of a certain amount of opposition, Paul Bishop regards mediate auscultation as an idea whose time had come – such was the clinical utility of the stethoscope and the authority with which Laënnec advocated it.[5] Bishop notes that Laënnec's *De l'auscultation médiate* evoked an overwhelmingly enthusiastic response from British reviewers. To him the story of the adoption of stethoscopy is thus essentially the story of the diffusion of information about the new technique.[6]

The apparent contradiction between these accounts of the reception and adoption of Laënnec's work springs from them referring to different processes and to different groups of people. Firstly, it should be noted that historians have not paid sufficient attention to the fact that, to many of his contemporaries, Laënnec's *De l'auscultation médiate* was more a text on pathological anatomy than one on diagnostics. A reader might thus respond positively to one aspect of the treatise without necessarily endorsing the other. Secondly, due importance has not been accorded to the crucial distinction which must be made between *academic* and *practical* knowledge of the techniques of physical examination. As will be illustrated below, when we are speaking of the diffusion of knowledge about the stethoscope, it is vital to differentiate between, on the one hand, physicians who knew enough about the stethoscope to write about it intelligently and coherently, and, on the other, physicians who could successfully apply the techniques of stethoscopy in the clinical context. In other words, we must distinguish between two groups of nineteenth-century commentators on stethoscopy – those whose senses were educated in the use of the instrument and those whose senses were not.[7]

I will argue that the successful adoption of percussion and stethoscopy was dependent not only upon the diffusion of academic knowledge of the techniques but also upon an experiential, learning process being undergone by prospective exponents. In other words the ears of the participating doctors had to be retrained. Moreover, not all British physicians and surgeons were equally eager to learn. There were, in other words, foci of enthusiasm for, and of reaction against, the innovation of mediate auscultation. In understanding the reception given to the new technique in the major British medical centres, we must consider not only the intrinsic merits of mediate auscultation as a clinical technique, but also the institutional contexts and cognitive frameworks of medical practice and pedagogy.

Andrew Duncan and thoracic percussion

One way of illustrating the importance of the distinction between academic and practical knowledge is to consider the history of thoracic percussion in

Edinburgh. In William Cullen's *First Lines of the Practice of Physic*, in the edition of 1784, there is a passing mention of Auenbrugger's innovation: 'How far the method proposed by Auenbrugger will apply to ascertain the presence of water and the quantity of it in the chest, I have not had occasion or opportunity to observe.'[8] Exactly the same statement occurs in the 'corrected and enlarged' edition of 1789, and in several subsequent editions.[9] As far as is known, Cullen never did take the opportunity to acquaint himself more closely with the diagnostic potential of the new procedure.

Following Cullen's equivocation as to its value, eighteenth-century Edinburgh doctors seem to have taken little further interest in thoracic percussion. There are very few other mentions of the technique in Edinburgh sources until 1811, when a review of Corvisart's *Essai sur les maladies et les lésions organiques du coeur et des gros vaisseaux* appeared in the *Edinburgh Medical and Surgical Journal*.[10] Jean-Nicolas Corvisart was one of the leading figures of the innovative Paris School.[11] One of the principal purposes of his book on the diseases of the heart was to demonstrate the clinical utility of percussion and to revive interest in Auenbrugger's diagnostic innovation. Although the 1811 review is unsigned, it seems likely that it was written by Andrew Duncan junior, who was then the editor of the *Journal* and Professor of Medical Jurisprudence at the University of Edinburgh.[12]

In his account of the *Essai*, the reviewer explained the new diagnostic technique in considerable detail and with admirable clarity:

> our author ... places much confidence in the information obtained from the percussion of the thorax, in the way recommended by Auenbrugger. This consists in striking the different parts of the chest with the ends of the fingers. If the lungs be sound, and if the cavity of the thorax be occupied by no foreign body, solid or fluid, the sound occassioned by this percussion has been compared ... to that of an empty barrel; on the contrary, when a solid or liquid body occupies any part of the thoracic cavity, the side of the thorax, or that part so occupied, gives a duller sound, compared to that yielded on striking the thigh in the same manner. Such, says Mr Corvisart, is the precision of this method, that I have often determined, with great exactness, the degree of dilation of the heart, by measuring it, as it were, upon the extent of the chest over which percussion yielded no sound, or only an obscure one; often after the death of the subject, I have verified the fidelity of my diagnostic ...[13]

The reviewer also quoted the details of several of Corvisart's clinical cases, indicating how percussion had aided the French author in the differential diagnosis of several chest ailments. It is evident that he had read Corvisart's treatise with some attention. No doubt he could have given a good lecture on how to percuss. But we cannot conclude from this that the reviewer was skilled in the employment of the technique in the clinical situation.

There is, in fact, strong presumptive evidence to the contrary. Five years after the review of Corvisart's *Essai* appeared, Duncan published a long article reporting the results of his own investigations on inflammation of the heart.[14] It was based on three cases admitted to the Edinburgh Royal Infirmary. In his description and interpretation of these cases, Duncan displayed his knowledge and appreciation of Corvisart's work. He followed his patients from the wards into the autopsy room in exactly the approved Parisian manner. In his understanding of their diseases, he employed much of the *theoretical* content of Corvisart's *Essai*. However, in two of the three cases, there is no mention of the patient having been examined with the new investigative technique of percussion. The clinical reports Duncan provided are so detailed as to leave little doubt that, if the patient had been percussed, the results of this examination would have been included.

The story of the third case sheds an interesting light on Duncan's diagnostic routines and his attitude to the practice of percussion. The patient, Mary Rickman, entered the Infirmary on 11 March 1815. On admission she complained of 'pain in the thorax, more particularly referred to the sternum'.[15] Duncan diagnosed pleuritis and prescribed a course of bleeding and blistering. The patient continued to complain of severe pain in the centre of the chest. On 5 April, Duncan decided to try the experiment of percussing the chest. He noted that the 'sternum, when struck, does not emit a hollow sound and the pulsation of the heart is very distinctly felt lower than the ensiform cartilage'.[16] Rickman died on 13 April, apparently not having been percussed again. Autopsy dissection revealed enlargement of the heart and inflammation of the pericardium.

Duncan explained his failure to apprehend the true nature of the case in terms of its not displaying the recognized general signs and symptoms of carditis:

Rickman had not the *pulses inequalis, palpitatio et syncope,* of Cullen; nor the constant vomiting of Darwin; nor the palpitation, faintings, quick and unequal pulse of Sauvages; nor the very intense thirst of Burserius; nor the hydrophobia of Daniel; nor the delirium of Davis.[17]

However, he admitted that, even in this confusing and anomalous case, his diagnosis could have been more acute:

And yet the intensity of pain ... in the region of the heart, combined with the comparatively natural state of respiration during the inflammatory stage, might have directed me to the heart. Add to this ... when it was discovered, the total want of resonance from the percussion of the sternum. Even this symptom did not undeceive me, for I had previously supposed a purulent collection to have been formed under the sternum, which was the reason for my making the trial ...[18]

It is clear from this example that Duncan had, by 1815, not adopted percussion as part of his routine clinical practice. His diagnosis of carditis was still based entirely upon gross observation of the patient's behaviour. Two of his three patients suffering from inflammation of the heart were not percussed. The third was percussed only once – some twenty-five days after her admission. Moreover, even having departed from his normal procedures to undertake the percussion in this case, Duncan was unsure how to interpret and weigh the results he obtained.

Duncan remarked that the value of the percussion sound 'as a diagnostic symptom, is, I think, very apparent from this case'.[19] But even such a relatively positive experience with the technique did not persuade him to employ percussion more intensively. This is evidenced by the *Reports of the Practice in the Clinical Wards of the Edinburgh Royal Infirmary* which Duncan published in 1819.[20] Here Duncan provides a tabulated record of the cases admitted to the Infirmary in late 1817, and early 1818, during which time he was in charge of the clinical wards. Thirty-one cases are described in detail.

Among these thirty-one cases, there is again only a single mention of the employment of percussion. It is recorded that a young woman, suffering from 'anomalous fever', was percussed after having been in the Infirmary for four days. Duncan noted that the 'thorax on percussion sounds well, except at the lower part of the sternum, where it seems to cause pain'.[21] The woman died and was dissected, but the account of the post-mortem examination does not indicate that any attempt was made to correlate the percussion sounds with pathological alteration of structure. Several other thoracic cases are fully described in the *Reports* but none of these would seem to have been percussed even when the condition was puzzling and the diagnosis problematic.[22] In other words Duncan's *Reports* provides no evidence of percussion having been routinely or even regularly employed in the Royal Infirmary at the end of the second decade of the nineteenth century, by Duncan or anyone else.

We may conclude that Duncan, in 1818 as in 1811, had a good academic, theoretical knowledge of percussion. He was capable of demonstrating how to percuss. We have, however, no good grounds for believing that, by the end of the second debate of the nineteenth century, he had developed much practical experience with the procedure. Percussion had certainly not become a standard part of his clinical routine. Nor had his knowledge of the technique caused him to modify his conceptions of thoracic disease. His clinical and cognitive procedures in such cases were still firmly traditional. In other words, accurate descriptions of the techniques of physical diagnosis, such as are to be found in the 1811 review of Corvisart's *Essai*, are not essentially evidence of developed clinical expertise in those techniques.[23]

Nor can Duncan be regarded as atypically conservative in this respect. In fact it is probable that other Edinburgh doctors were behind, rather than ahead, of him in their adoption of Auenbrugger's method. Andrew Duncan senior, for example, published in 1816 his *Observations on the Distinguishing Symptoms of the Three Different Species of Pulmonary Consumption*.[24] This text contains no mention of percussion or any other technique of physical diagnosis.

The employment, by Duncan junior, of Corvisart's work in particular, and the French anatomico-clinical exemplar in general, is a striking example of how selective the process of cultural transfer and adoption of innovation can be. As we have seen, Duncan knew the French work well, admired it, and utilized it extensively in his own clinical research. But his use of it was conditioned by his own concerns and interests, the routines and priorities of his own characteristic forms of practice and enquiry, which were, of course, the product of his being based in Edinburgh and not in Paris.[25]

The literary reception of *De l'auscultation médiate*

As Paul Bishop has noted, virtually all the British reviews of Laënnec's *De l'auscultation médiate* were favourable.[26] Most, indeed, were enthusiastic. It is, however, important to note that this positive response was not necessarily based upon an appreciation of the practical value of stethoscopy. Many critics reviewed Laënnec's book as a text on pathological anatomy, granting only secondary significance to the diagnostic innovations which he had proposed. Indeed, more than one commentator expressed regret that Laënnec had obscured the value of his investigations into pathological anatomy by constantly relating his results in the autopsy room to clinical diagnosis.[27] These reviewers thus identified as a weakness precisely what later commentators and historians have come to regard as the great strategic strength of Laënnec's research enterprise.[28] In other words, there is no simple identification to be made between our present-day enthusiasms for Laënnec's work and the enthusiasms of his British contemporaries.

The conviction that Laënnec had diminished the impact of his pathological anatomy by not dividing it from the discussion of diagnostics was shared, at least initially, by Laënnec's translator, John Forbes. A desire to remedy this defect led Forbes radically to alter the ordering of the text for the English edition:

By this means, the work, in place of appearing, as in its original form, a system of Diagnosis, with the pathological part subservient to, and partly concealed by it, is now restored to what I humbly conceive it ought always to have been, viz. two independent treatises, – one on Pathology, the other on Diagnosis . . .[29]

Forbes did not, however, value the two sections equally when he planned the rearrangement of the text. He originally conceived of the English translation principally as a contribution to the literature on pathological anatomy. It was not until after he had begun the translation that, at the instigation of James Clark, he made a trial of the stethoscope in his own practice.[30] The results of this experiment caused him to revise his opinion of the value of Laënnec's diagnostic suggestions. In the light of a growing conviction of the utility of mediate auscultation, Forbes undertook some further alteration of the text:

The truth is – that when I began my translation I was too little impressed with the importance of the diagnostic measures recommended in the work; and my object was rather directed to improve the pathology at the expense of the diagnosis. In consequence of this, I must admit that several of the cases . . . are too much abridged; and that some valuable diagnostic details are thereby excluded. With a view of making all the amends in my power, I have given several of the more important cases thus abridged, more at length in the appendix; and have added several others not translated in the body of the work.[31]

It is evident therefore that the favourable reception which British medical commentators gave to *De l'auscultation médiate* cannot be taken as a whole-hearted endorsement of stethoscopy. It is true, of course, that some early commentators did respond to Laënnec's diagnostic suggestions with interest, even with enthusiasm.[32] However Laënnec had not necessarily added, actually or even potentially, to the diagnostic repertoire of these authors.

This holds true even in Edinburgh where, as we shall see, practical trials of stethoscopy were very promptly initiated. One of the earliest mentions of the stethoscope in an Edinburgh source is to be found in an M.D. thesis written by Charles Locock in 1821.[33] But Locock merely recorded and repeated what other authors had already written about the clinical value of mediate auscultation. He mentioned nothing of his own personal experience with the instrument and we have no grounds at all for assuming that he had any. It is worth noting that, in 1821, Locock had not yet seen a copy of Laënnec's book – he confessed that his account of its contents was drawn from a review lately published in a London medical periodical. Locock's thesis therefore contains textual commentary rather than evidence of the clinical utilization of mediate auscultation.[34]

A very similar story may be told with regard to another, rather more famous, early Edinburgh text on stethoscopy – that written by the later-to-be-eminent physician, William Stokes, while he was in the final year of his medical studies in Edinburgh. Stokes's book was published in 1825 and is entitled *An Introduction to the Use of the Stethoscope with its Application to the Diagnosis in Diseases of the Thoracic Viscera.*[35] Unlike Locock's thesis, Stokes's account of stethoscopy was impressively furnished with clinical cases and examples. However, Stokes's work in preparing the text was again wholly that of a compiler. Every one of the clinical examples he cited had been derived from the published French sources.[36] None of them was of a Scottish subject, far less having been drawn directly from Stokes's own clinical experience. His description of the clinical use of the instrument was largely derived either from

Laënnec directly or from Collin's *De diverses méthodes d'éxploration de la poitrine*.[37] The appendix consists of an abridged translation of Andral's thesis on expectoration.[38] Stokes's own views were made explicit only in three footnotes, none of which related directly to the clinical use of the stethoscope.[39] *An Introduction to the Use of the Stethoscope* is, thus, best regarded an an exercise in medical literary scholarship. It demonstrated Stokes's interest in the development of the anatomico-clinical method and his acquaintance with the French literature but said nothing at all about his own clinical expertise.[40]

Thus, while we may agree with Bishop that the initial British response to Laënnec's book was overwhelmingly favourable, we must bear in mind that the response was not necessarily based upon a positive evaluation of the book's suggestions in diagnostics. And even when it was, as in the two Edinburgh examples, a positive response to Laënnec's diagnostic innovations is not evidence that the commentator's own clinical practice had been modified in the manner Laënnec proposed. It was to take more than reading books, more than favourably responding to them, to achieve the transfer of a practical clinical technique from Paris to Edinburgh. The senses of the participating personnel had to go through the difficult process of being trained.

Contemporary observers were well aware of the crucial distinction to be made between academic, theoretical knowledge of Laënnec's text, on the one hand, and clinical experience with the stethoscope, on the other. They knew that stethoscopy was not to be established in British clinical practice by a few favourable book-reviews. In 1824, Forbes wrote:

when the work of M. Laënnec was first introduced to the knowledge of the profession in this country, it appeared from the reports of the Medical Journals ... that a very considerable impression had been made on the public mind, in favour of the diagnostic measures therein recommended. Since that time, however, if we may judge from the same journals, the impression then made seems to have been productive of few practical results; as I am not aware that even a single case, illustrative of the use of Auscultation, has appeared in any one of them. From this circumstance, and from not having heard of its employment in any hospital, or indeed by any individual practitioner in this country (with the exception of my friend Dr Duncan Jun. of Edinburgh), I am led to fear that the impression made was more lively than profound, and that through the influence of prejudice, theory and indolence ... the greatest medical improvement of the present age, is in danger of sharing the fate of those thousand idle and useless projects which daily spring up among us, and which, after obtaining a temporary notoriety through the patronage of inexperienced and over-zealous individuals, soon sink into merited oblivion.[41]

The remainder of this chapter will be devoted to following up Forbes's suggestion that something different from the general pattern was indeed happening in Edinburgh.

Practical trials with the stethoscope

Edinburgh doctors began experimenting with the stethoscope very early in the 1820s, even, indeed, before Locock produced his thesis. On 12 November 1820, John Lane, assistant to Andrew Duncan in the Royal Informary, recorded the following account of a clinical examination:

The right side of the thorax is very sonorous and by means of the stethoscope the air is very distinctly heard penetrating the air cells (puerile). But the left side gives on percussion a dull sound and an obscure sense of fluctuation. The entrance of the air into the lungs on this side is indistinctly heard in all parts, a little more distinctly along the side of the dorsal vertebrae . . . The action of the heart is faintly heard in the praecordial region but is very evident in the right side of the sternum.[42]

In a clinical lecture on the same case, Duncan remarked:

I have noticed, by the stethoscope, under the sternum, a singular sound, which I cannot compare to anything more accurately than the fall of a heavy drop of water . . . At another time it resembled the sudden separation of moist surfaces, as in the smacking of lips.[43]

Some years later, Duncan again referred to his examination of this patient: 'At this time I was not acquainted with the *tintement metallique*, of Laënnec; but I have now no doubt that it was the phenomenon which I attempted to describe.'[44]

Lane made several observations, similar to the above, in November and December, 1820. However, it should be noted that, while his notes show that he was already able to exploit some of the clinical potential of percussion and mediate auscultation, Lane used the stethoscope only to listen to the respiratory murmur and to locate the apex beat of the heart. In other words he employed it only in relatively straightforward clinical tasks, which required relatively little in the way of experience or developed expertise with the instrument. He cannot be said to have fully developed the *auditus eruditus*, the educated ear necessary to exploit the stethoscope to the full. As we have seen, Duncan was aware that his and Lane's early efforts to emulate Laënnec's example left much to be desired. He did not publish their results until 1827, and then only, it would appear, to establish a priority claim.[45]

The *Edinburgh Medical and Surgical Journal* did not review Laënnec's book until the appearance of the first edition of Forbes's English translation in 1822.[46] This is, at first sight, surprising since Duncan prided himself on the full coverage which the *Journal* gave to foreign work. If however one looks at the review of *De l'auscultation médiate* which eventually appeared, one gets a hint as to what might have been the cause of this delay. Unlike nearly all the London reviewers, the Edinburgh reviewer had tried out the stethoscope for himself.[47] The Edinburgh reviewer, again possibly Duncan himself, can assess *De l'auscultation médiate* in terms of personal, practical experience of the diagnostic innovations which Laënnec proposed.

There was no doubt that the Edinburgh trial had been, within limits, a successful one:

Anyone who will take the trouble to apply the cylinder with tolerable attention ... to the chest of half a dozen patients in a hospital will easily satisfy himself of the great diversity to be observed in the action or rhythm of the heart, and in the sounds caused by respiration, and as these depend upon the physical state of the organs, the one is a certain indication of the other.[48]

It is noteworthy, however, that the Edinburgh reviewer did not claim that he had himself completely mastered the art of correlating the stethoscopic sounds with the physical state of the internal organs. He had been convinced, 'from considerable experience' as he put it, of the diagnostic potential of the stethoscope.[49] But he acknowledged that the clinical decisions he had made on the basis of the stethoscopic sounds had not always been reliable: 'we readily admit, that, from deficiency of skill and knowledge, we have been occasionally deceived in our diagnosis and prognosis deduced from the method of observation'.[50] Moreover much still had to be taken on trust from Laënnec: 'the observations we have had opportunities to make induce us to place implicit confidence in the finer distinctions mentioned by Laënnec which we have not yet acquired skill enough to reach'.[51]

Not only was the Edinburgh reviewer having trouble educating his own ears, it would seem that his students, or perhaps his colleagues, were experiencing difficulties too. He noted that 'it requires attention and some adroitness to apply it [the stethoscope] properly at one end to the chest of the patient, and at the other to the ear of the observer'. He complained that 'the awkwardness of some persons in so simple an operation is incorrigible'.[52] This sounds, to the present reader, like the *cri de coeur* of an exasperated teacher.

The 1822 review provides us with the first Edinburgh, indeed perhaps the first British, account of a full trial of the stethoscope in the clinical situation. The trial had been very positive but, at the same time, very limited. It is apparent that the reviewer was not, at this time, wholly competent with the stethoscope. He was having some difficulty learning the technique and teaching it to others. It is evident that the new diagnostic technique had not yet become fully naturalized within Edinburgh clinical practice.

This conclusion is substantiated by evidence from other sources. A very valuable, but as yet little exploited, resource for the history of Edinburgh medicine is the probationary essays demanded of prospective members by the College of Surgeons. Of great interest, in the present context, is an essay, dating again from 1822, by William Cullen, the grand-nephew of the more famous bearer of that name.[53] Cullen described the usefulness of the stethoscope in the diagnosis of 'peripneumony', in a manner which suggests that he had had some experience of the use of the instrument. However, no specific or original clinical information was presented. Moreover, a probationary essay on emphysema by James Russell dating from the following year, 1823, contains, amid quite detailed clinical descriptions, no mention whatsoever of stethoscopy.[54] If the instrument had been in general use in Edinburgh at that time one would certainly have expected to find mention of it in such a context.

The impact of trained stethoscopists

This situation was to change quite rapidly. We know, from Laënnec's own records, that Cullen studied under him in Paris for several months, probably late in 1822. In a note made in 1824, Laënnec wrote that Cullen 'today teaches the stethoscope in Edinburgh'.[55] This is corroborated by John Struthers, who, in his *Historical Sketch of the Edinburgh Anatomical School*, stated that, sometime about 1824, William Cullen began to give a series of special lectures on the stethoscope.[56] These classes were attended both by students and by his fellow members of staff – Cullen being, at this time, a house surgeon to the Royal Infirmary. We also have the testimony of J. P. Kay, a contemporary of Cullen and a clinical assistant in the Infirmary, who recorded that Cullen's audience included two of the clinical professors.[57] Thus, from 1824, stethoscopy was being proselytized for in Edinburgh not only by the self-taught Lane and Duncan but also by an exponent who had had his senses trained in Paris by the Master himself. Nor was Cullen for long alone in this distinction – in 1824 James Crauford Gregory also went to study under Laënnec, returning to take up a position as physician to the Royal Infirmary in 1826.[58]

We know nothing of the content of Cullen's lectures but other evidence suggests that the influence exerted by his advocacy of stethoscopy was considerable.[59] The M.D. thesis submitted by James Hope in 1825, for example, is quite different in character both from Stokes's literary efforts published in the same year and from the probationary essays of 1822 and 1823.[60] Its accounts of stethoscopic investigations also represent a considerable advance in sophistication upon Lane's clinically useful but technically rudimentary work. In 1825 Hope was, like Cullen, a house surgeon in the Royal Infirmary. He was, of course, later to become famous for his investigations into the diseases of the heart.[61] He is also remembered for his determined advocacy of the stethoscope, particularly in London.

Hope's thesis describes a trial of the potential of the stethoscope in the diagnosis and investigation of arterial disease. It was based upon a series of six case histories, each of a named patient from the Royal Infirmary. The patients were examined with the stethoscope in the wards and the results were correlated with autopsy observations. The names of Hope's patients may be found in the patient register of the Infirmary and the diagnosis and outcome of each case checked against Hope's account.[62] Thus, the investigations described in Hope's thesis, unlike those in Stokes's book, actually took place in Edinburgh. In other words, Hope's M.D. thesis undoubtedly describe a genuine anatomico-clinical investigation using the stethoscope, rather than being merely a literary or translation exercise.

It will be remembered that the 1822 Edinburgh reviewer had to take a great deal on trust from *De l'auscultation médiate*. Likewise, Duncan, Lane, Locock, Cullen and Stokes all had, by 1825, added little or nothing to the technical content of the continental authors. Hope, on the other hand, was able explicitly to contradict and correct Laënnec on a crucial point relating to the clinical application of the stethoscope. Laënnec had maintained that the stethoscope would be of little use in the diagnosis of aortal aneurysms.[63] Hope argued that in fact it was of considerable use in such cases. Laënnec had believed that the noises associated with thoracic aneurysm would generally be impossible to distinguish from those of the heart itself. Hope demonstrated that this distinction could often be achieved: the aneurysmal murmur diminishes as the stethoscope is moved toward the heart while the heart sounds become louder.[64] He conjectured that the reason why Laënnec had thought differently was that his experience of cases of aortic aneurysms had not been sufficient for him to attain the requisite degree of acuity in the discernment of the distinctive aneurysmal sounds.[65]

This aspect of Hope's work is most significant, not only because it vividly demonstrates how far skill with the stethoscope had improved in Edinburgh since Lane began his investigations, but also (and primarily) because it illustrates the existence of a new independence from the French sources on the part of Edinburgh academic physicians. It also indicates that, from 1825, the stethoscope had research potential as well as diagnostic utility for this group of practitioners. For example, Hope's work on the use of mediate auscultation in cases of aortic aneurysm was shortly followed up and augmented by Robert Spittal, also a house surgeon to the Royal Infirmary.[66] Spittal argued that one of the reasons that the stethoscopist failed to diagnose aneurysm correctly was that, in mature cases, the deposition of 'fibrine' in the aneurysmal sac rendered the distinctive noises obscure.

Hope's development of Laënnec's legacy was bold and original. It was not, however, the only or even the most radical of the departures from the French exemplar being undertaken in Edinburgh in the 1820s and 1830s. For example, in 1828, John William Turner, Professor of Surgery, dissented from Laënnec on an even more fundamental question of the physiological and pathological meaning of the noises to be heard with the stethoscope. Laënnec had described the normal heart as producing two distinct sounds, followed by a pause. He attributed the first sound to the contraction of the ventricles and the second to the contraction of the auricles. Turner pointed out that Laënnec had ignored the experimental work of Harvey and Haller on the motion and rhythm of the heart. According to these earlier authors, the contraction of the auricles occurred after the long pause and before the contraction of the ventricles. Turner suggested, *contra* Laënnec, that the second heart sound was produced as the heart fell back into the pericardium, following diastole.[67]

This view of the second heart sound did not however achieve widespread acceptance in Edinburgh academic circles. In 1828, Matthew Baillie Gairdner read a paper to the Royal Medical Society of Edinburgh in which he argued that the second sound of the heart was produced by the closure of the semilunar valves.[68] This view was later corroborated by experimental work undertaken by James Hope and by C. J. Williams, likewise an Edinburgh graduate and a famous advocate of auscultation.[69] In 1830, Spittal used several cases from the Royal Infirmary to illustrate that refinement in the understanding of the heart sounds could be translated into a greater clinical acuity in the localization of structural alterations of the heart.[70]

Other Edinburgh personnel worked not to develop the theory underlying mediate auscultation but to improve the instrument itself. N. P. Comins, a physician to the Royal Infirmary, was concerned at 'the great difficulty of attaining the accurate knowledge of which it [the stethoscope] is the medium of communication, notwithstanding the numerous cases of thoracic disease that have been treated in the Infirmary'.[71] The root of this difficulty lay in the fact that the application of the cylinder was often uncomfortable to the patient, who had to change his or her position to accommodate the stethoscopist and who had to submit to a rigid cylinder of wood being pressed against the skin. In 1828, in an attempt to alleviate these problems, Comins designed a 'flexible' stethoscope which would enable the examiner to 'explore any part of the chest, in any position, and in any stage of disease, without pressure or inconvenience to the patient or to himself'.[72] The new instrument had, Comins wrote, 'for some weeks been successfully used in every case of thoracic disease in the Royal Infirmary'.[73] (The fact that all thoracic cases were now being examined with the stethoscope indicates, of course, that a considerable change had occurred in Edinburgh hospital practice in the five or so years since Russell had written his probationary essay.)

Comins presented his flexible stethoscope as having other advantages to the physician: 'As it does not require the head of the stethoscopist over the chest of the sick person, and as another tube may be screwed to the instrument, it can be used in the highest ranks of society without offending fastidious delicacy.'[74] Nor were its benefits confined to the doctor's intercourse with the more elevated social orders:

Timidity or disgust is unpardonable on the part of the physician when engaged in the discharge of his duty. But, as it is often necessary in contagious disease to explore the chest of the poorest individuals, may not reasonable precaution and the feelings of a gentleman be so far complied with as to use the cylinder with the additional tube, in cases manifestly contagious or miserably wretched?[75]

Another virtue of the new instrument lay in the assistance it gave to those learning stethoscopy. The drawbacks of the rigid cylinder were most obvious when it was in the hands of large numbers of inexperienced users:

This difficulty arises from the great numbers of medical students who prosecute their studies in Edinburgh; and who, from their anxiety to attain facility in auscultation, are often denied permission to use the instrument, in consequence of the torture unavoidably inflicted by repeated attempts, and by the frequent change of posture necessarily required of the afflicted persons.[76]

Comins stated that the utility a flexible stethoscope would possess for the inexperienced student constituted his principal reason for developing such an instrument.

From innovation to standard practice

By 1825, the use of the stethoscope was being taught in Edinburgh, if, perhaps, not quite routinely. As we have seen, it was, according to Comins, being regularly employed in clinical investigation and instruction in the Royal Infirmary by 1828. It is, of course, often very difficult for the historian to ascertain exactly when an innovation attains the status of standard practice. However, one datum which is always relevant to such an assessment is when the novelty in question appears in the general textbooks. Again, this happens surprisingly quickly in the case of the introduction of stethoscopy to Edinburgh.

The dominant Edinburgh textbook of the latter half of the eighteenth century was the elder William Cullen's *First Lines of the Practice of Physic*. This text remained in regular use well into the nineteenth century. In 1829, upon the appearance of a new edition, the *Edinburgh Medical and Surgical Journal* described it as 'not ... displaced as a textbook in the hands of the lecturer and the student'.[77] Revision for the new edition was begun by the younger William Cullen, who died in 1828 while the work was still in progress. It was continued by his colleague and fellow pioneer of stethoscopy, James Crauford Gregory.

Cullen wrote the section on diseases of the chest for the new textbook and Gregory wrote the section on catarrh and similar conditions.[78] In revising these sections, both authors took the opportunity to demonstrate the utility of the stethoscope, giving detailed instructions as to how it was to be used in distinguishing one disorder from another. Especially in the younger Cullen's

case, but to a large extent in Gregory's as well, such a revision entailed dis-
mantling large parts of the structure of the original author's nosology and
introducing new categories and new distinctions between old categories. In
particular the elder Cullen's union of pneumonia and pleurisy was proclaimed
to be erroneous in the light of the information furnished by the new instrument.[79] In other words the stethoscope had by 1829 radically and irreversibly
changed the medical theory that was being taught to undergraduates in
Edinburgh.

Clinical lecture courses from this period contain many references to the
stethoscope, indicating that its clinical use was now being routinely taught.[80]
In the published accounts of interesting clinical case histories we can also see a
significant change. In the publications of the Edinburgh pioneers of stethoscopy which appeared between 1820 and 1830, those of Hope, Gregory and
Robert Spittal, the point is explicitly, ostentatiously one might say, to demonstrate the value of the instrument. But, even as early as 1831, examples of
another way of describing the clinical application of the stethoscope may be
found.

Here is an extract from a case history published in the *Edinburgh Medical
and Surgical Journal* of that year:

Having stripped the patient I made a careful examination of the chest ... The left side
of the thorax sounds perfectly clear even in its most inferior position and in the situation naturally occupied by the heart. Respiration of the puerile character and mixed
with some bronchial râles is to be heard over the entire lung and is as distinct in the
mammary region as in the other portions.[81]

Much of the information presented here could only have been gained by the
use of the techniques of percussion and auscultation. 'Respiration of the
puerile character' and 'bronchial râle' are technical terms for auscultation
noises, established in medical discourse by Laënnec. The reference to the
sounding of the left side of the thorax indicates the use of a percussive technique. But neither auscultation nor percussion is explicitly mentioned in the
text. At least in the context of research publications, the utility of these techniques no longer has to be argued for or displayed. Their application has
become routine and unremarkable, if not in every case, at least in these
especially interesting cases.

Thus, by 1831, transfer of the innovation of stethoscopy from Paris to Edinburgh had been successfully accomplished. Moreover, this reform of the
clinical practice of Edinburgh's academic doctors seems to have occurred with
a minimum of controversy. Indeed it is difficult to find any opposition being
voiced to the introduction of the new techniques. Duncan wrote of having
persevered with his early experiments with the technique 'notwithstanding the
ridicule and sneers of the ignorant'.[82] George Julius, a classmate of James

Hope, recorded that his friend had not been discouraged from taking up stethoscopy '[n]otwithstanding the indifference with which it was treated at that time by some, even of the Professors of the Colleges'.[83] But both these observations were made some years after the event and may reflect only the tendency of pioneers to exaggerate the magnitude of the obstacles they had to overcome. Neither author, moreover, unequivocally locates the opposition within Edinburgh.

Apart from the above, the present author has come across only a single instance of criticism of the stethoscope in Edinburgh and that a brief paragraph in a private letter. This one hostile comment is, however, particularly interesting since it contains a very clever theoretical argument against the stethoscope. It occurs in a letter written to William Stokes by John Nimmo in 1825. He is referring to the proposed use of the stethoscope to detect the foetal heart-beat:

The various media through which the pulsations have to pass are perfectly inelastic and I would as soon expect to be sensible of the [word illegible] motions of a number of fishes in a glass jar by applying the Stethoscope to a dozen folds of flannel cloth covering the surface of the jar as to be able to discover the undulating movements of the foetus in the way which has been proposed.[84]

Nimmo's letter indicates that the intellectual resources for mounting an attack on the validity of the stethoscope sounds were available to Edinburgh commentators. But as far as I have been able to ascertain (it is, of course, difficult to confirm a negative conclusion), such opposition was neither institutionalized nor sustained. Thus what seems to the twentieth-century observer to be change of the greatest magnitude and significance, the crossing of the divide between ancient and modern clinical practice, seems to have been achieved in Edinburgh quickly, harmoniously, even consensually.

Conclusions: Edinburgh and London

The introduction of stethoscopy to Edinburgh might thus seem, at first sight, to fit Bishop's account better than those of Reiser and Bluth. Bishop, however, is right for the wrong reasons. He points to the overwhelmingly favourable reception of *De l'auscultation médiate* but, as we have seen, this is not sufficient evidence that the process of naturalizing the stethoscope into clinical practice had begun. Moreover, whatever happened in Edinburgh, Stanley Reiser and Edward Bluth are certainly correct in their contention that the introduction of mediate auscultation to Britain was marked by controversy. The stethoscope was indeed heartily opposed – in London, for example. Many Edinburgh graduates met such opposition when they went south to take up practice.[85]

The contrast between attitudes to the new techniques in the two major medical centres was very apparent to contemporary observers. When, in 1827, Andrew Duncan announced he had 'now the satisfaction to see that [percussion and stethoscopy] are duly appreciated by the whole profession, even by those who at first opposed them',[86] a London correspondent was forced to contradict him:

Softly, friend Duncan! These means are very far from being duly appreciated by the whole profession, or by one half of the profession . . . What will Duncan say, when we inform him that, on the day we received his journal . . . a professor of physic, and a public lecturer in this metropolis . . . publicly denounced the stethoscope as a . . . piece of quackery, which he never could countenance! There are many of the most eminent physicians and surgeons in this metropolis who entertain the same sentiments . . .[87]

In the 1830s and even the 1840s, London commentators can still be found bemoaning the existence of considerable ignorance of, and opposition to, the stethoscope among the metropolitan medical profession.[88] What is remarkable about events in Edinburgh is not that the French literature on stethoscopy was initially well received but that the subsequent and potentially more problematic process of reforming clinical procedures happened so quickly and smoothly.

Why was a consensus as to the value of stethoscopy arrived at so much faster in Edinburgh than in London? It might first be noted that, in Edinburgh, the ground was laid for the stethoscope by the growing interest in pathological anatomy which had been a conspicuous feature of Scottish medicine in the first two decades of the nineteenth century.[89] Many of the academic Edinburgh physicians had followed the new work of the Paris School very closely and had themselves endeavoured to undertake autopsy investigations with a rigour seldom seen among their eighteenth-century colleagues.[90] They were thus cognitively well prepared to appreciate the possibility of 'anatomizing the living' which was offered by physical methods of diagnosis. Moreover the Scottish tradition of clinical teaching, however inadequate subsequent developments might have made it seem, undoubtedly helped prepare students to benefit from visits to the Paris hospitals.

It is also possible that Scotland's traditionally stronger cultural links with France were a factor in promoting a more positive attitude to the Parisian innovation of mediate auscultation in Edinburgh than in London. In the period immediately after the Napoleonic Wars, the Scots were perhaps more receptive to French developments in scholarship and science than were the English.[91] Even in the late 1820s there was a conspicuous element of Francophobia in some of the pronouncements made about the stethoscope by older London physicians. The instrument was called a 'French bauble' and an 'insult to John Bull'.[92] As one of the stethoscopy's principal supporters, James Forbes was convinced that the adoption of the instrument in England was handicapped by the fact that 'its whole hue and cry is foreign'.[93] He considered that only the publication of 'original English cases' would suffice to persuade an English audience. Such sentiments are absent from the record of events in Edinburgh.

Furthermore, it should be noted that, unlike some leading London-based early advocates of stethoscopy, Andrew Duncan was an active teacher of medicine. He had plenty of students whom he could encourage to take an interest in learning and developing the new techniques. Moreover, the more favoured among his students had the facilities of the Edinburgh Royal Infirmary at their disposal, providing them with an invaluable supply of clinical and pathological material. It is undoubtedly true that, as many of Duncan's contemporaries observed, mediate auscultation could be learned much more easily in a hospital than in private practice.[94] Thus the conversion of Duncan to mediate auscultation was a crucially important event in the history of its adoption within British medicine in a way that, for example, the conversion of James Johnson or Sir Charles Scudamore was not.[95]

It must also be remembered that in medicine, as in much else, Edinburgh was, by the early nineteenth century, a small town compared to the Metropolis. Edinburgh medical pedagogy was dominated by one institution, the University's Medical School and its extension, the clinical wards of the Royal Infirmary. As far as the development of a programme of anatomico-clinical research is concerned the Edinburgh medical faculty can, therefore, be regarded as virtually a single research school. Thus, the character of Edinburgh medicine could be determined by a relatively small group of individuals. The medical scene in contemporary London was, as Susan Lawrence has recently revealed, very different.[96] London in the 1820s had several teaching hospitals, of which none could truly be said to be *primus inter pares*. There were also as many as twelve private medical schools, each of more or less equal status. In other words London, unlike Edinburgh, was a nexus of competing medical institutions, with little in the way of an organized hierarchy existing among them. The social dynamics of achieving a general consensus in favour of an innovation must, correspondingly, have been much more complex and problematic in the English centre than the Scottish one.

Furthermore, the introduction of mediate auscultation was one area in which the continuing practice of family patronage and filial preferment, so often cited as a factor in the decline of Edinburgh's Medical School, perhaps worked to its advantage. In many places, it took until the 1840s and 1850s for the stethoscope to become fully established. As Segall has put it, this was 'just enough time for those who ... chose to learn the new method to displace from the centre of the stage those who could not or would not learn it'.[97] But, in Edinburgh, the full acceptance of the innovation did not have to wait upon generational succession. The Scottish old guard seemed to have embraced stethoscopy simultaneously with, or only very shortly after, their junior colleagues. There are several accounts of established professors learning auscultation from younger men or, alternatively, asking junior colleagues to auscultate their patients for them.[98] But it should be noted that the young pioneers of the stethoscope, Cullen and Gregory for example, often bore the names of famous Edinburgh medical families. There is little doubt that a dignified Edinburgh professor would have found it easier to appear dependent upon a younger man who was bound to him by strong ties of pedagogical patronage and social allegiance and who was, in effect, more of a protege than a rival. The structured dependency of the young upon the old, so characteristic of Edinburgh medicine, may have worked, in this case, to facilitate a free exchange of opinion and expertise among a relatively tightly-knit and hierarchical group of practitioners.

Another point to be made with regard to the story of mediate auscultation in Edinburgh is that it supports the argument, made by Reiser and Newman among others, as to the central importance of the stethoscope within the development of modern clinical procedures.[99] There was never an Edinburgh vogue for the older technique of immediate auscultation, the placing of the ear directly against the patient's chest. The adoption of percussion was slow and uncertain before 1820. Palpation and succussion were known but their clinical potential was not being systematically exploited. But, as we have seen, once the stethoscope came into general use, the rapid development and application of a variety of techniques of physical diagnosis was stimulated. It is important to note, however, that this maieutic role of the stethoscope has little to do with any technical superiority of mediate auscultation. It is likely that, as many nineteenth-century physicians maintained, a skilled examiner could hear as much, or very nearly as much, with the unaided ear as with the instrument.[100] It would seem rather that it was the physical barrier of a few inches of wood which the stethoscope interposed between the physician's head and the patient's body that was its crucial advantage.

Early nineteenth-century Edinburgh doctors complained frequently about how physical examination was disagreeable to the physician and often offensive to the patient.[101] As we have seen, one of the major advantages of mediate auscultation over other techniques of physical diagnosis was that it offered physicians a means to undertake examinations without compromising their professional dignity. The fact that stethoscopy did not involve direct bodily contact was considered to be very helpful, both when one's clientele were the unwashed poor of the hospital or dispensary and when one was consulted by modest ladies in one's private practice. In other words, the stethoscope respected the social niceties of the practice of elite physic. With that degree of protection accorded to his sensibilities and those of his patients, the physician could safely undertake the education of his senses. He could set about converting his academic knowledge of physical diagnosis into practical expertise.

9

Educating the senses: students, teachers and medical rhetoric in eighteenth-century London

SUSAN C. LAWRENCE

Teaching about sensations is fraught with ambiguities. Words serve uneasily to reify experience. Language pretends to define, structure and codify sensory data, but ever falls short of the Enlightenment philosophers' dreams to construct a perfectly transparent symbolic system in which words, things and ideas march in one-to-one correspondence. Medical instruction, like that in other subjects centred on objects and experiences, has always had to cope with the tensions between tacit and verbal knowledge. This chapter focuses on medical teaching at a time when many still hoped that a 'scientific' language could be unambiguous, yet lecturers struggled to convey what they could not, in fact, *say* about the body and disease.[1] Specifically, it examines how late eighteenth and early nineteenth-century London medical men instructed pupils who came from a broad range of backgrounds to use their senses to acquire knowledge from objects (such as the dead) and patients.

Based on a reading of advice manuals and over fifty sets of students' manuscript lecture notes dating from 1750 to 1820, this study concentrates on three of the common medical subjects taught in London: anatomy, surgery and physic.[2] Exploring both the explicit and implicit injunctions about the senses offered to young men entering the professions allows a closer look at two of the intertwined themes that run through eighteenth-century medicine and surgery. First, lecture notes carry a host of assumptions about the relationships between language, objects, knowledge and authority, in particular the role of formal medical systems and the place of the 'surgical point of view' in organizing medical perceptions.[3] Second, they reveal much about the encounters between practitioners and their patients, which in turn shaped the contours of appropriate clinical experience.[4]

Examining how, and what, medical men taught provides a limited, yet fruitful, perspective on the intellectual and social relationships that structured late eighteenth-century English medicine. Whatever the epistemological orientation of the London teachers, which in itself is difficult to categorize,[5] lecturing demanded that knowledge be verbalized. The strategy of demonstrating objects, particularly anatomical preparations, partially bridged the gap between sensory experience and the inadequacies of language. In the clinical subjects, however, lecturers sometimes found themselves at a loss for words when they attempted to descend from the abstract to the particular, and could only urge their auditors to connect the terms that they defined or used with sensations acquired outside the lecture rooms. As argued below, London lecturers were in the business of educating – not training – the senses, and hence in structuring their pupils' experiences through the authoritative weight of their own scholarship and clinical acumen. The didactic, 'academic' lecture itself centred on offering pupils a formal, institutionalized vocabulary of theoretical terms with which to deal with patients. Yet, while students were told that there were two obvious sources of sensory knowledge, what was 'either felt by the patient [or] observed by the physician',[6] as actually taught these two realms were inseparable when identifying and treating illness in the late eighteenth century. The practitioner constantly translated the patient's account into symptoms with professional and lay meaning, at the same time that he transformed his own sensations into perceptions intelligible within commonly accepted medical and surgical categories.[7]

An analysis of London teaching about the use of the senses suggests that the simplistic contemporary and historical division of the medical domain into 'internal' illnesses that the physician prescribed for, such as fever, gout, rheumatism and diabetes, and 'external' conditions that the surgeon treated, such as wounds, hernias, fractures and visible tumours, obscures their shared assumptions about medical knowledge.[8] In broad terms, elite physicians are often portrayed as relying heavily on the patient's 'subjective' accounts, together with visual inspection of the clothed body, judicious observation of urine, faeces, blood and sputum and a delicate hand on the pulse.[9] As Nicholas Jewson has argued, the highly passive, scholarly physician provided an individualized explanation and treatment of disease, essentially in subservience to the patient's own assessment of his or her condition. Competing theoretical systems, attention to the patient's account and the lack of physical examination nicely follow from this patron-dominated view of the clinical encounter, for the practitioner – in theory – had little social or intellectual authority to violate the patient's physical privacy and much to gain by providing acceptable explanations of illness and therapeutic regimens.[10] The craft-oriented (and socially inferior) surgeons, in contrast, were much more closely tied to the 'objective' experience obviously offered by a deep knowledge of anatomy and the need to touch their patients to identify conditions and to operate. For surgeons, what the patient said would supposedly be of less importance than what the practitioner saw or felt. A major 'problem' in the history of medicine has concerned how, when and why the boundaries between these realms of experience were constructed and changed. As some scholars have noted, only since the rise of modern medicine and the thorough disjunction between 'objective' and 'subjective' clinical knowledge, has the patient's account become of secondary, if not peripheral, importance in identifying and treating organic disease.[11]

Yet, at least in London teaching, the traditional 'internal' versus 'external' dichotomy transcended the usual professional and rhetorical distinction between the practice appropriate for the physician and that of the surgeon. (The man-midwife already violated this polarization.) Both physicians and surgeons taught that 'internal' disorders were identified primarily by visual inspection and the patient's report, while 'external' diseases could be further elucidated through the practitioner's and patient's touch. The overlapping realms of information garnered from sight, from touch and from the patient's reports were mediated by social, professional and intellectual criteria underlying what could be known in the clinical encounter. Which methods were used probably depended upon whether the patient and the practitioner initially categorized the disorder as 'internal' or 'external'.

The ideas and relationships that London medical lecturers presented were certainly neither unique to London nor, in some areas, to eighteenth-century knowledge. It is not yet possible to date specific changes in the perceptual orientation of London physicians and surgeons, however. Any attempt to locate trends reveals more hindsight than historical sensitivity, given the wide range of men who lectured and the multiplicity of their sources, goals and approaches. The following discussion, therefore, does not attempt to reveal a conception, gestation or birth of 'the clinic' in late eighteenth-century London. Despite what might appear to be very promising developments in clinical instruction, such precursor-searching obscures the nuances of eighteenth-century medical knowledge and experience.[12] Finally, as a last caveat, at this stage it is premature to make any overt claims about the impact that London teaching had on how medical men actually shaped their perceptions and used their senses in medical and surgical practice. The instruction offered to students, from prosaic directions about setting simple fractures or bleeding in inflammatory fevers, to complex anatomical demonstrations and detailed discussions of the stages of labour, probably had, nevertheless, a significant role in structuring the day-to-day encounters that practitioners had with their patients. While the chasms between what was said, what was learned, and what was done inevitably remain, we can carefully construct a few platforms to narrow these gaps.

Although impossible to document through the lecturers' self-conscious

admissions, what they said – and how they said it – was surely shaped in part
by their need to attract a paying audience. London medical education emerged
during the eighteenth century as a competitive and potentially lucrative private
enterprise. Whether on hospital grounds or in extramural rooms, lecturers
offered their knowledge on a fee-for-course basis, outside the umbrella of any
university degree requirements or (before 1815) licensing regulations. From the
early decades of the century, but especially from the 1770s, medical men advertised dozens of courses in nearly all the branches of medicine – anatomy,
chemistry, botany, materia medica, midwifery, the theory and practice of
medicine and the theory and practice of surgery. London also offered considerable opportunities for clinical experience in its large general and specialized
hospitals. By the late eighteenth century literally hundreds of men signed up to
walk the wards at these charitable institutions, primarily as surgeons' pupils,
and so formed a potential audience for the courses offered either at the hospitals or in extramural rooms.[13] Advice books, student accounts and several
manuscript compilations reveal that pupils routinely followed a broad curriculum, attending medical, surgical and midwifery courses, while following hospital men on their rounds.[14]

Neither courses nor hospital experience were explicitly required before the
second decade of the nineteenth century for certification by the Royal College
of Surgeons, the Society of Apothecaries or the Royal College of Physicians.
The lecturers' audiences were, therefore, entirely voluntary ones in the sense
that their efforts and payments were not imposed by official mandates. The
pupils came to fulfil their own expectations about the education necessary for
successful practice. Scattered supporting evidence from the hospitals' pupil
registers and students' letters and diaries, suggests that a considerable majority
intended to practise as surgeon-apothecary-man-midwives, rather than pro-
ceeding to earn the M.D. degree and establish physicians' rounds, or to limit
themselves to surgical treatments. Many of the students, moreover, had
already served an apprenticeship and were thus seeking the additional knowledge, experience and polish the metropolis offered.[15] The enterprising lecturer
needed to attract and retain young men with some prior experience with
patients and treatment, not just professional neophytes.

Quite a few hard-working students approached their London courses con-
scientiously, as the large number of surviving manuscript notes attest. Not
only did taking notes and transcribing them into fair copies produce introductory texts, to which the new practitioner could later refer, but, as William
Hunter emphasized, the process itself also gave the pupil 'a facility of writing
upon subjects in his profession ... and of expressing them in the most clear
and proper language'.[16] As a genre, lecture notes deserve a serious and
extended study, particularly to analyse more deeply their social, professional
and pedagogic functions in the eighteenth century.[17] Like so many historical

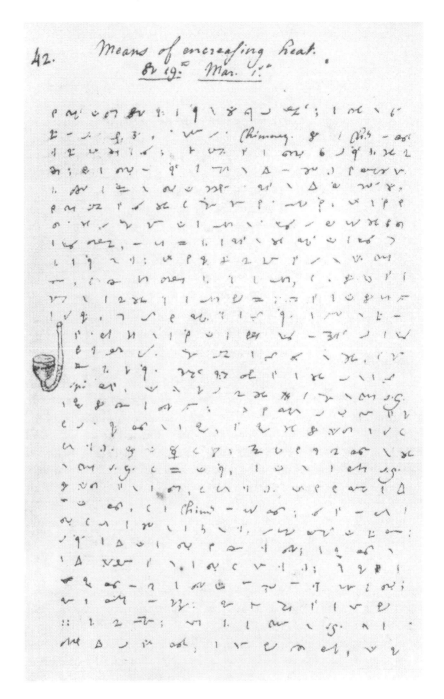

Fig. 47. 'Means of encreasing heat', in George Fordyce [1736–1802], Lectures on chemistry, in shorthand, p. 42.

records, they are not unproblematic sources. Neither reflections of what was said nor necessarily accounts of what the pupil learned, these texts only tentatively support broad generalizations about late eighteenth-century teaching. Hence a few cautions are in order.

First, the surviving notes unevenly reflect the diversity of lecturing that occurred.[18] In general, notes from anatomy and surgery courses outweigh those from chemistry, materia medica and the theory and practice of medicine, perhaps partially reflecting differing enrolments, but also corresponding to the later image of London as a centre for surgical instruction.[19] Notes from hospital lecturers also far outnumber those from extramural teachers, except for a few extremely influential or popular men such as William Hunter and Colin Mackenzie.[20] This uneven distribution unfortunately puts disproportionate weight on hospital men's instruction during a period equally rich in teaching by non-hospital entrepreneurs.

Second, as records of what was spoken in lecture theatres, manuscript notes lie open to all sorts of possible criticisms. Many are undated; a large number unsigned; some do not even record the name of the lecturer. These obviously must be used with caution. More important, however, is the fundamental relationship between what was said and what the student wrote. Very few of the men who made lecturing a business in eighteenth and early nineteenth-century London either published their complete lectures[21] or composed introductory texts. Even fewer left their own copies of lecture material.[22] Comparison, therefore, with what the lecturer thought he said and what the students wrote is, in most cases, impossible.[23] One striking early exception to this generalization is the posthumous publication of William Hunter's *Two Introductory Lectures, Delivered to his Last Course of Anatomical Lectures* (1784), which he left in manuscript apparently corrected for the press. This text, with 114 pages for two lectures, has a pale reflection in pupils' notes. At least one student recorded several of the basic points in 1779, but his thirteen pages omit most of the details and flourishes Hunter included in the published version.[24]

Students used shorthand (fig. 47), rough non-verbatim comments and hurriedly scribbled longhand to capture their lecturers' words. The unknown student who attended John Abernethy's lectures in 1813 (fig. 48) mentioned the key anatomical terms associated with Abernethy's demonstrations and several of his lecturer's remarks on their clinical significance. Yet he also clearly went back to his notes to emend and embellish some points, interjecting either his own observations or ideas that he later remembered. In contrast to such manuscripts, where the student conspicuously interacted with the subject, most surviving pupils' notes appear to be fair copies of condensed accounts of what they thought the lecturer said, ideally written out cleanly in complete sentences. The anonymous student who attended Percival Pott's

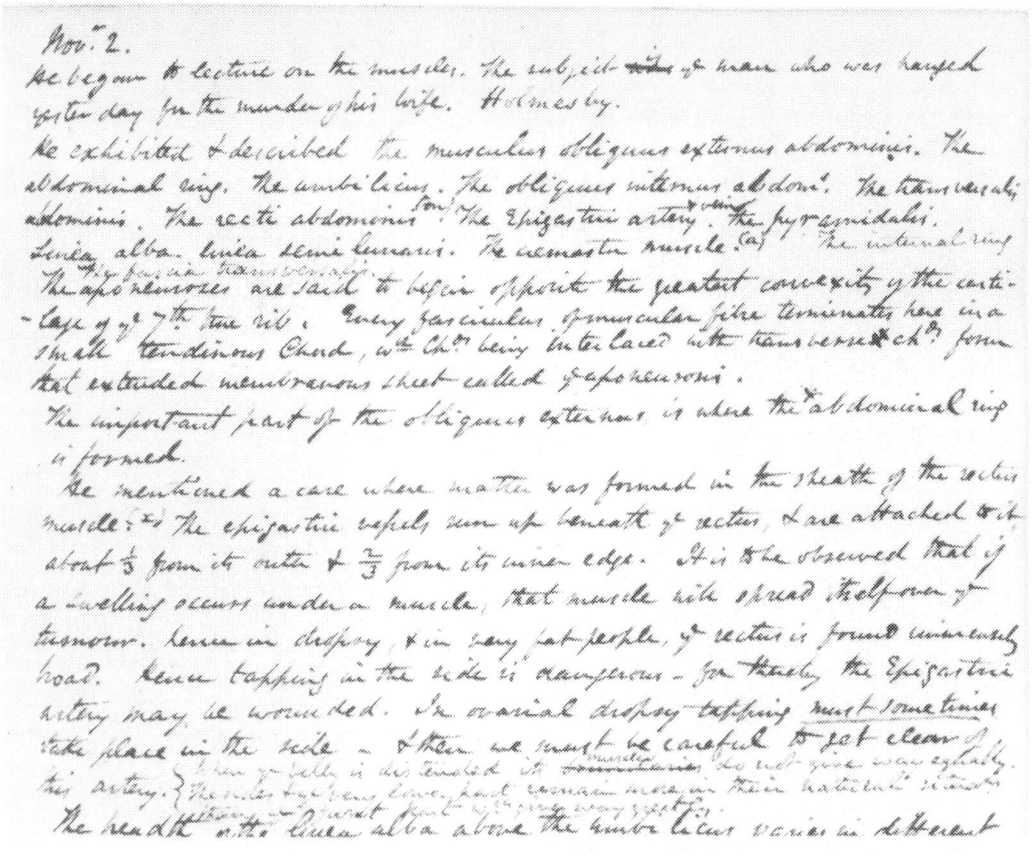
Nov.r 2.
He began to lecture on the muscles. The subject of man who was hanged yesterday for the murder of his wife. Holmesby.
He exhibited & described the musculus obliquus externus abdominis. The abdominal ring. The umbilicus. The obliquus internus abdom.s The transversalis abdominis. The recti abdominis. The Epigastric artery. The pyramidales. Linea alba. linea semilunaris. The cremaster muscle. The internal ring
The aponeuroses are said to begin opposite the greatest convexity of the cartilage of ye 7th true rib. Every fasciculus of muscular fibre terminates here in a small tendinous Chord, wh Ch.ds being interlaced with transverse ch.ds form that extended membranous sheet called ye aponeurosis.
The important part of the obliquus externus is where the abdominal ring is formed.
He mentioned a case where matter was formed in the sheath of the rectus muscle: the epigastric vessels run up beneath ye rectus, & are attached to it about 1/3 from its outer & 2/3 from its inner edge. It is to be observed that if a swelling occurs under a muscle, that muscle will spread itself over ye tumour. hence in dropsy, & in very fat people, ye rectus is found uncommonly broad. hence tapping in the side is dangerous – for thereby the Epigastric artery may be wounded. In ovarial dropsy tapping must sometimes take place in the side – & then we must be careful to get clear of this artery.
The breadth of the linea alba above the umbilicus varies in different

Fig. 48. Entry for 2 November, in John Abernethy, Notes of lectures on anatomy, *c.* 1813, unpaginated.

lectures around 1770 (fig. 49) typically polished his notes using Pott's voice, as though giving a verbatim report. (Note the use of the first person in the third line of fig. 49. This convention regularly lead to syntactical contortions when the pupil decided to interject his own 'I'.) Among the London manuscripts, moreover, even those with the closest similarities reveal enough variation to suggest that the students put the information they heard into their own words and were not simply copying others' notes.[25] Certainly the accuracy of the end result also depended heavily on the pupil's intelligence, skill and dedication.[26]

Lecture notes thus reflect an interaction between the instructor and the student. They are neither sources for what the lecturer necessarily said or did, nor accounts of what the pupil understood, but an amalgam of statements and interpretations. At a deeper level, too, the lecturers themselves constructed their courses as a synthesis of their own reading, education and experience. Some of the medical courses, in fact, were obvious derivatives of Boerhaave or

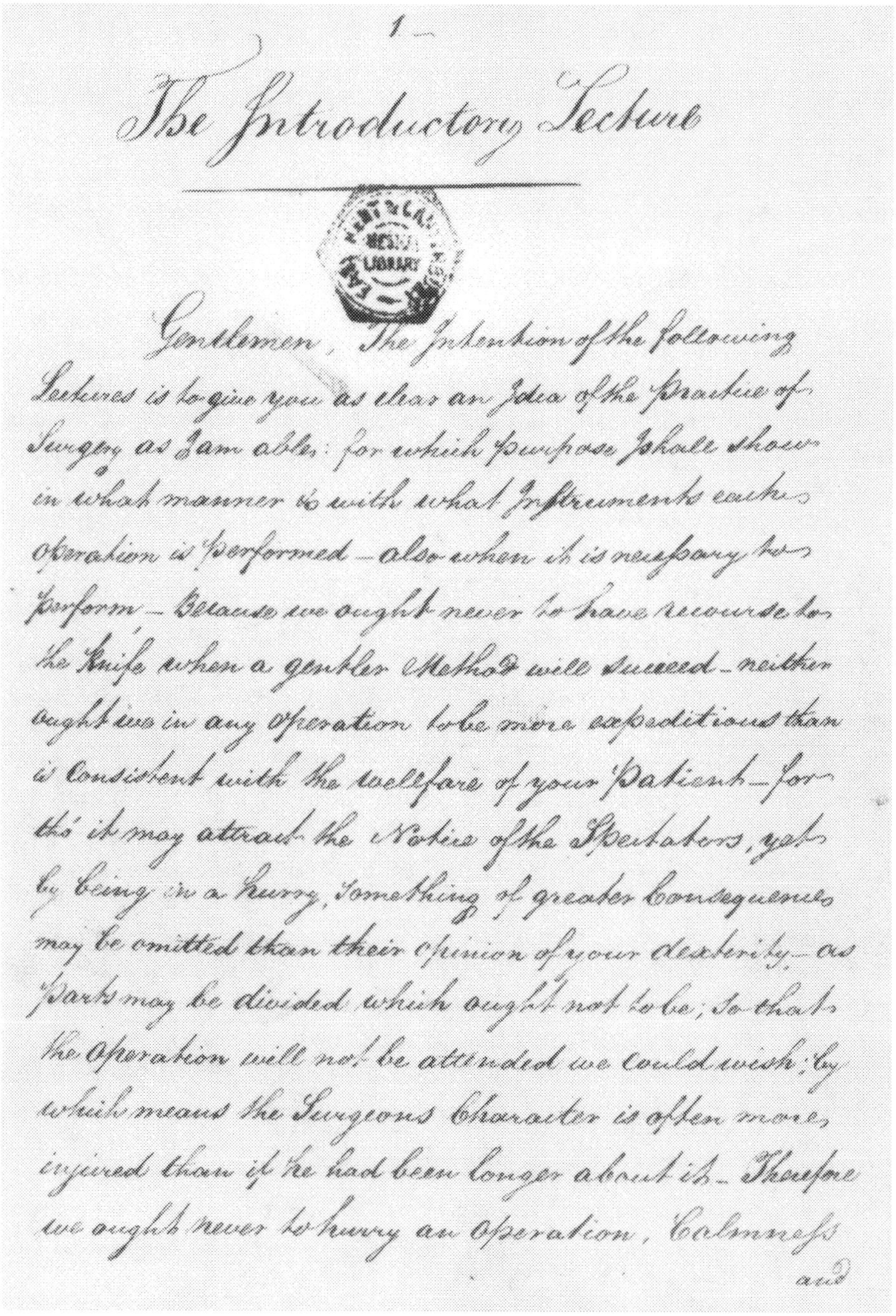

1

The Introductory Lecture

Gentlemen, The Intention of the following Lectures is to give you as clear an Idea of the Practice of Surgery as I am able; for which purpose I shall show in what manner & with what Instruments each Operation is performed — also when it is necessary to perform — Because we ought never to have recourse to the Knife when a gentler Method will succeed — neither ought we in any Operation to be more expeditious than is Consistent with the welfare of your Patient — for tho' it may attract the Notice of the Spectators, yet by being in a hurry, Something of greater Consequence may be omitted than their opinion of your dexterity — as Parts may be divided which ought not to be; So that the Operation will not be attended we could wish; by which means the Surgeons Character is often more injured than if he had been longer about it — Therefore we ought never to hurry an Operation, Calmness and

Fig. 49. Introductory lecture, in Percival Pott [1714–88], The surgical lectures, p. 1.

William Cullen; others, more complicated blends.[27] The lecturers' reliance on other scholars' work affects what they said about using the senses. On one hand, it can be argued that what they taught was merely a rhetorical repetition of familiar homilies, and can tell us nothing about what the lecturer might have done in his practice.[28] On the other hand, for students who transcribed points about, for example, physical examination, there was always the possibility that even classical instructions could have been taken literally, especially in conjunction with the skills and ideas learned from other courses.[29]

Whether they took it seriously or not, London pupils frequently heard how important 'observation' was to acquire and to advance medical knowledge. All of the authors who prepared or published texts about medical education in the eighteenth and early nineteenth centuries noted that students, no matter what their formal instruction, would ultimately need to learn how to identify and treat illnesses by observing the sick and practising themselves. From Sir John Floyer in about 1720, to James Lucas and James Parkinson in 1800, moreover, authors urged the young practitioner to acquire his initial experience at hospital patients' bedsides.[30] Yet their recommendations were simple programmatic statements, for they did not specifically discuss how the pupil should use his senses once he got there.

Similarly, in their general discussions, London lecturers upheld the significance of personal observation, but rarely explicitly addressed sensation as a distinct topic or problem. At an ideological level, they glorified the benefits of direct experience. They often devoted the first, introductory lecture in many subjects, for example, to presenting a brief history of anatomy, surgery or medicine. One purpose then, as now, was to promote professional bonding by linking the student to an intellectual tradition. But these historical sketches served other rhetorical functions, not the least of which was to portray the disciplines as both sciences and arts, as the fruits of judicious reason and careful observation. Hippocrates, Harvey, Bacon and Sydenham were the acknowledged heroes; those who merely speculated and spun fantastic theories, the villains, blinded by prejudice.[31] The lecturers, nevertheless, upheld the role of reason, of course, for that divided the man of science from the mere quack or unthinking empiric.[32]

The London teachers obviously adopted a didactic tradition that justified presenting knowledge in lectures rather than simply by direct experience. They were educating the senses, not training them. Although lacking a university's elitist prestige and social cliquishness, London's courses probably succeeded in part because they appealed to those seeking an 'academic' distancing from apprenticeship. To the surgeon or apothecary who hoped to present himself as a respectable, learned practitioner instead of an ignorant craftsman or shop-keeper, lecturers offered the language and theoretical frameworks that had previously been the grounds separating the elite physician from the lower ranks.[33] One of the most overt testimonies to this professionalizing function of lectures came, not surprisingly, from a physician, William Graeme, who wrote in 1729 to justify his proposal to lecture on physic in London. To those who claimed that 'the only way to give Instructions in Physick, is to carry the Student to the Patient's Bed-side, and there shew him the Disease and the Practice', Graeme responded that the pupil 'cannot be the better for what he sees, but rather the worse', if he has not already learned the rationale of practice.[34] As Dr William Hamilton put it in 1787, in theoretical courses 'diseases are represented as they occur in general, divested of those peculiarities which we observe in every particular instance of them'. The abstract method, so familiar in eighteenth-century medical systems, gave physic 'all the graces of science'.[35]

The didactic formalization that structured medical lectures also characterized other subjects and probably influenced practitioners seeking to enhance the scholarly image of their disciplines. Some surgeons and anatomists, in particular, appear to have tried to make their courses, as William Cheselden put it in 1721, suitable for 'gentlemen'.[36] The emphasis on constructing a theory of surgical diseases, especially on creating new physiologies to account for morbid changes, such as inflammation, well known in John Hunter's work, made surgery respectable by giving it an abstract foundation. In the process, the senses could not be given the free rein associated with empiricism, but had to be disciplined and ordered by a rational system.[37] In 1790–1, for example, John Pearson dubbed his lectures 'Chirurgical Institutes'. After an extended theoretical introduction, Pearson discussed surgical diseases according to their genera and species, often latinizing their names. Although he ridiculed medical nosologies based on collections of symptoms, calling them 'nothing more than Medical Vocabularies', he revealingly claimed that his own lectures offered 'a sort of Grammar of the Art'. He ended up creating a surgical nosology as abstract and artificial as the physicians' medical ones.[38]

Yet even this formal level, centred on mastering a vocabulary for disease and treatment, implied the constant use of sensory data. The pupils needed to learn a wealth of definitions and distinctions which, ideally, they would ultimately observe in their patients. The 'putrid' breath, spongy gums, lassitude and shortness of breath indicating scurvy; the 'copper color'd … dry, scurfy scab' of the venereal eruption; the 'sighing & sobbing inspiration … unequal pulse', cough and fever of peripneumonia vera; the 'impeded and difficult respiration, attended with fear of suffocation' marking asthma; or the 'bloody, sanious mucous [stools] often in the state of putrid fermentation and mixed with fleshy, skinny fibrous matter' found in acute dysentery are only a few examples of the symptoms the practitioner would need to note on seeing his patients or having their conditions reported to him.[39] Students' lecture notes forcibly testify to the complex range of clinical detail that the eighteenth-century practitioner had to master. Much of it is both visual and closely connected to what the patient reported, yet at the same time presented in such abstract terms that it is difficult to read from it any special or personal hints on how to use the senses in clinical encounters.

In several instances, however, lectures implicitly acknowledged that they could not convey the clinical sensations associated with the words they used. When some lecturers attempted to describe non-visual perceptions, often in the context of specific cases, their efforts frequently resulted in instructions to touch, smell, taste or listen rather than in coherent verbal accounts of distinguishing experiences. The occasional references to smell, as in the 'putrid' breath of scurvy already mentioned, or to taste, as in the sweetness of diabetic urine, presupposed either prior or future clinical contact with these sensations. Lectures on the pulse especially demonstrate the instructors' limitations with language. Dr George Fordyce, for example, like most physicians in the late eighteenth century, emphasized the importance of measuring the number of pulse beats per minute. Yet he also tried to characterize the qualitative variations for his students. He described a full pulse as 'whn ye Arteries act strongly the Pulse is hard feeling like a Cord high braced & having a Thrill under ye finger at ye beginning of ye Contract[ion]'. He went on to note 'whn ye Vessels are very full they have not room to play the Pulse is small & called oppressed'.[40] Clearly dissatisfied with his efforts to render such distinctions verbally, Fordyce declared (according to his auditor): 'These we cannot convey to you by Words, there are not Words expressive of their feels [sic] or sensations ... you are to learn them by actually feeling the Pulse of the Patient'.[41] Most lecturing physicians and surgeons simply used the common terms for clinical variations in the pulse, such as 'hard' or 'small and low', without attempting to describe how these felt to the observer. It was enough for them that the student simply learn that the 'small & frequent' pulse indicated a low fever, or that the 'strong hard pulse' was found in rheumatism.[42]

Faced with failure to describe the complex nuances of non-visual sensations, some London lecturers, notably George Fordyce, became increasingly frustrated with formal, abstract 'systems', and yet could not escape them when teaching courses on the theory of medicine. As already suggested, Fordyce urged his pupils in no uncertain terms to attend clinical lectures and walk the hospital wards.

I have seen a young man perfectly instructed (& old men too sometimes) in all that knowledge [of genera and species] & brought them [sic] into St Thomas's Hospital & set them into a ward to give names to diseases & they did not know one single disease that affected the Patients, nor how to name it at all, because it was not exactly according to the Definitions laid Down in these books.[43]

Such comments only reiterated the fact that what the student learned on the wards, while shaped by the formal discourse given in lectures, was up to him to acquire. The paucity of surviving notes known to have been taken by either physicians' or surgeons' pupils in the hospitals leave us in the dark about what they actually experienced at the bedside.

One of the major purposes of lectures was, thus, to provide a shared technical vocabulary which, as much as clinical acumen, both set the practitioner off from the layperson and allowed him to converse intelligently with educated patients.[44] This verbal instruction was to precede contact with patients, although in the case of students who had already spent time as apprentices, it also served to organize and codify previous experience. Yet, while a glance at almost any set of manuscript notes confirms this formal goal, lecturers also instructed their students in how to use their senses and to interpret their patients' accounts in several intertwined ways. Their advice and approaches appear in the methods they used to teach and the implicit models of clinical experience they presented.

Demonstrating objects was one of the most obvious techniques used to bridge the gap between words and things. Throughout the eighteenth century, lecturers in materia medica relied on collections of simples and compound medicines to aid instruction.[45] Midwifery teachers, such as Colin Mackenzie, used both anatomical preparations to show foetal development and a 'machine' representing the pregnant uterus to demonstrate difficult births.[46] Within medical teaching, anatomy has long been recognized as the paradigm for instruction through the use of an increasingly complex array of preparations, from freshly dissected parts to intricate specimens of injected arteries and veins. Accompanying the development of techniques for preserving anatomical material came the well-known emphasis on individual dissection by students. Hands-on experience, it was repeatedly argued, provided a knowledge of natural and morbid body structure far deeper than that acquired by merely seeing demonstrations and hearing the associated terms. William Hunter's role in proselytizing (if not introducing) the importance of dissection does not need to be repeated here; after mid-century nearly all London anatomy teachers had dissecting rooms distinct from their lecture theatres and students had numerous opportunities to attend a dissecting course, for which they paid separately.[47]

The emphasis on individual dissection, however, should not be seen as a glorification of simply learning by experience, with the young man tossed among the corpses to recapitulate centuries of investigation and discovery. William Hunter argued that the student who begins to dissect too early 'will be so much at a loss in his work, and recover so little instruction or satisfaction, that at least it will be so much time almost thrown away'.[48] Only after at least one, or preferably two, demonstration courses would the pupil be ready to take up the knife himself. During formal anatomy lectures, instructors, from William Hunter to Henry Cline, John Abernethy, Henry Watson and Joseph

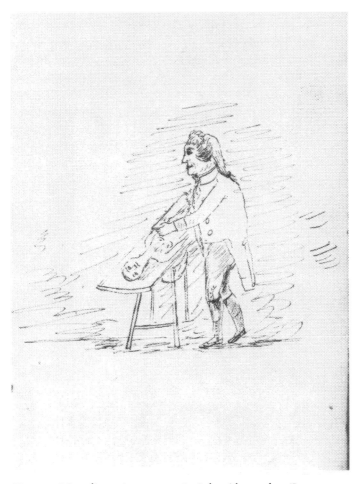

Fig. 50. Man dissecting corpse, in John Abernethy, 'Lectures on anatomy, physiology, etc.', notes made by D. D. Dobree, *c.* 1814, last flyleaf and drawing.

Else, showed a wide range of preserved and fresh preparations.[49] (See fig. 50, a student's sketch of a be-wigged and frock-coated surgeon lecturing over a corpse.) 'What the student acquires this way, is solid knowledge, arising from information of his own senses: thence, his ideas are clear and make a lasting impression on his memory.'[50] When the student came to dissect on his own, he would thus have an entire system of anatomy 'deeply impressed' in his mind by a series of class sessions where the senses (particularly vision) had been rigorously disciplined.[51]

Most students who referred to preparations simply noted that they were 'exhibited' (as in fig. 48, line 3) and concentrated on mastering the technical anatomical vocabulary associated with the part. Only a rare few embellished

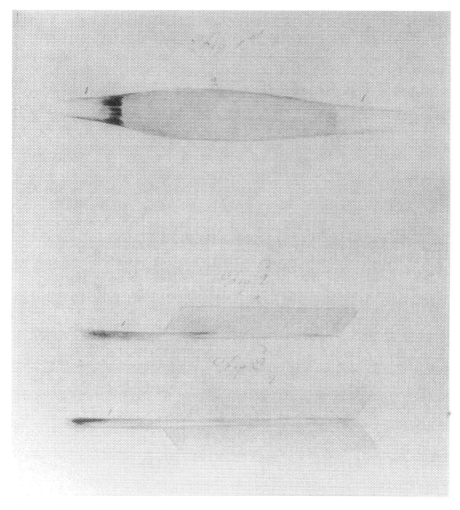

Fig. 51. Coloured drawing of muscle fibres, figs. 1–3, in Henry Cline, 'anatomical lectures', vol. 1, at St Thomas's Hospital, n.d. [late eighteenth century], unpaginated.

their notes with sketches that attempted to record visual instruction in visual form. In some cases, pupils prepared illustrations when working on their fair copies and apparently translated abstract points into diagrams, rather than working to capture the immediacy of parts displayed. (See figs. 51 and 52, where the manuscript describes types of muscles and the coloured sketches at the end of the volume support minor points in the text.) Daniel Dobree, in contrast to most of his peers, relatively lavishly illustrated his notes of John Abernethy's anatomy lectures and Astley Cooper's lectures on surgery. Tellingly, however, the drawings accompanying Abernethy's lectures were those that showed 'The exact representation of the sketches used by Mr A

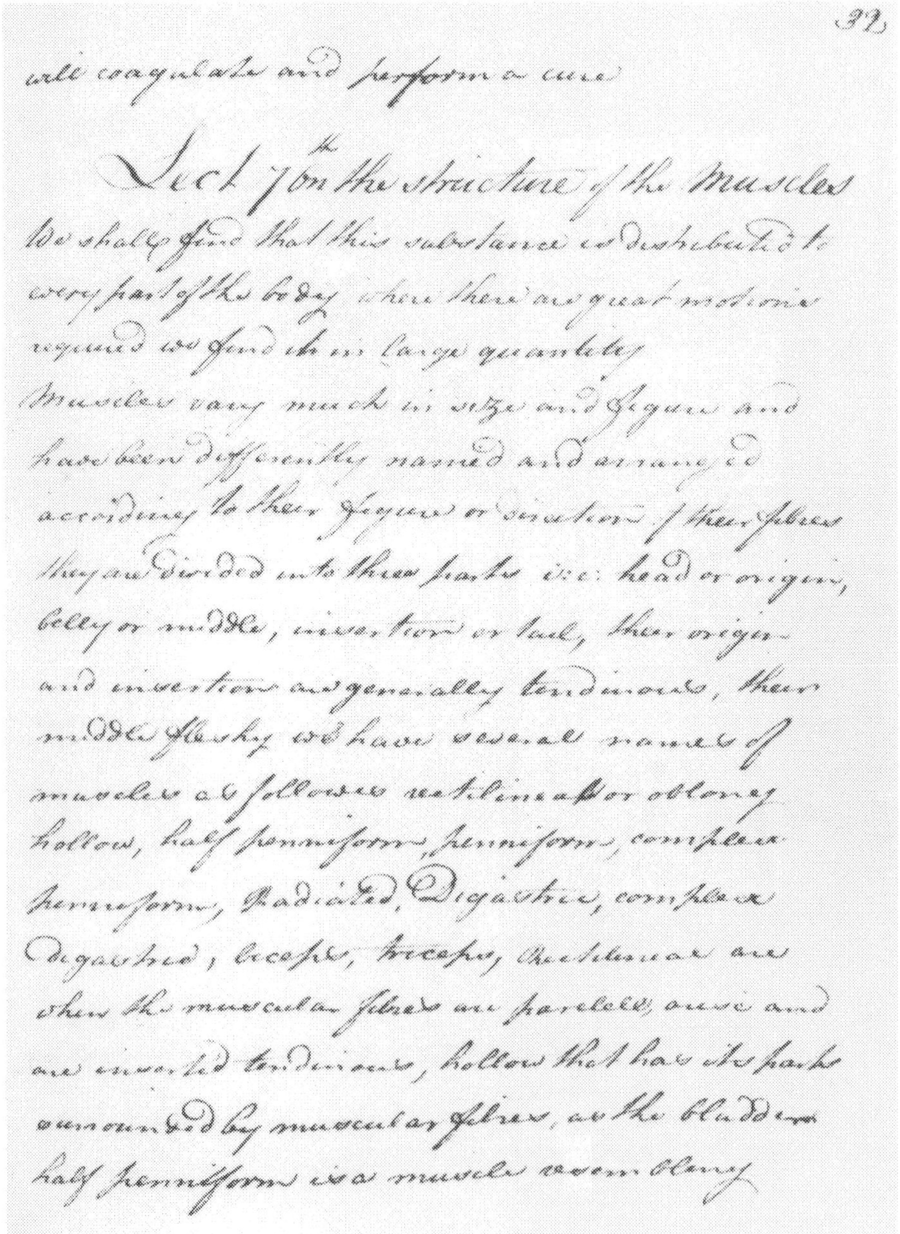
32

will coagulate and perform a cure

Lect 7th on the structure of the muscles

We shall find that this substance is distributed to every part of the body where there are great motions required we find them in large quantity

Muscles vary much in size and figure and have been differently named and arranged according to their figure or direction of their fibres they are divided into three parts viz: head or origin, belly or middle, insertion or tail, their origin and insertion are generally tendinous, their middle fleshy we have several names of muscles as follows rectilinear or oblong hollow, half penniform, penniform, complex penniform, Radiated, Digastric, complex digastric, biceps, triceps, Rectilinear are when the muscular fibres are parallel, arise and are inserted tendinous, hollow that has its parts surrounded by muscular fibres, as the bladder half penniform is a muscle seem oblong

Fig. 52. On the structure of the muscles, in Henry Cline, 'Anatomical lectures', vol. 1, at St Thomas's Hospital, n.d. [late eighteenth century], p. 32, seventh lecture.

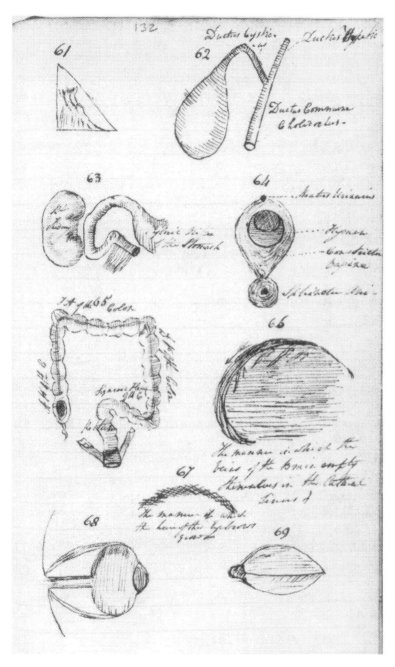

Fig. 53. Anatomical drawings, in John Abernethy, 'Lectures on anatomy, physiology, etc.', notes made by D. D. Dobree, *c.* 1814, p. 132.

to illustrate his lecture' (see fig. 53). While Dobree's comment shows that Abernethy supplemented his use of anatomical preparations with illustrations, likely to focus on particular points not easily seen in the flesh, the student only copied information that someone else had transferred to a two-dimensional medium. For the vast majority of students, whatever their talent for sketching, their notes confirm that even learning by demonstration centred on translating sensations into words, however inadequate those might be, rather than on transcending language.

Physicians adopted the rhetoric of demonstration subjects when introducing clinical lectures.[52] As James Parkinson put it in his advice to students in 1800: 'Clinical lectures are, to the practice of medicine, what dissection is to anatomy – it is demonstration. By clinical lectures, disease is, as it were, embodied and brought before the student, as a subject for his leisure examination.'[53] Clinical lecturers generally assumed that the student had already taken courses in the theory and practice of medicine. The structured contact with cases, then, had the primary pedagogic value not only of discussing particular instances of disease but also of connecting sensation with what was already formally known. William Hamilton explained that when confronted with the clinical patient

you are made immediately judges of the accuracy of the representation [given in systems], a deeper impression is made on the mind, than by any description, and at the same time that knowledge may be communicated, your faculties of observation are exercised and improved, and you are thus able to acquire future knowledge without aid of instruction.[54]

Hunter and Hamilton both used the central image that being shown the 'object' made the 'impression' formed on the mind by direct observation somehow 'deeper', hence longer lasting. At one level, then, pervading Lockean sensualist philosophy supported and informed the epistemological justification for demonstration courses. As long as the senses were in good working order, the mind would receive clear and distinct impressions which were the basic foundation of ideas upon which the mind operated.[55]

Although touch was sometimes considered rhetorically as the primary sense, since it worked by direct contact, vision preoccupied most eighteenth-century philosophers. Eyes were effectively the most important organs for knowledge of the external world.[56] Commonplace metaphors linking light to reason bear out the primacy of vision as the sense at the pinnacle of the hierarchy, with touch, hearing, taste and smell of quite secondary importance.[57] To teach sound knowledge, therefore, the instructor linked correct terms with what the pupil *saw*. The other senses, such as touch in anatomy or smell in materia medica, certainly provided data supporting the impressions given by sight, but these secondary sensations were rarely discussed or described explicitly during the lectures.

Underlying all the demonstration courses, however, was the assumption that the lecturer prepared the students' senses by explicit association with appropriate vocabulary, showing an object, patient or procedure and leading him to experience a controlled 'sensation' for which he already had conceptual knowledge; that is, he learned to fit the appropriate categories (words) to what the lecturer presented for him to perceive. Examined from this perspective, London lecturers both acknowledged that words alone were inadequate as a basis for sound knowledge, yet would have heatedly denied that a correct medical education could be constructed from experience alone.

Lecturers used a second technique to illustrate how knowledge emerged from controlled experience: they discussed either experiments they had performed or cases they had seen. This method allowed them to filter out extraneous data, to present a purely verbal and structured model that the student might follow. In these discussions, the instructor indirectly demonstrated the (correct) source of knowledge through sensory experience. John Hunter's and John Haighton's detailed descriptions of their experiments exemplify this procedure. Both bombarded their audiences with the image of a practitioner who would hardly accept what anyone else had observed without repeating the experiment for himself. Reported accounts and 'speculation' were thus officially undermined in favour of direct personal observation, ironically distant from the pupils, who had no chance to sharpen their own perceptions or to form their own judgements.[58]

Illustrating general points about diseases or injuries with case histories that the lecturer had personally encountered offered a much more convoluted approach to how the student could link conceptual, verbal knowledge with sensory experience. As emphasized above, most eighteenth-century teaching focused on abstract definitions, not depictions of the conditions actually seen in the idiosyncratic patient, although it required a complex 'sensory' vocabulary. Turning to the comments which overtly or implicitly reveal how students were to deal with living patients thrusts us into the nuances of eighteenth-century clinical relationships. Lecturers on both medical and surgical topics offered 'clinical' instructions, usually through case-exemplars, which suggest that the traditional 'internal' (or medical) versus 'external' (or surgical) division between illnesses did not strictly separate physicians from surgeons, but rather represented a spectrum of conditions, in part defined by how they could be recognized by the practitioner and his patient. As London teaching from the mid-eighteenth century centred around educating the *de facto* general practitioner, the elite dichotomy between physician and surgeon was increasingly unrealistic. The eighteenth-century surgeon-apothecary-man-midwife already practised in multiple realms of conditions and treatments. Unless we imagine him metaphorically changing hats when asked first to set a fracture and then to prescribe for a fever, we need to view eighteenth-century medical and surgical knowledge as forming a consistent system.

If we take 'external' to refer not to what surgeons did, but more generally to conditions giving rise to perceptible, localized changes on the body's surface and accessible orifices, then both surgical and medical lecturers agreed that 'external' conditions came most directly under the practitioner's senses. In 1758, Dr Donald Monro, physician to St George's Hospital, summed up a prevailing eighteenth-century opinion in his bald statement: 'internal diseases are of the same kind to external only they can't come under the notice of the senses'.[59] Or, as Dr Fordyce later put it more carefully:

The nature of the disease must be known by its external appearances, as pleurisy is known from a pain in the side, owing to some inflammation on the pleura . . . Now we can't see the pleura or the lungs, but there are symptoms attending the disease, namely the pain accompanied with a cough, a hardness and fullness of pulse and an increased circulation, which are all evident to the senses.[60]

Here 'the senses' clearly refer to what the practitioner and patient perceived as indirect indications of the disorder which, if external, would be far easier to grasp; for, as Fordyce remarked, in such cases 'the parts become visible'.[61] William Hunter pessimistically reminded his students 'it is very hard to guess at the nature of internal disorders whatever some people may pretend to do'.[62] When Astley Cooper, surgeon to Guy's Hospital, instructed his auditors that the pulse provided an important clue to the seat of inflammation, being 'small, contracted & quick' in abdominal inflammations, but 'full and hard' in thoracic ones, he clearly articulated how surgeons also relied on common medical signs in their clinical encounters where the suspected disorder was not patently external.[63]

Certainly lecturers covering surgical conditions routinely mentioned the key symptoms offered by the practitioner's visual inspection and touching of parts normally hidden or clothed. Their advice amply confirms that the 'surgical point of view' was focused on organic changes the surgeon (and his patient) must perceive. Henry Thompson, in his 1759 lectures on surgery, for example, declared that 'wounds are distinguished by the Sight–Touch–Smell etc.'. Looking showed the type of wound and its location; touch revealed the wound's depth, direction and the presence of foreign bodies; 'cadaverous smell' suggested gangrene, while an unspecified odour would indicate if the intestines were injured.[64] Dozens of examples would unnecessarily confirm that surgeons coupled touch with sight both to distinguish surgical conditions and, of course, to operate. Henry Cline provided typical remarks. In 1788, he described the early diagnosis of a scirrhous tumour in the breast by noting 'if we place the hand on any part of the breast, one part will feel harder than the other'.[65] Cline's vagueness about the details of this examination points to the trouble several lecturers had in describing the sensation offered by touch.

For external conditions such as wounds, fractures, visible tumours and ulcers, both practitioner and patient expected the surgeon to inspect and touch the parts involved. But several London physicians also taught this approach, referring to physical examination in certain very specific contexts. Dr Donald Monro, in his course on the practice of physic, took 'physic' to cover all medical and surgical conditions. When dealing with head wounds, for example, he stated 'the first thing to be done is to examine the extent of the wound' and gave a detailed description of moving the fingers carefully across the skull, feeling for fractures. To diagnose a bladder stone, he emphasized that the decision was not positive 'until we feel it by A catheter or examining by Anus with our finger'.[66] Dr Fordyce detailed how the practitioner could distinguish inflammation of the cellular membrane lying under the psoas muscle from 'a local external abscess'. He instructed: 'lay the patient on his back and squeeze the Tumour if it be a Lumbar Abscess the matter will be pressed into the cavity of the Abdomen, but if it be on the part itself, no alteration takes place'.[67] In these examples, and similar ones, physicians followed what were recognizably surgical procedures on understood external disorders. Similarly, in dealing with childbirth or women's diseases, vaginal examination by surgeons, man-midwives and physicians was widely accepted and taught, although hedged with advice on appropriate times and procedures. Henry Cline, for example, emphasized how to pass a catheter in the female *without seeing the parts* it being more decent and agreeable to the patient'.[68]

Beyond the realm of clear-cut surgical conditions, students were also taught that investigating by touch could be problematic. When William Hunter discussed the diagnosis of uterine cancer in the 1770s, he noted that one should suspect this condition when the patient had 'tiresome gnawing pain, sallow look & foetid discharge'. He went on to attempt to describe the examination:

you examine & feel there is a cancer (ie) you perceive all the parts about the vagina are bloody & unequal & if you touch them it brings blood or you only feel that the uterus is schirrous [*sic*]. As to ye cancerous feel when the Parts are spongy & uneasy I have never been deceived, but as to schirous [*sic*] I have several times (ie) I have imagined a woman to have a schirus [*sic*] which I thought in ye end would become a cancer, but yet it subsided, so that altho' there has been considerable hardness, yet I have been deceived.[69]

Hunter could not quite convey precisely how a scirrhus felt and, although he clearly upheld the importance of the examination, it was obviously of equivocal utility even for someone with his expertise.

Hunter's example demonstrates the area of ambiguity where 'external' diseases and procedures overlapped with anatomically 'internal' ones. Here pupils frequently found that physicians and surgeons agreed that examining by touch often gained only a little additional information on the seat of the disease over what could be learned by close attention to the patient's general symptoms, discovered by sight and the patient's account. Inflammations in the abdomen or thorax, dropsies and fluid in the chest particularly fell into this grey area.[70] Henry Cline, for example, discussed the identification of general versus encysted dropsy. In general ascites, 'we may feel the fluctuation' of the fluid, a well known diagnostic technique. Yet the typical fluctuation could occur when manipulating a large cyst, as in ovarian dropsy. Cline went on to argue 'we are only able to distinguish the disease by attending to the patients general health which is very good in the encysted Dropsy or Dropsy of the ovary' while quite poor in a general dropsy.[71] Dr Monro noted 'the water collected in one or both cavities of the chest is difficult to discover, because the Bulk etc. prevent its pushing or feeling of fluctuation with your finger'. He then stressed that the important signs were the patient's 'difficulty of breathing in a lying posture & when erect a difficulty toward ye Diaphragm' without evidence of inflammation or fever.[72] Similarly, Percival Pott, surgeon to St Bartholomew's Hospital, detailed the diagnosis of hydrops pectoris according to how the patient breathed in various postures, lack of expectoration and heart palpitations. He told his students: 'it has been asserted by writers that you may know this disease from the fullness of the thorax, but I was never able from any such appearances to ascertain the existence of this disease'.[73]

In these discussions, surgeons did not present a distinctly 'surgical point of view' in the sense of upholding physical examination – or 'objective' practitioners' accounts – as the key diagnostic technique for all disorders. Visual inspection of the clothed body and the patient's reports served both the surgeon and the physician to distinguish many 'internal' conditions. The patient's description of pain, in particular, was among the 'internal' sensations that eighteenth-century medical men of all stripes assumed gave objective knowledge, even though not directly perceptible to the practitioner. Pain, with its teleological function of naturally revealing injury and disease, has, of course, a long clinical pedigree.[74] Each generation of students, nevertheless, had to be taught to interpret the particular significance of this uneasiness, ranging from the pricking pain sometimes associated with pleurisy to the unmistakable agony caused by the descent of a kidney stone through the ureter. Pain, in fact, provided considerable data about the seat of a disease or injury, whether known only from the patient's description or used in conjunction with physical examination. In thoracic diseases, for example, lecturers routinely emphasized that inflammation of the liver could be distinguished from pleurisy partly by the obtuse pain felt in the former compared with the acute pain in the latter, presumably carefully elucidated through questions.[75] Similarly, pleurisy gave rise to a sharper pain than pneumonia, and the practitioner could track its dispersion along the membranes in part according to the spread of the pain.[76]

Both William Hunter and Dr Fordyce pointed out that one (of the many) uses of a thorough knowledge of relational anatomy was the consequent ability to localize patients' internal sensations. Hunter commented 'in considering what viscus is affected, when the patient shows us the place of his pain we must remember that the Viscera ascend & descend or go to one side with the different positions of the Body'. Fordyce, in recounting a case of inflammation of the intestines, praised anatomy for helping the practitioner rule out other conditions, such as a stone in the bile duct, according to the differing sensations of pain.[77] Surgeons regularly reported how pain provided a key guide to localized injuries as well as internal disorders. Henry Cline, for example, while discussing skull injuries that brought on general symptoms of febrile inflammation, noted that if there is no 'external mark we ought to press in various parts about the skull and if the patient cries out more at any one part in particular there the operation [of trephan] should be performed'.[78]

In general, physicians and surgeons thus presented the same views about what could be learned about disease by rudimentary physical examination and patients' accounts. Surgical courses clearly contained far more references to touching than those on physic did, but when it came to diseases often taught by both kinds of practitioner (such as dropsy), the approaches to identifying (and explaining) the conditions were often quite similar. No distinctly 'surgical' approach – beyond, not surprisingly, more descriptions of morbid anatomy – fundamentally distinguished the eighteenth or early nineteenth-century surgeon from his medical counterpart.

As the discussion of the spectrum between external and internal conditions suggests, the student was instructed to use his senses in the complex context of interaction with the patient. What the practitioner perceived was constantly tempered by the patient's account of his or her internal sensations and previous symptoms. For the eighteenth-century pupil, the patient's responses – unless he or she were delirious or unconscious – were vital for the entire process of interpreting what he learned visually. In several courses, lecturers taught students how to question the patient and to integrate all the parts of the clinical encounter into a coherent picture of the patient's past, present and anticipated condition.

Physicians, not surprisingly, more frequently gave the most explicit advice on how to question the patient. In his clinical lectures, for example, Dr Fordyce told his students to keep the rules of evidence in mind. For him the patient did not necessarily know the truth about his condition and was often beset by the peculiar ideas he had of an illness, such as fever or venereal disease. 'It is with the utmost difficulty', he noted, 'that this kind of Prejudice can be overcome & in many cases it cannot.' For Fordyce, the famous story of Galen's perspicacious diagnosis of Glaucon, in which Galen deduced by subtle clues the patient's liver disease and asked only confirmatory questions, was hardly a model to follow. 'The Patient finding his Physician has found out several of his Complaints, thinks he knows them all.' Instead, Fordyce advised, let the patient talk at length about his symptoms without asking leading questions. 'You ought never to ask him if he has a Pain in such a Situation, or in such a Place, excepting after he has given you the whole Description of the disease as far as he is Master of himself.' Then the practitioner can ask about other feelings of 'uneasiness', but without using any manner which would lead the patient to answer what he thinks the practitioner wants to hear. The account the patient gives, moreover, must certainly not be taken at face value. Fordyce summarizes his cautions by saying 'such bad evidence Patients are'.[79] Other lecturers similarly warned their pupils that patients sometimes dissembled or lied.[80] In several instances, teachers stressed conditions, often illustrated by particular case histories, where the patient might in fact feel better and claim recovery, while the practitioner would know full well that relief was an illusion often portending death.[81]

At every stage of the clinical encounter, therefore, London lecturers taught that both the practitioner's and the patient's sensations were to be interpreted in light of medical and surgical theories and formal vocabularies. Social assumptions about appropriate methods of diagnosis, moreover, also cut across the presumed boundaries between physicians and surgeons. This point is best illustrated by a close look at how lecturers discussed specific cases. In his surgical lectures, for instance, John Abernethy offered numerous examples from his own practice. Many of these were clearly designed to display particular methods, techniques and treatments; they also obviously served to highlight Abernethy's own elite surgical status and clinical acumen. Yet these reports further demonstrated the varying relationships that Abernethy had with his patients and, as models for his pupils, suggested that a successful surgical practice required the practitioner to listen and interrogate as much as to touch and to operate. Abernethy, one of John Hunter's students, emphasized constitutional, or non-localized, causes for surgical conditions. For him, disordered digestion was the root of nearly all systemic evil and he regularly urged his pupils to enquire about the patient's diet, lifestyle and evacuations, very much as physicians did.[82]

For external, obviously surgical conditions, Abernethy was as ready as the next man to exert the surgeon's authority to see and to touch all parts of the body. Yet his sensitivity to the patient's willingness to be examined appears strikingly in several cases he described to his pupils. He recounted how women suffering from painful or difficult urination could become so desperate that they would even 'consent to exposure' to be sounded for a bladder stone. This, Abernethy urged, was often quite unnecessary. A lady 'of rank' once consulted him at last for this procedure. She had pain and the desire to make water, but, according to Abernethy's account of her report, urination 'was not succeeded by that horrible pain, as in the case of Stone'. He continued: 'Her tongue was furred, and Bowels as wrong as possible. I said to the other Medical Attendants that there was no necessity for exposure, but advised them to give her the Blue Pill, and Decoction of Sarsaparilla.' The lady became well in a short time, having suffered from a constitutional disorder consequent upon poor digestion.[83]

The lessons here for Abernethy's students are unmistakable. A properly educated surgeon, well versed in medical as well as surgical knowledge, would know when to forgo physical examination. Understanding the nuances of pain and recognizing the symptoms of disordered functions that the patient reported encouraged the practitioner to see certain conditions as 'internal'. Identifying such illnesses with the preferable repertoire of polite visual inspection (of, e.g., the tongue) and verbal interrogation clearly pleased the refined client. Only when both patient and practitioner agreed that a disorder was 'external' or surgical, did the broadly educated medical man put on his surgeon's hat and cross the social boundaries to discover what he could by intimate observations and his own hands-on manipulation.

London lecturers in the eighteenth and early nineteenth centuries thus offered their students a wide ranging rhetoric on how to use their senses both to learn medicine and to practise it. Faced with many pupils who came from apprenticeships and intended to practise as surgeon-apothecaries, these teachers had two sometimes conflicting goals. They wished to glorify observation and sensually based knowledge, yet, at the same time, to uphold the formal, didactic presentations that gave them part of their incomes and enhanced the professional status of non-university-educated practitioners. While demonstration courses nicely combined the visual display of objects with disciplined words, they were designed to structure sensations through verbal discourse. Case reports and clinical advice similarly offered models of how to acquire knowledge by sight, touch and judicious questioning from recalcitrant patients at the same time that they depicted the understood social context in which the practitioner used his senses.

Patients' accounts of their symptoms were so intertwined with practitioners' observations in the lecturers' clinical descriptions and case examples that it is quite anachronistic to seek to untangle the 'subjective' from the 'objective' data informing medical knowledge, misleading to assert that physicians necessarily relied on verbal interrogation more than surgeons did, and dangerous to assume that the patient's understanding of his or her illness was more crucial for dealing with 'internal' than 'external' diseases. In both surgical and medical courses, pupils learned that the patient's responses contained much information that was as important and 'real' as that available to the practitioner's own senses. From this perspective, London medical teaching highlights the shared spectrum of assumptions about how both the patient and the medical man could discover and treat 'internal' and 'external' disorders. The complex social and intellectual relationships between the ill person and the medically trained individual tempered the supposedly positivistic and progressive role of 'the surgical point of view' in the late eighteenth and early nineteenth centuries.

10

The rise of physical examination

Roy Porter

It is revealing of both the preferences and prejudices of medical historians, and the random survival of evidence, that we know so little about the conduct of routine consultations between practitioners and patients in earlier centuries. Taking eighteenth- and nineteenth-century England as its focus in time and place, this chapter will explore – and hopefully help to explain – the part physical examination played within such clinical encounters. Above all, it will address the puzzle of why a technique destined to become the cornerstone of modern clinical practice traditionally had such a limited significance. Over the last hundred years, the sick have so far come to expect being physically examined, that they regard the doctor who omits 'hands-on' examination as negligent. Their predecessors of two hundred years ago, by contrast, would have found the physician who routinely laid hands upon them at least eccentric, and possibly offensive.

As it has emerged from the nineteenth century, the examination revolves around a series of highly stylized acts performed by the doctor – feeling the pulse, sounding the chest, taking the blood pressure, peering into the eyes, inspecting the tongue and throat, and so forth. The patient will commonly be made to lie on a couch and loosen or remove clothing. Other diagnostic tests may be initiated, for example, through taking a urine sample.[1]

Many of the procedures involve the touching of body zones not normally exposed or handled, though the use of diagnostic instruments perhaps reduced the sense of violation and provides legitimation. Often the doctor is aiming to garner information about a particular condition; but the ensemble of procedures and tests also serves to corroborate the diagnostic act as such. The examination thus forms a ritual enactment of the identities of being a doctor and being a patient, confirming *inter alia* the fact that the doctor's role confers special privileges – the right to ask intimate questions, and, above all, to touch and penetrate the body.[2] Without such reassuring ritualized, consensual sanctions, what the doctor does would be taken at least as unusual, embarrassing, intrusive or offensive, and would perhaps constitute assault.[3]

The ritual of the physical examination appears to have developed in the Victorian age, aided by the popularization of the stethoscope, discussed elsewhere in this volume by Malcolm Nicolson.[4] The Queen herself, however, held out against this trend. Sir James Reid, her last personal physician, noted her 'great aversion' to the stethoscope. In all the twenty years he attended her, 'the first time I had ever seen the Queen ... in bed' was when she was actually dying, and it was only after her death that he discovered that she had a 'ventral hernia, and a prolapse of the uterus' – surely proof that he had never once given her a full physical examination.[5]

We know, however, all too little about pre-Victorian practice, or even precept. As Susan Lawrence demonstrates in her contribution to this book, lectures for medical students did not prescribe in detail how they should comport themselves with patients; presumably they were expected to pick that up by watching and doing.[6] Manuals of medical ethics and etiquette, such as Percival's *Medical Ethics* (1803) similarly have little to say about precisely how to conduct a consultation. What seems to have marked the difference, however, between what we may conveniently call the 'pre-modern' and the 'modern' eras is that traditional physicians did not routinely carry out extensive physical examinations. Take the case of the philosopher, David Hume.

In 1775 Hume fell into a rapid decline, and required multiple consultations with a gaggle of leading physicians. Their unintelligible jargon and inveterate differences of opinion became the topics of his genial correspondence. 'You have frequently heard me complain of my physical Friends that they allowed me to die in the midst of them without so much as giving a Greek Name to my Disorder', he bantered to his friend, the Rev. Hugh Blair,[7]

a Consolation which was the least I had reason to expect from them. Dr Black, hearing this Complaint, told me, that I shou'd be satisfy'd in that particular, and that my Disorder was a Haemorrhage, a word which it was easy to decompose into αιμοξ and ρηγνυμι. But Sir John Pringle says, that I have no Haemorrhage; but a Spincture in the Colon, which it will be easy to cure.

For that relief, much thanks, was Hume's response: 'This Disorder, as it both contained two Greek Appellations and was remediable, I was much inclined to prefer'.[8] But his delight in the disease that had been diagnosed was short-lived:[9]

when behold! Dr Gusthart tells me that he sees no Symptoms of the former Disorder, and as to the latter, he never met with it and scarcely ever heard of it. He assures me, that my Case is the most common of all Bath Cases, to wit, a bilious Complaint, which the Waters scarcely ever fail of curing; and he never had a Patient of whose Recovery he had better hopes.

Hume's banter was a smokescreen concealing his exasperation at the physicians' fundamental disagreement over his diagnosis. Indeed, despite Gusthart's euphoria, Hume proved to have just two months to live. His account of subsequent treatment by his physicians for the terminal cancer which they had failed to diagnose makes pitiful reading. He tried the waters at Bath, which 'did not agree with me'. Nevertheless, 'Since that time, I have been prevailed on by Importunity and Teazing, contrary to my Reason, and very much contrary to my Inclination, to delay my Departure [from Bath] some time'.[10] This was because the ever-optimistic Dr Gusthart, perhaps disingenuously, wanted a second chance at a diagnosis (he had suspected a liver complaint, but 'not caring directly to oppose Sir John Pringle, he said nothing of the Matter'). Eventually, the great sceptic's uncertainty was ended by the greatest surgeon of the age:[11] 'John Hunter ... coming accidently to Town, and expressing a very friendly Concern about me, Dr Gusthart proposed that I should be inspected by him: He felt very sensibly [i.e. palpably] as he said, a Tumor or Swelling in my Liver.' True to his philosophical stance as an anti-rationalist truster to experience, Hume placed his faith not in his physicians' theories but in the surgeon's fingers:[12] 'this Fact, not drawn by Reasoning, but obvious to the Senses, and perceived by the greatest Anatomist in Europe [i.e. Hunter], must be admitted as unquestionable, and will alone account for my Situation'. As if Hume had not suffered enough from overweening physicians, that were worse to come. 'They kept, very foolishly, this Opinion of Mr Hunter's a secret from me till Yesterday': was ever a philosopher so insulted? Worse, they still seemed to the sufferer to be advancing an utterly fatuous prognosis:[13] 'and now they pretend, that the Tumor, being small, may be discussed [sic] by Medicines and Regimen: A very silly Expectation, that an inveterate Disease of long Standing and in a vital Part, will yield to their feeble Remedies, in a man of my Years'. *Le bon David*, however, displayed his habitual good grace: 'To avoid, however, the Reproach of Obstinacy, I delayed my Journey'.

Hume's narrative makes it clear that his physicians diagnosed his condition without giving their patient a physical going-over. Yet it would be wrong to interpret this as a mark of negligence or ineptitude. In so doing, they were merely following the normal and approved practice of the physic of the day. For it was not believed that physical examination was a necessary or a sufficient procedure for diagnosing internal conditions. Rather the *sine qua non* of traditional diagnostics was the relating by the patient of his own 'history'.[14] He would tell the doctor what was wrong: when and how the complaint had started, what events had precipitated it, the characteristic pains and symptoms, its periodicity. The patient would also describe to his physician key lifestyle features – his eating and sleeping habits, his bowel motions, recent emotional traumas and so forth, not to mention the perhaps slightly indelicate matter of his indulgence in home-made, quack, or patent medicines.[15]

The politics of Georgian medicine meant that many patients did not merely list their pains but (as Dr James MaKittrick Adair wearily complained) confidently enunciated their own diagnosis.[16] As can be inferred, for instance, from many of Samuel Johnson's letters recording his medical encounters, the old bear typically formed a self-diagnosis, leaving it to Lawrence, Brocklesby, Heberden, or one of his other physicians to *confirm* the diagnosis – or, were he very brave, to challenge it – and then recommend treatment.[17] (Indeed, Johnson often also outlined the treatment he wanted as well. In 1783 he told Mrs Thrale that he had just 'bullied, and bounced . . . and compelled the apothecary to make his salve according to the Edinburgh dispensatory [i.e., a leading pharmacological manual] that it might adhere better'.)[18]

If some patients 'knew' too much, a far more serious diagnostic difficulty was that others, apparently, stymied the physician by saying too little. 'Some patients think it is the business of the doctor to find out their disorders, without being told any thing about them', grumbled Buchan. Such want of candour was hopeless:[19]

They treat physicians as conjurors, and think they need no information. A patient, who wishes for a cure, cannot be too open and explicit with his doctor. He should not only impart every circumstance he knows concerning his disease, but follow the doctor's directions, as far as it lies in his power.

But in the Georgian high noon of hypochondria, all the signs are that garrulity rather than taciturnity marked the consultation. Bernard Mandeville's brilliantly penetrating *Treatise of the Hypochondriack and Hysterick Diseases* (1730) constitutes a reconstruction, in the form of a 350-page fictional diagnostic dialogue between a doctor ('Philopirio') and a patient ('Misomedon'), of 'history taking' as a prophecy of the 'talking cure' two centuries before Freud.[20] Merely through conversation, the complaint is diagnosed and, it seems, a cure effected, though the ironist in Mandeville leaves it studiedly ambiguous as to whether this diagnostic logorrhoea is authentically therapeutic, or serves primarily to pander to hypochondriacal tendencies.[21] Whichever, his book perfectly exemplifies how a series of clinical encounters with a sick person could proceed expeditiously without the prospect ever arising of the sufferer being physically examined.

The practitioner would thus listen to the patient's 'history' – a process which might be lengthy: a correspondent wrote in 1721 of a 'thoro' enquiry' of a patient conducted by Hans Sloane which had lasted over half an hour.[22] He would, it should be added, also make some kind of physical scrutiny of the body; but, by today's standards, this would be extremely perfunctory. It would be conducted primarily by the eye – not by touch – paying attention to skin discolouration and lesions (e.g., spots and rashes as indices of fever), to the colour of the eyes, and so forth. Physicians would commonly take the pulse, although typically making a qualitative assessment (was it languid or racing, regular or erratic?), rather than timing its beats. They would also perforce listen to coughs, wheezings and eructations, just as they would sniff the odour of putrefaction.

The physical examination, however, was quite secondary (as is proved by the perfect willingness of top practitioners, such as William Cullen, to diagnose by post).[23] For one thing, Georgian medicine had no diagnostic technology to aid and objectify the senses. Stethoscopes, ophthalmoscopes and so forth were not introduced until the nineteenth century, and then not without meeting considerable resistance, from patients and practitioners alike.[24] For another, systematic and trained use of the senses, apart from the eye, for diagnostic purposes was rather rudimentary. As late as 1800, he was probably still a rather advanced doctor who would tap the body with his finger (percussion), listening for tell-tale evidence as to whether the internal cavities were full of fluids or not (auscultation).[25]

Seeing that, during the nineteenth century, the physical examination became the *pièce de résistance* of the bedside encounter, it is natural to ask why earlier physicians were apparently disinclined to engage in physical contact with the body. To some degree, this may be *une question mal posée*, smacking of anachronism. For the reliance upon 'taking the history' was a positive mark of the confidence felt by the expert clinician in his personal ability to assess a case solely from the patient's story and gross visible signs. The fame of great clinicians hinged upon their sagacity at 'history-taking'. The renowned William Heberden excelled in this probably by virtue of his well-ordered memory.[26] Erasmus Darwin, by contrast, dazzled as a diagnostician because of his penetration in quizzing his patients and reading between the lines of what they said.[27] Anna Seward criticized him in his respect for being a brow-beating bully; she was nevertheless intrigued by his clinical acumen. 'Extreme was his scepticism to human truth', she reported:[28]

From that cause he often disregarded the accounts his patients gave of themselves, and rather chose to collect his information by indirect inquiry and by cross-examining them, than from their voluntary testimony. That distrust and that habit were probably favourable to his skill in discovering the origin of diseases, and thence to his pre-eminent success in effecting their cure.

Even so, Miss Seward thought Darwin only half-successful, for as a result of being needlessly blunt with his patients, he was:[29] 'apt to wound the ingenuous and confiding spirit, whether seeking his medical assistance, or his counsel as a friend. Perhaps this proneness to suspicion mingled too much of art in his wisdom'. (Complaints against verbally intrusive doctors seem to have grown more frequent. Elizabeth, Lady Holland, noted in 1839, that 'Lady F.' was 'in a dreadful state of health':[30] 'The Doctor seems to be chiefly to blame. He is a vain, presumptuous, meddling man, like most modern medicos, much inclined to meddle with the private concerns of patients, from the days of poor Farquhar down to his day.') Mary Anne Schimmelpenninck, by contrast, believed that Darwin's bold and frank manner was just the ticket, inspiring confidence in his patients:[31]

the doctor's eye was deeply sagacious, the most so I think of any eye I remember ever to have seen; and I can conceive that no patient consulted Dr Darwin who, so far as intelligence was concerned, was not inspired with confidence in beholding him: his observation was most keen; he constantly detected disease, from his sagacious observation of symptoms apparently so slight as to be unobserved by other doctors.

Darwin stood out because of his skills in verbal and visual, not physical examination. It was perfecting the former which preoccupied Georgian clinicians. Thus, discussing the problems of dealing with hypochondriacal patients, Thomas Trotter suggested that verbal interrogation needed to be especially alert and tactful, for that 'class of diseases, so variable in appearance, and equivocal in their symptoms, requires a full share of experience and discernment, and not a little patience in actual attendance':[32]

The physician must often take a very circuitous route to put questions to his patients, that he may learn the real genius of the distemper. He must in many cases be guarded in his inquiries, lest he excite fears and suspicions in the irritable mind, which is observant of every trifle, jealous of a whisper, and when once alarmed, however falsely, not easily quieted again.

Overall, the hallmark of the distinguished practitioner was thus his skill in managing patients through words (there is a similarity to moral management and moral therapy in the treatment of the mentally ill). Thomas Withers, physician to the York Hospital, waxed lyrical over the healing power of physicians blessed with 'an humane and generous disposition':[33]

Their conversation, which is manly, rational, and untainted with the low deceits of a craft, both soothes and animates the mind. It affords at once entertainment and instruction, social pleasure and rules of health. The physician should study and humor the different dispositions of his patients.

Yet, referring back to the serious misdiagnosis of Hume, it still seems important to ask why *such* little recourse was had to physical examination. Professional demarcations certainly played their part. The physician – whose province by definition was internal medicine – wished to differentiate himself clearly from the surgeon, whose terrain comprised the externals of the body, and whose skill lay at his fingertips not in his mind. The physician by contrast was a thinker not a toucher. Hume's case shows that Dr Gusthart did not dismiss or disapprove of physical examination. It was merely not for him to perform. He was perfectly happy for the surgeon, John Hunter, to try his hand. And the job of the surgeon, of course, routinely involved touching the patient on any number of occasions, from lancing a boil to fixing a plaster, treating a skin abrasion or amputating a leg. His business, after all, was with external medicine. The physician, by contrast, would not want to be seen to be stooping to the manual operations which were the surgeon's bread and butter. The science of physic was not only different, but more dignified, being the work primarily of the head not the hand.[34]

It is important thus to recognize the impact of the medical division of labour, because it will prevent us from automatically assuming that the prime reason why physical contact between physicians and patients was so minimal must have been a matter of prudery. In other words, it might be tempting to presuppose that the sick would not wish, or even permit, their bodies to be inspected, and, above all, *felt* by their physicians (especially in the case of the female patient and the male physician), precisely because this would have involved a transgression of etiquette or decency, and constituted an act which was immodest, immoral, or (to use a term introduced into the English language during the eighteenth century) *tabu*.[35]

Clearly, the play of prudery cannot serve as a full and final explanation for the minor role played by physical examination, for surgeons at least were habitually involved in physical contact with their patients, often of an intimate kind. Skin diseases – scurvy, scrofula, ulcers – were extremely common in earlier centuries, and surgeons made a speciality, as Margaret Pelling has stressed, of treating physical blemishes and disfigurements. Not least, the cure of venereal conditions became a major department of seventeenth- and eighteenth-century medicine (one practised, as Bynum has noted, by both physicians and surgeons), and this necessarily involved inspections of private parts.[36] Above all, perhaps, the eighteenth century saw the rise of man-midwifery.[37] Had overwhelming and inviolable *tabus* operated against having one's body seen or touched by other people (particular in the case of a woman being touched by a male physician), these developments would be hard to explain; it would, above all, be inconceivable that so many mothers-to-be (and their husbands) would have drawn upon the services of the new accoucheurs with such eagerness.

Yet it would be equally simplistic to suppose that the practice of physicians was governed solely by the dictates of medicine, and that issues of prohibition and permissibility (whose lengthy history is surveyed in Sander Gilman's contribution to this volume)[38] played no part in shaping clinical protocols. After all, recent histories of the body have emphasized that, in many ways, the flesh was becoming progressively enveloped in privacy during the early modern centuries – for instance with the development of underwear or the individual bedroom.

Perhaps people had traditionally been rather uninhibited about displaying their bodily functions.[39] Samuel Pepys, visiting Lord Sandwich, entered a public room only to discover the Duchess 'doing something upon the pott',[40] and even in the early nineteenth century we encounter Anne Lister, a member of the Halifax gentry, noting in her diary how on one occasion she got into a coach and 'sat down or squatted, in the bottom & made water, so that it ran out'.[41] Yet, as Elias and others have demonstrated,[42] there was a growing sense that it was improper and shameful to be seen to be performing intimate bodily functions. Early in the nineteenth century, the governess Miss Weeton perhaps recorded such change in process. 'I like to be alone when I dress and undress', she insisted, admitting, however, that she was somewhat exceptional:[43]

many people have no scruples of delicacy in this respect. My excellent mother was strict in this part of our education; for my brother was taught to have as great a regard for personal modesty as I was, and never were we exposed to each other in washing and dressing, as I see most families of children are.

As a result of this very proper upbringing, which she utterly endorsed:[44]

From a child, I could never bear to suffer any one to be witness to my preparing for bed at night, or to quit my room in a morning, nor any exposure of person at any other time . . . For the above reason, I like to bathe alone, and a private bath is just to my taste.

Others, of course, were happy to transgress norms, or to create new norms of their own – as, for example, ladies at the leading edge of fashion who would receive callers while performing their *toilette*. John Evelyn was perhaps both titillated and shocked when attending Charles II at court:[45]

Following his Majesty this morning through the gallery, I went with the few who attended him, into the Duchess of Portsmouth's *dressing-room* within her bed-chamber, where she was in her morning loose garment, her maids combing her, newly out of her bed, his Majesty and the gallants standing about her.

There were many ways in which display of, and discussion about, the flesh became rather indelicate.[46] We are familiar with the epidemic of euphemisms introduced by 'Victorianism before Victoria' (in the end menus could not even announce chicken breasts).[47] Yet not only prudes became squeamish. In his *Memoirs*, that free-thinking man of the world, Edward Gibbon, professed his disgust for the minute cataloguing of physical ailments which had marred the autobiographies of earlier writers such as Cardinal Quirini and Montaigne.[48]

Given that sensitivity surrounded the presentation of the body, it should be no surprise that the uniquely privileged position of the doctor, succouring the sick when at their most vulnerable, at the bedside to which strangers would not normally be admitted, was at least felt to be highly charged, and at worse open to abuse. Above all, as I have argued in detail elsewhere, a shock-wave of moral outrage – from moralists and critics, though not, it would seem, from mothers themselves – went up in particular against the opportunities for impropriety afforded by the new speciality of man-midwifery.[49] Given that obstetricians were apparently being summoned at an early stage to conduct breast and genital examinations to test for pregnancy, what scandalous opportunities were afforded (critics intimated) not merely for mutual lewdness and arousal, but for a few months' deliciously safe adultery. As Philip Thicknesse insinuated, such practitioners would engage in a little 'touching' (slang for sexual contact) to see if 'any emotion arise in the touched lady's breast, that the doctor may take advantage of'.[50]

Tongues wagged about rum goings-on. Thus the Duchess of Devonshire commented, *à propos* of the recent miscarriage suffered by Lady Clermont: 'to tell you the truth, as it is pretty certain Mr Morden the apothecary was the father, I fear some wicked method was made use of to procure abortion, and that is more likely as Mr Morden might bring the drug from his own shop'.[51] As Peter Wagner had documented, one genre of erotica, verbal and visual, which never flagged throughout the eighteenth century, was the depiction of the surgeon-accoucheur as a sexual predator, his syringes and other instruments serving as standing erotic *doubles entendres*; the doctor as marauder was a theme illustrated by Rowlandson.[52] The doctor might be envied for the erotic opportunities which came his way. 'Luellin and I to my Lord's and there dined', recorded Pepys:[53]

He told me one of the prettiest stories; how Mr Blurton, his friend that was with him at my house three or four days ago, did go with him the same day from my house to the Fleece taverne by Guild Hall and there (by some pretence) got the mistress of the house, a very pretty woman, into their Company. And by the by, Luellin, calling him Doctor, she thought that he really was so, and did privately discover her disease to him – which was only some ordinary infirmity belonging to women. And he proffering her physic – she desired him to come some day and bring it, which he did; and withal hath the sight of her thing below, and did handle it – and he swears the next time that he will do more.

Thus public opinion voiced fears lest prescribed physical barriers might break down in doctor–patient encounters, and, with them, moral barriers too. Usually, the anxiety concerned female patients, but not exclusively: in the early eighteenth century, ribald pamphlets exposed Dr John Woodward as a notorious pederast, ever eager to insert his instruments into male patients' orifices and sometimes making 'evacuations' upon them.[54] It was thus crucial that rules of propriety should effectually govern what was spoken, seen and done at the patient's bedside. These clearly varied with circumstances and social status. A pauper was doubtless handled with less circumspection than a dowager (in Percival's axiom, 'greater *authority* and greater *condescension* will be found requisite in domestic attendance on the poor').[55] Yet even here practice was perhaps ambivalent: might the very superior patient have been supremely nonchalant about revealing his or her body to a doctor, precisely because of the great, and hence safe, social distance involved; after all, lords and ladies habitually performed intimate functions in front of the servants, precisely because such distance created a kind of two-way invisibility.

What is clearly true is that doctor–patient etiquette was not an island entire of itself; rather it was determined by the broader norms of body propriety operative throughout society at large. Yet these were themselves not clear-cut and stable, but in a state of confusion and contention. For the period from the Restoration to the accession of Victoria saw powerful currents and cross-currents, some repudiating existing norms, some demanding a new liberty, others an end to licentiousness.[56] The Restoration itself rejected the demureness demanded by the Saints; the Enlightenment simultaneously derided Christian sexual taboos yet – remember Chesterfield! – deplored the gross corporeal habits of the vulgar;[57] Evangelicalism campaigned for a new purity. Fashion itself became the dictator of décolletage, legislating for the bagginess of britches and the tightness of trousers. And such differences themselves provoked a literature arguing that the entire rigmarole of directives about decency was at best utterly artificial and at worst arrant hypocrisy. All was relative, argued the spokesmen of the Enlightenment. As Joseph Banks, back from the South Seas, reflected, to display one's private parts might not be provocative in Polynesia; to show an ankle would be sinful in Spain.

The Enlightenment debate about nature and culture was a theme enlarged upon by Samuel Rolleston, archdeacon at Salisbury Cathedral, in his whimsical *Philosophical Dialogue Concerning Decency* (1751). What was our sense of decency and disgust but mere habit? After all, Diogenes masturbated in the street, following the needs and calls of nature, and many peoples, past and present, went near naked and even fornicated in public. 'Custom has a very great influence, for *nature* no more requires that a woman's legs should be cover'd than a man's, and therefore it can be no dictate of *nature* that a lady should be asham'd, if she discovers as high as her calf, which every modest woman in England is'.[58] In time, fashions went full circle: 'In one century our English Ladies conceal not only their breasts but their very necks ... now in another century the stays are made low, and the whole snowy bosom is laid open *ad umbilicum fere*, pray does nature make that immodest? ... Can that be indecent in itself now, which was very decent only five and thirty years ago?'[59]

The same relativism, Rolleston argued, applied not merely to exposure of the body, but to the sense of *pudor* attaching to bodily functions. 'Our Ladies in England are asham'd of being seen even in going to, or returning from, the most necessary parts of our houses, as if it was in itself shameful to do even in private, what nature absolutely requires at certain seasons to be done'.[60] They ordered these things better in the Netherlands. 'I have known an old woman in Holland set herself on the next hole to a Gentleman, and civilly offer him her muscle shell by way of scraper after she had done with it herself'.[61]

Rolleston, however, was no radical. Having exposed that the mores governing the body were conventional rather than natural, he then argued it was, after all, natural to obey convention. Bernard Mandeville – himself a doctor – was, as ever, more provocative, contending in *The Virgin Unmask'd* that such conventional 'delicacy' might itself conceal something more sinister than the flesh: an underlying Machiavellian hypocrisy. The sophisticated *grande dame* understood only too well that she could captivate the men more effectively by demurely concealing, rather than revealing, her charms.[62] Boswell seems to have been of the same mind. He demurred from the 'established opinion' about female modesty, holding instead 'my private notions as to modesty of which I would only value the *appearance*; for unless a woman has amorous heat she is a dull companion'.[63]

As these examples hint, Georgian culture operated a complex sign-language, verbal and visual, governing propriety in the presentation of the body. Foreigners often found the peculiarities of the English, their mixture of permissiveness and prudery, quite paradoxical. 'These Englishwomen are incredible', exclaimed Dorothea Lieven, after a session with the Marchioness of Worcester:[64]

That little woman is a perfect compound of prudishness and English freedom. She would blush to hear anyone say in the company of men that a woman had just had a baby; yet the other day she did something quite incredible. We were talking I don't know why, about Lady Castlereagh's thin legs; and Princess Esterhazy said that she had never been so astonished as when she saw what sturdy calves I had – a discovery she made staying with me in the country when I was climbing over a hedge. The little Marchioness says at once that she was just the same, and that, although she was very slight and delicate, she had a well-turned leg. Immediately, Princess Esterhazy proposed showing our respective legs, and began displaying hers – heavens, what solid pillars all the way down! The little Marchioness was not slow in following her example, clumsily enough to let us see her garter; it must be admitted it was a very pretty sight. For my part, I informed the inquisitive that they must wait for the first hedge I had to get over.

In polite society, behaving too 'stiffly' could be no less a breach of good breeding than being too 'loose'. And so it was, in a modified form, with clinical interpersonal relations. The young Fanny Burney disliked being treated by the eminent Quaker practitioner, John Fothergill, because his demeanour was cold, formal and intimidating. Yet she complained that taking the waters in Bath was an indelicate business – though by then the ladies wore not merely shifts but bonnets too, whereas, little more than a century earlier, sufferers had gone into the public bath nude.[65] Adroitness in the little courtesies of address might contribute more to making a doctor's reputation than his success rate.

Thus we cannot properly understand the moral charge surrounding physical examination, except in context of the wide issue of the protocols of contact between doctor and patient – always delicate matters, governed by unwritten rules of etiquette individually applied. So how were consultations transacted? The problem is that, as mentioned at the outset, we know almost nothing about what routinely transpired, because nobody troubled to record the trivial commonplaces. Doctors' casebooks and patients' letters, diaries and journals tell us a great deal about personalities, sicknesses and therapies, but very little indeed about exactly how normal consultations proceeded.[66] Often hints have to be gleaned from passing comments, made *à propos* of something else, as when William Buchan records – expressing a disapproval clearly medical not moral – that[67]

Many physicians affect a familiar way of sitting upon the patient's bedside, and holding his arm for a considerable time. If the patient has the small-pox or any other infectious disease, there is no doubt but the doctor's hands, clothes, &c will carry away some of the infection.

But in general, the information we have mainly surrounds exceptional cases, the instances in which norms were transgressed – and especially ones in which sexual danger arose. I shall conclude this chapter by addressing some of these rather anomalous situations, and assessing their possible significance.

Healing by touch

Folk and religious remedies commonly make much of the claims of certain individuals to harness healing power in their own hands. Above all, the thau-maturgical force of the healing touch was one of the appurtenances of the English and French royal houses, marks of their divine right.[68] A culture which permits or encourages healing by laying on of hands clearly invests touching with tremendous potency while regarding contact not as contagion – a touch of danger – but as a helping hand.

Matthew Ramsey and Judith Devlin have recently suggested that healing by touch continued to exert a considerable hold in French rural society throughout the eighteenth and nineteenth centuries – affording roots for dynamic psychotherapeutics from Mesmer to Charcot.[69] It is hard to discover any equivalent in England. After the career of Valentine Greatrakes at the Restoration, there was no eminent amateur healer by touch.[70] Quack publicity likewise makes hardly any claims for special personal healing powers (though of course bone-setters, etc. were believed to possess a special wisdom of the hands).[71] Why this absence?

It is possible that in the atmosphere of the Enlightenment, thaumaturgy was simply intellectually discredited. Once the Hanoverians had disdained to heal by touch, no one else could or did. But it is also possible that the sexual frisson of such healing practices had grown so overt as necessarily to be discordant with proper doctoring. Already, allegations were being made against Greatrakes – who appears to have been an utterly proper man – that when curing women and children, his patients 'unlaced and untied their Petticoats, and he followed it [the pain] on their bare bodies till 'twas gon . . . There were many children that had the Rickets he stroked naked all over'.[72] Similarly, over a century later, English Mesmerists were the subject of ribald satire implying that the Mesmeric 'crisis' was orgasm induced by the healer's hand.[73] The signs are that healing by touch had become altogether too explosive.

It is thus specially interesting that the peasant poet, John Clare, writes of a mountebank called 'Doctor Touch', who itinerated around the rural East Midlands in the early nineteenth century. Clare condemned the man, alleging that he would 'boast of his ignorance' and claim he was 'born a docter by being the seventh son of a parent who was himself a seventh son' – such a person 'is recknd among the lower orders of people as a prodigy in medicine who is born to perform miracles'. He 'got into fame amongst them till 2 or 3 patients dyd under his hands'. He bragged he could heal by laying on of hands, but, Clare stresses, 'the fellow did not cure them by touch but by blisters which he laid on in unmercifull sizes at half a guinea a blister', to be paid in advance.[74] Thus even in folk practice, the healing touch appears to have become obsolescent.

Women patients, physical examinations and embarrassment

An extensive trawl of such sources as letters and diaries has uncovered hardly any evidence that articulate women found *talking* to doctors about medical problems, however intimate, emotionally trying.[75] On Friday 3 August 1821, Anne Lister, the Halifax gentlewoman mentioned earlier, felt 'a queer, hottish, itching sensation tonight, about the pudendum'; she assumed it was a venereal infection, picked up from sleeping with one of her female lovers, M—.[76] The next day she took the bull by the horns, and consulted the local general practitioner: 'A few minutes conversation with Steph before breakfast. Mention M— & my suspicion of venereal'.[77] She proved right: 'He said he was treating her [i.e. M—] as for this & suspected it, tho' there were certainly some symptoms against it. I hinted that some latent principle of the disease might have broken out in C— [i.e. M—'s husband]. He answered no, but it might or must be some late imprudence'.[78] Miss Lister then resorted to the time-honoured device for obtaining medication: 'Said I knew someone in the same situation. A young married woman, poor, who had tried much advice without relief & therefore asked Steph for the prescription he gave M—, which he promised'. Having got the script, she then ordered the local apothecary[79]

to make me up Steph's prescription for venereal & what I copied from Mr Duffin long ago for an injection. A scruple of calomel gradually mixed in a marble mortar with an ounce of sweet oil. Two or three drops to be injected two or three times a day after making water generally cure in two or three days. Asked Suter [the apothecary] if he had ever made up Steph's prescription before. 'Yes', said he, 'very frequently'.

Miss Lister then proceeded to inject herself with the medicines, using an ivory uterine syringe which she owned.[80]

When she was still not recovered some time later, Miss Lister visited Dr Simpson 'about my complaint & the consequent discharge. Said I had caught it from a married friend whose husband was dissipated'.[81] The next year, she 'told my aunt about my complaint, that I thought it venereal'; 'my aunt took it all quite well. Luckily thinks the complaint very easily taken by going to the necessary, drinking out of the same glass &.'.[82] It would thus appear that Miss Lister suffered no emotional traumas over consulting male doctors about her condition, partly because of her superior rank, but surely not least because her consultations remained entirely verbal (and clearly dominated by herself).

It is equally clear, however, that women found having to undergo physical examinations a source of deep embarrassment (fig. 54). 'Doctor Williams called', wrote Harriet Wynne in 1803, 'and made me undergo a *blushing* examination. He finds me about the same and I had to rub my side with Mercury which was very nasty work. I took an immense dose of Calomel'.[83] Doctors experienced the same response. A lifetime later, in 1881, Conan Doyle recorded how, *en voyage* for Madeira, he had to deal with a 'frightful horror' of a patient. 'She won't let me examine her chest. "Young doctors take such liberties, you know my dear."' Doyle was less compliant with 'Mrs MacSomething' than Sir James Reid had been with the Queen: 'I have washed my hands of her'.[84]

The signs are that situations involving direct physical contact between doctors and female patients often sent waves of anxiety rippling out from the patient's bedside into wider circles. Elizabeth Pepys had a long-lasting disorder affecting what her husband called her '*chose*' – it seems to have been an abscess in the vulva, which developed into a fistula. It interfered with their sex life. On 17 November 1663, Pepys – who of course himself had been cut for the stone just a few years earlier – summoned his friend, the trusted surgeon Mr Hollyard, to see her. Interestingly, Hollyard examined her in bed, with Pepys present, but without Elizabeth's maid (one surmises that this was at Pepys's own insistence). Both Pepys and Hollyard had originally been disposed

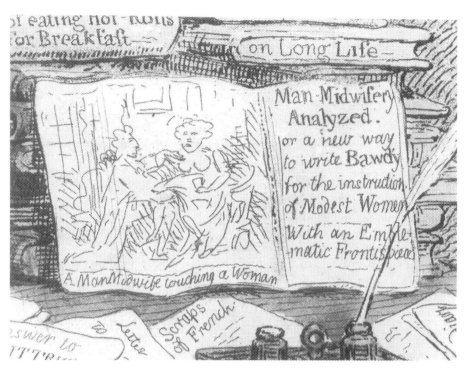

of eating not-roits
for Breakfast —
on Long Life —
Man-Midwifery
Analyzed.
or a new way
to write Bawdy
for the instruction
of Modest Women
With an Emblematic Frontispiece
A Man-Midwife touching a Woman
Scraps of French
swer to
1778

Fig. 54. Coloured etching: 'Lieut. Gover. Gall-stone, inspired by Alecto', caricature of Philip Thicknesse; by James Gillray [1757–1815] after himself, 1790.

towards surgery. On further reflection, Pepys was pleased to find it could be avoided, for:[85]

> though it would not be much pain, yet she is so fearful and the thing will be somewhat painful in the tending, which I shall not be able to look after but must require a nurse and people about her; so that upon second thoughts, he [Hollyard] believes that a fomentacion will do as well; and though it will be troublesome, yet no pain, and what her maid will be able to do without knowing directly what it is for, but only that it may be for the piles – for though it be nothing but what is very honest, yet my wife is loath to give occasion of discourse concerning it.

Reading between the lines, it sounds as though Pepys himself, presumably as well as his wife, was perturbed – jealous even – about exposing her to a more public gaze, not least for fear of gossip. One imagines he feared that it would be said that she had been venereally infected – by himself (as may well have been the case).

The diary of Thomas Turner, the mid-eighteenth century Sussex grocer, presents a comparable example of the tensions arising from intimate contacts between practitioners and female patients in gynaecological matters. After a long and agonizing illness, Turner's wife died, it would seem of some disease of the womb. Soon afterwards, his antennae picked up a whispering campaign:[86]

This day I was informed of the ill-nature and cruel treatment I have privately received from malevolent tongues, who have made, propagated and spread with indefatigable industry and diligence a report that Mr Snelling [the surgeon] at my request (and by force) castrated my wife, which operation was the immediate cause of her death.

Turner was scandalized at how such an irresponsible, groundless rumour had spread like wildfire through the locality:[87]

there is hardly a child of four years old or an old woman of four score within ten miles of the place but has it at their tongue's end, and even so credulous as to give sanction to it; that is, if they do not directly believe it they will by no means let it die with them, but still continue to circulate it about, so vile and envious is man to man. Now from what occasion this palpable falsehood could take its rise I am quite at a loss to guess; as to my own part I know myself thoroughly innocent, therefore I defy and despise the malice of the vulgar multitude.

He concluded with hardly convincing compassion: 'if I know my own heart I sincerely forgive them; neither have I in the least any anger against them for it'.[88] Thus direct relations between female patients and male practitioners may have been fraught; but the ambiguous role of the husband, and then the community at large, could make an embarrassing situation ten times worse. No wonder, perhaps, that one of the trump cards often played by Stuart and Georgian quack doctors – one not available to regulars – was to claim that a female patient hesitant about consulting with the empiric himself could discuss her ailments instead with his admirably experienced and utterly sympathetic wife or sister.[89]

Intimate physical proximity between doctor and female patient was increasingly recognized as posing severe problems not least because doctors themselves grew more insistent, in the nineteenth century, that good medical practice demanded that they be interventionist. The solution, Victorian medical men insisted, lay in the integrity and standing of the profession and the imperatives of science. As professional men, they had an entitlement to be treated as above suspicion, and granted full 'confidence'. 'It ought to be fully understood', insisted John Haslam, apothecary to Bethlem,

that the education, character and established habits of medical men, entitle them to the confidence of their patients: the most virtuous women unreservedly communicate to them their feelings and complaints, when they would shudder at imparting their disorders to a male of any other profession; or even to their own husbands. Medical science, associated with decorous manners, has generated this confidence, and rendered the practitioner the friend of the afflicted, and the depository of their secrets.

The Cleland case

But the eighteenth-century medical profession had been less certain of its professional right of entry. This is demonstrated by one of the rare instances in which the uncertainties as to the liberties and limits of physical examination were debated and documented. In 1743, the Bath General Hospital had a scandal on its hands. It surrounded Archibald Cleland, a former army surgeon, who had been appointed assistant surgeon to the hospital in the previous year.

Two female patients, Mary Hook and Mary Hudson, both of Princess Ward, made depositions against him, in writing, that he had behaved improperly to them, by subjecting them to internal examinations without their consent. Cleland was called upon to answer their charges before the Governors of the hospital, meeting as a court. The outcome was that Cleland was dismissed from his post.[90]

Cleland exonerated himself in print in his *Appeal to the Publick or a Plain Narrative of Facts Relating to the Proceedings of a Party of the Governors of the New General Hospital at Bath against Mr Archibald Cleland (One of the Surgeons of the Said Hospital)*. He did not deny that he had carried out internal examinations upon both patients. He stated that he had first conducted such an examination upon a certain Sarah Appleby, a former patient in the hospital, recently deceased. His clinical judgement told him that Appleby (who was venereally infected) had earlier been pregnant, had induced a miscarriage, and as a consequence had suffered from convulsive fits. After expelling a retained part of the placenta, she had been much better. In order to ensure that every scrap of the offending placenta was expelled, Cleland had made injections into her uterus, though first obtaining the permission of Dr Rayner.[91]

Thereupon Cleland had examined the dropsical Mary Hook, first externally and then internally, upon her bed,[92] in the presence of Sarah Appleby and with patients and nurses in the ward as usual. Cleland claims he did this 'with great ease and no pain to her'.[93] When she later developed fever (one suspects by consequence of his examination) and complained of a stoppage of urine, he had carried out a further examination 'taking some Oil upon my Hand'. For this examination, she was standing.[94] His only motive was 'charity, and the desire of relieving the afflicted'.[95]

Mary Hudson had a swollen belly. He had examined her externally and had subsequently performed an internal examination, testing her uterus 'in the presence of the nurses and patients in the ward'.[96] He suspected that, as with Appleby, a damaged uterus was the cause of her fits. He had undertaken all this, Cleland insisted, 'in so Publick and Open a Manner, and in Presence of so Many People', as to create no possible ground for offence. Such examinations were vital to good diagnostic practice and the advance of physical knowledge. 'Without diligent Inquiry, accurate Observations, frequent Examinations and close Attendance', how would it be possible to have a 'rational Method' of relieving the sick? The truth was, he assured the public, that all the charges against him were trumped up: the two Marys – Mary Hook in particular – hardly had spotless characters, and had been put up to making false charges by a cabal of the hospital practitioners, engaging in 'back-biting and calumny' and plotting to get Cleland removed.[97]

The hospital produced its own counterblast, *A Short Vindication of the Proceedings of the Governors.*[98] This in no way alleged that Cleland had been guilty of exploiting these patients for the gratification of any 'immodest intention'.[99] It rested content with arguing that such internal examinations, because of their delicate nature with regard to female modesty, ought to be regarded as rather exceptional procedures. Cleland had conducted them unnecessarily, primarily for the gratification of his own intellectual curiosity in pursuit of a private hypothesis about the patients' conditions (which in any case had turned out to be mistaken).[100] He should at least have discussed their cases, and his diagnostic surmises, with the senior surgeon, and only then have sought full permission to examine, as the Hospital rules prescribed.[101] A further pamphlet, treating the whole case with an air of ribaldry, dismissed these arguments as specious special pleading, and thought it preposterous that a surgeon should be dismissed for thrusting his fingers into 'two nasty pocky Wenches'.[102]

Here, in a nutshell, we see a crucial juncture in the development of physical examination. A surgeon treats it as his prerogative to follow purely medical imperatives in the investigation of cases; a board of practitioners, in the public limelight, and conscious of the 'trust' lodged in them, regards such a course of action as intrusive, the product of private ambition, and in breach of good public practice. Restrictions of this kind, Cleland alleged, would make the practice of medicine impossible. He noted that one member of the committee, the apothecary, Mr Bush, had confessed 'if he was a Surgeon, he wou'd never examine any patient of the Hospital (let their disorder be what it would) above the Shoe-strings or below the Necklace'.[103] Such debates were to be held time and time again during the following century, but the balance steadily swung in favour of the rationale advanced by Cleland.[104]

In conclusion, it is clear that this chapter has raised more problems than it has resolved. It has sought to demonstrate that the early history of the physical examination should be understood as no mere narrow, technical matter of medical progress; rather it was inextricably bound up with profound ambiguities inherent in our culture concerning the sense of touch – according to Condillac, the father of all senses. Touch is simultaneously healing, yet (with its echoes of 'noli me tangere') it also violates and spells sexual danger.

At the same time, the chapter has aimed to show the part played by conven-

tion. The same physical act – say a male hand placed upon the female breast –
will have radically different meanings and resonances depending upon whether
it is a lover's or a physician's. It is the threat of surreptitious slippage from one
code into another that leaves clinical practice so subject to the anarchy of
double entendre.

11

Touch, sexuality and disease

Sander Gilman

Theoretical considerations

Much of the scholarly interest in the recent past in the history of touch has been, whether intentionally or not, focused on the biology of touch, rather than in its representation. Indeed, the major book on touch by that most insightful anthropologist Ashley Montague, seems, on its surface, to be more interested in describing the 'real' physiology of touch, with its importance for human development, than the culture of touch.[1] Thinkers as diverse as Michel Serres, Desmond Morris and Marielene Putscher, who write well on the cultural implications of touch, tend to return over and over again to the physiological 'realities' for their understanding of the history or culture of touch.[2] My interest in this chapter will not focus overtly on the physiology of touch, but rather the construction of the representation of sexualized touch with all of its implications for our understanding of the medicalization of touch.

Our construction of the social implications of touch is facilitated, however, by an understanding of the ambiguity inherent in the physiology of touch. All of the senses are not alike – either in their physiological 'realities' or in their social construction. The physiology of touch provides a matrix for an understanding of the representation of the sexualized touch from the Renaissance through to the twentieth century. The ambiguity inherent in the sense of touch permits the greatest latitude in the construction of its representations. But the very nature of 'representations' of touch demands that we understand the interaction of the very senses in creating, storing and retrieving their image. To comprehend the social construction of 'touch' and its relationship to sexuality, we must take into consideration the fact the representation of touch is always in the realm of another sense, that of sight, whether it is the 'seeing' of the text representing sexuality, or the 'seeing' of touch. Since culturally we do not record our icons on our skin but only through the organ of sight we need to link these two senses to write our history of the erotic touch. Thus the status afforded sight and touch, most often considered the highest and the lowest of the senses, is not random. These two senses are inexorably linked within the social construction of their history, just as they are linked within the internalized construction of the erotic gaze.

There are two moments of splitting in the social construction of touch. The first is the separation of two major constructions of touch – the erotic and painful – and the second, the separation between 'good' touching and 'bad' touching, between the touching of the opposite-sex Other and the touching of the self (and its powerful homologue, the touching of the self in the form of the same-sex Other). Both of these divisions are represented in the iconography of touch, an iconography which incorporates not only the representation of the sense of touch but also the iconography of the organ of touch, the skin. This seems evident in any discussion of the iconography of the other senses; think, for example, how closely the phenomenology of transcendentalism is linked to Emerson's caricature of the human being as a walking eye. However, the iconography of touch seems to be alienated from its sensory organ, the skin. Thus any critical history of the representation of the sense of touch must be closely linked to the iconography of the skin.

The study of touch is made difficult because it is at the same time the most complex and the most undifferentiated of the senses. Sight, hearing, smell and taste all have specific, limited sensory organs, all of which have specific limited functions. The eye is placed at a specific point in the skull and it 'sees' – whatever we wish to understand under the act of seeing. Touch seems to be an undifferentiated quality of the entire body but it is, in fact, a multifunctional aspect of the skin.[3] Touch is indeed the complex sensory response of sensors which judge pressure, temperature and vibration. But the receptors are not clearly differentiated by function. Ruffini's corpuscle, for example, responds to pressure and warmth, while Meissner's corpuscle responds to pressure and vibration. Because of this complexity our response to 'touch', i.e., to the inter-relationship of all of these sensations over the entire envelope of the skin (with, of course, great concentrations of certain receptors in specific areas), is much less focused than our response to the other senses. The skin, which functions within other semiotic systems (such as physiognomy) is thus not only an organ of sense but it serves as the canvas upon which we 'see' touch and its cultural associations. The skin is understood simultaneously as such an organ, transmitting heat, cold, vibration and pressure/pain, and as the blank page upon which the signs associated with these sensory impressions are written. In addition, while we can 'see' ourselves or 'hear' ourselves, such an act is purely an act of reception; when we touch ourselves, we respond both as object 'touched' and the subject 'touching'. And this is especially true in touching one area of greater sensitivity, such as the genitalia, with another, such as the hand. It is not merely the genitalia which are touched and stimulated, but also the hand, so that the erotic touch is double-edged.

The religious origins of the image of the sexualized touch

The primary formulation of the sexualized touch for Western culture lies (at least initially) within the world of religious representations of Christ's sexuality.[4] The iconography of touching the same-sex in the touching of the self is linked in religious iconography in the Middle Ages and early Renaissance to two icons of the sense of touch, the image of the pain of the crucifixion and that of the pleasure of the infant Christ's touching of his genitalia.[5] (Both of these aspects of human experience are associated with Eve in her traditional role as the icon of the sensorium.)[6] Here the ambiguity of the touching (and, therefore, the representing) of the genitalia, with its link to pleasure and pain, becomes evident. The touching of the genitalia represents the touch of pleasure; the stigmata, the touch of pain. Each are aspects of the human nature of Christ. Pleasure and pain are aspects of the body, of the sense of touch which recalls the Fall. This is the image of touch which is standard in medieval representations of touch.[7] It is a Christian reworking of the Platonic view as expressed in the *Phaedo* that pleasure and pain are as closely connected as if they were two bodies attached to the same head.[8] This wholeness, without any of the negative associations of the Fall and the debased nature of human sexuality, echoes the image, found in the *Symposium*, of the entire body before its division into male and female segments. Pain and pleasure thus become analogues to the male and female aspects of human nature for Plato. They are divided but closely, indeed necessarily, linked. In the iconography of the New Testament, they both serve as references to the debased nature of post-Edenic sexuality.

In the medieval and Renaissance understanding of the model-character of the life of Christ, all aspects of Christ's life, from the pleasurable touching of the infant Christ's penis to the suffering mirrored by the crucified Christ are inexorably interlinked. St Teresa evoked this sense of the link between the painful and the pleasurable (which assumes the form of the erotic) when she wrote:

for an arrow is driven into the entrails to the very quick, and into the heart at times, so that the soul knows not what is the matter with it, not what it wishes for. It understands clearly enough that it wishes for God, and that the arrow seems tempered with some herb which makes the soul hate itself for the love of our Lord, and willingly lose its life for Him. It is impossible to describe or explain the way in which God wounds the soul, nor the very grevious pain inflicted, which deprives it of all self-consciousness; yet this pain is so sweet, that there is no joy in the world which gives greater delight. As I have just said, the soul would wish to be always dying of this wound.[9]

The image of the arrow, with its representation of penetration and pain, is associated with Christ as the erotic metaphor for the *Unio Mystica*, the mystic union between the human and the Godhead. This is not the female mystic speaking, desiring to be pierced by the arrow which is Christ, for the central image of this passage is taken by St Teresa from St John of the Cross. The image of painful penetration, which biologically should be a sexual reference for the female, has, of course, through the iconography of Christianity, been extended to Christ, the masculine representation of the Godhead in which masculine and feminine aspects are merged. It is the linking of the erotic and the sensual with the senses, especially with the sense of pain and pleasure of touch, which is present in the representation of the Christ crucified. This tradition is itself a religious reworking of the inherent relationship between pleasure, pain and Eros which can be found even in Lucretius when he writes of touch as:

> the sense of the body: whether it be
> When something from without makes its way in,
> Or when a thing, which in the body had birth,
> Hurts it, or gives it pleasure issuing forth
> To perform the generative deeds of Venus.[10]

Indeed, it marks the return to a continuous understanding of touch such as that mirrored in Alain de Lille's *Anticlaudianus* of 1183, where touch is understood as that primary force which 'the Mother of the Gods gave to Nature and with it the Knot of Love was tied tighter and bound their vows'.[11] From the early Middle Ages touch had been the sense of the 'libido'.[12] Touch is not a neutral sense for the Renaissance but is closely associated with brute sexuality rather than love in any of its forms. Marsilio Ficino, in his commentary on the *Symposium*, gives the link between the senses and desire. He sees the senses as able merely to generate qualities of objects (such as cold, softness, hardness). None of the senses provides the totality of human beauty, which demands a sense of the harmony of the higher senses, of sight and hearing, and it is this which generates love ('amor'). The lower senses, such as touch, for Ficino, are the sources of 'lust or madness'.[13] Touch is the erotic sense, and Eros is the equivalent to the antithesis of rationality, madness. Both lust and madness may be states beyond language, but not beyond the representational systems of the culture in which they are conceptualized.

The seeing of the sexualized touch: disease and fantasy

By the seventeenth century the fantasy of 'seeing' the sense of touch had already become a commonplace within the tradition of the visual representation of the senses. Following the Renaissance the sexualization of the representation of touch, with its linkage of pain and pleasure, the material and the transcendental, becomes part of the standard repertoire of systematic images of the macrocosm (along with the seasons, the ages of man, etc.) in the fine arts.[14] Within the tradition of the emblem, touch, as part of the model of the five senses, becomes a standard aspect of the repertoire of icons. Touch, as we can see in the Cluny 'unicorn' tapestries, traditionally is feminized as well as traditionally sexualized. In the Renaissance, touch and Eros are closely related. But between the Middle Ages and the Renaissance lies a major shift in the social implications of the association between sexuality and touch. For the great syphilis epidemic of the late fifteenth and early sixteenth centuries made the sexualized touch also the sign of death. What had been in Christian iconography an association between the sense of touch, the materiality of Christ and the act of crucifixion (and eventual resurrection), was secularized as the association between images of touch, images of disease and images of polluting sexuality. In two images by Agnolo Bronzino, from the first half of the sixteenth century, we see Venus holding Cupid's arrow.[15] In the first version of the painting (*c.* 1540) Cupid moves to seduce her, but does not touch her. In the second image it has reached the point in his seduction where he is touching her (fig. 55). In the first image, sexuality is still held at bay in the process of Cupid's seduction of Venus. A dark figure lurks in the background.[16] It is a male in the prime of life, his skin darkened; in a pose redolent of pain and distress he presses his hands to his head. His eyes are reddened and we observe that he has lost some teeth. His fingers are swollen and his hair, falling out in clumps, lies loose on his right shoulder and upper arm. It is the *morbus gallico*, Syphilis the shepherd present in the background of the seduction of Venus. And it is a *black* Syphilis. For, at least in the Latin tradition, syphilis (like leprosy) was understood to turn one black, the syphilitic *rupia*. Francisco Lopez de Villalobos, court physician to Charles V, in his long poem on syphilis, observes that the 'colour of the skin becomes black'.[17] Blackness marks the sufferer from disease, sets him outside of the world of purity and cleanliness. It is also, of course, the sign of the inferiority of the Black, the object of the new colonial trading system, a sign which associates him with disease and corruption.

In the second image, the one of direct contact, the erotic touch on the breast, Venus holds the apple, not merely the apple of the Hesperides, but also the apple from the Tree of Knowledge. It marks the lascivious kiss and wanton embrace of mother and son, of Venus and Cupid. Present within the image, once the touch has occurred, are signs of vice and of lechery. The mask, so familiar from the traditional, emblematic appearance of Kakia, the attempted seducer of Hercules (fig. 56), appears here as the mask of beauty. But it is the mask of age and disease which lies at the feet of the beautiful creature with the

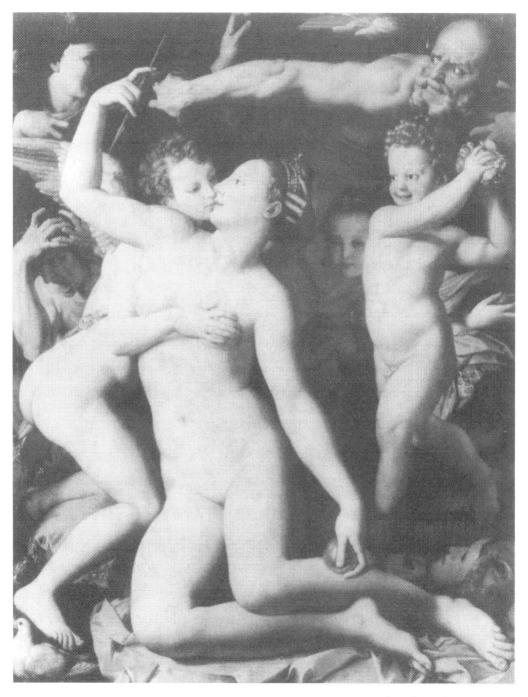

Fig. 55. The moment of contagion in Agnolo Bronzino, *Venus, Cupid, Folly and Time*, c. 1545.

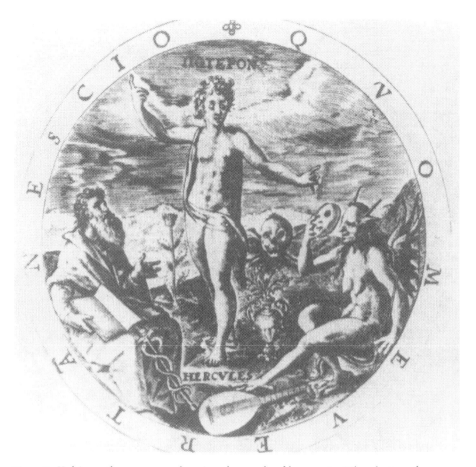

Fig. 56. Kakia as the temptress bearing the mask of beauty in 'The choice of Hercules', engraved by Crispyn van de Passe the Elder taken from George Withers' *A Collection of Emblems*, 1635.

clawed feet who offers pleasure in the form of the honeycomb – and at the left, the sting of the scorpion, the sign of the genitalia. In the second image we have, in addition, Venus' cuckolded husband, the fire-god Hephaistos. Immoderate, promiscuous, dangerous sexuality is linked to touch, disease and deception in these two images. The relationship of the senses, images of sexually trans-mitted disease, and the images of race and sexual deviancy are found, not only within Bronzino's work.

In Titian's *Venus and the Organ Player* (1550), of which there are six ver-sions (some with organ, some with lute), the association between the world of the senses, sexuality and touch adds a further dimension. For we again have Venus and Cupid in much the same iconographic position as does Bronzino, with Eros' hand on Venus' breast (fig. 57).[18] In only one of the versions of this

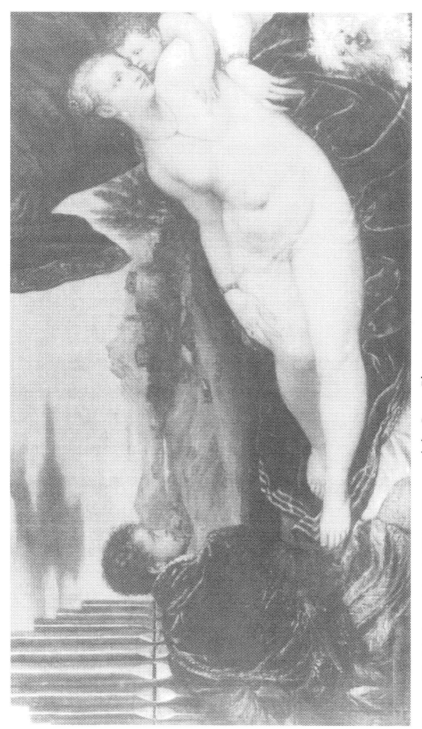

Fig. 57. The black musician in Titian, *Venus and the Organ Player, c.* 1550.

painting does Cupid rest his hand on (rather than near) Venus' breast. And in that one version the musician is clearly a Black, the sign of corruption and pollution. It is evident that these pictures all serve as comments on the role of the various senses in the act of seduction.[19] The musician also serves as the sign of promiscuous sexuality, in his role as the observer, the signifier that immodest sexuality is taking place. He is represented as playing the organ (with all of the puns associated with this act) but his action is also the creation of sound which reaches the body in immaterial form, it is the incitement of the senses without direct, physical contact between the players. This translation of the sufferer from syphilis as black into the image of the Black as the source of the sensuality which leads to disease is presented within Titian's image. The sensual (with all of its intimation of disease and the exotic) becomes the manner of evoking sexuality within the Italian sixteenth-century tradition.

Within the new tradition of the emblem books in the late sixteenth century there is a radically altered association between the feminized touch and pain. Touch is most often represented by an image of the woman bitten or pierced by a wild animal. This, in analogy to the icon of the wise and aged male's cutting open of the body of the dead prostitute (the source of the male's pain) exemplifies the opening of the female body in the frontispiece of many of the anatomies of the period (a tradition which begins with Vesalius). The pleasure of the sense of touch, the sense of the sensual and the sexual, which is clearly part of the medieval representation of touch is initially unrepresented in the Northern world of Dutch Protestant emblems. In the sixteenth century Hendrick Goltzius (1587) (fig. 58) and Frans Floris (1561) helped establish this tradition in their representation of touch within their series of the five senses.[20] (Note the abandoned boat in Floris's image. We shall see it again soon.) In 1611, Cesare Ripa, the great Italian emblemist, in what came to be the major handbook of icons, discusses touch solely within the tradition of the painful.[21]

The animal bite – either falcon or snake – comes to represent for the early emblem tradition the sense of touch, even in artists as complex as Caravaggio. With Caravaggio's image of the young boy being bitten by a lizard (fig. 59), of course, the homoerotic aspects of the image are overt specifically because he works against the tradition of having the painful touch, the equivalent of penetration, exemplified by a female figure.[22] For Caravaggio, touch, at least touch as exemplified by pain (and, as we shall see, by sexuality), is male. But in all of these images and counter-images, pleasure, or at least sensual sexuality, seems to have vanished or have been sublimated.

But while the emblem books place pain, the pain associated with penetration (and disease), in the forefront, the intimation of the erotic, the touching of the Other, is domesticated in the Northern, Protestant tradition by Dutch genre painters such as Dirck Hals, Louis Finson and David Teniers (fig. 60).[23] All of these images represent the world of the senses as social affairs, as parties

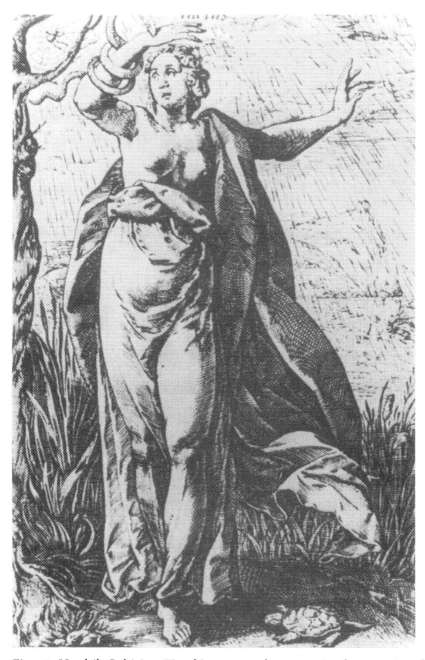

Fig. 58. Hendrik Goltizius, 'Touch', a copperplate engraving from a series of five senses, 1587.

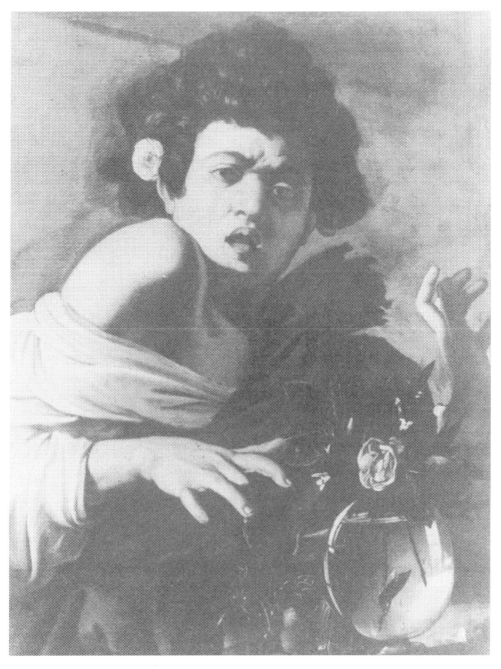

Fig. 59. The male responds to the painful touch in Caravaggio, *Boy Bitten by a Lizard*, 1594.

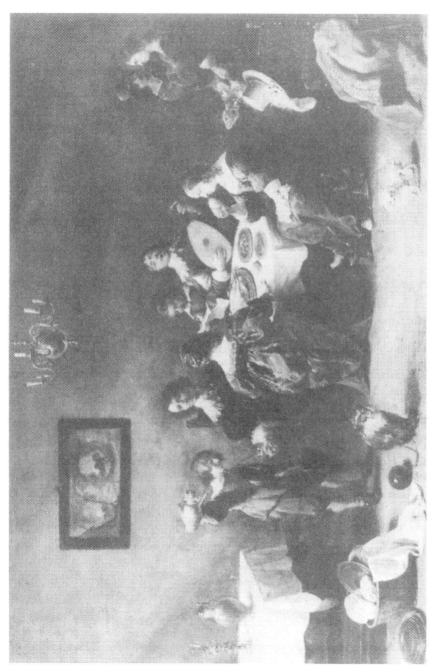

Fig. 60. Food as a context for the senses in David Teniers' mid-seventeenth century *Merry Company at the Table.*

in which the erotic is present but marginalized. In these three genre paintings
the representation of the erotic is literally reduced to a heterosexual kiss
without a heterosexual touch. The hand, the exemplary organ of touch, is
never sexualized. This signifies that the body remains inviolate and untouched, and therefore unpolluted. In this world all fear of disease and
deviance is banished, and the sense of touch is placed within rigid boundaries.
One may kiss, but one may not fondle. But touch also serves in this world of
images as the common sense – all of the individuals represented are touching,
if not one another, then objects within the world. And this universalization
works to counter the sexual associations inherent in the representation of
touch. What is missing is the heightened sense of the proximity of touch, an
absence which provides some of the hidden tension for these images. It is not
merely that these individuals interact in a heterosexual world whose link is the
seeing or hearing of the Other: they all interact through touching, but not
overtly through the erotic touch. Touch in this Dutch Protestant tradition is
desexualized, but in this desexualized form points even more strongly towards
the powerful tradition of the sexualized touch which it attempts to
neutralize.[24] This is to be seen in a contemporary allegorical image of the
senses, that of Henrick van Balen in which Touch is represented in the traditional manner by the bird's bite (and the feel of the turtle's shell), but the
response is clearly not pain but pleasure, the erotic being present subliminally
within the tradition of the painful.

At the very end of the sixteenth century Crispyn van de Passe the Elder, in a
more complex series relating the five senses to the four seasons, places the
sense of touch equivalent to summer (fig. 61). Touch, in the emblem books
always represented as a woman, her firm breasts bared, is about to be bitten by
the falcon; she strokes the turtle which is part of the standard tactile image in
the earlier emblematic tradition. To her right a crude heterosexual seduction is
taking place. The rude clothing of the two participants points towards a lustful
Arcadian tryst. (Sexuality is permitted in the 'unreal' world of the Dutch
iconographic emblem as it is banned from the 'realism' of Dutch genre painting.) To Touch's left, Christ is converting Peter, who walks toward him in the
sea (which explains the abandoned boat in Floris's earlier emblem). Most
important of the signs in the foreground are the figures of a lizard, the fabled
salamander, and the scorpion at Touch's feet. The magical salamander is able
to survive 'the consuming flames of amorous fire'.[25] The fire is both lust and
disease. And this is Caravaggio's reference. In his image, the youthful fear of
penetration is transferred to the young male, whose fear is both of the act of
penetration and sexually transmitted illness.

The scorpion, as we have seen, is the zodiacal sign that rules the male as
well as the female genitalia. The primary references of Touch are overtly
sexual. For the lying, base nature of the scorpion's appearance denies its

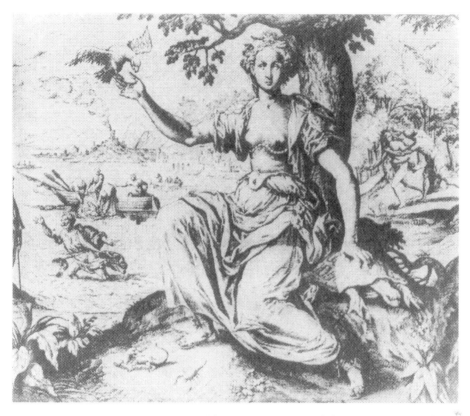

Fig. 61. Crispyn van de Passe the Elder, *The Seasons and the Senses*, engraved in Cologne between 1594 and 1610.

hidden, destructive potential. It is thus merely a woman in another form, carrying in its tail the sting of sexually transmitted disease, as in Ecclesiasticus 26. But the scorpion is also the sign of the Synagogue (as opposed to the Church). With the visual reference to Simon's conversion to Peter, the Jew's conversion to a Christian, placed parallel to a scene of Arcadian or primitive sexuality, the double referent of the scorpion, this image evokes one of the hidden messages in the icon of touch, the difference of the Jews' sexuality (exemplified through the image of the circumcized penis) as a marker of their separateness from Christ. It is through a specific form of touching, through baptism, that conversion takes place and the damaged is made whole. Van de Passe's image makes reference to these iconographic traditions, with the image of the conversion of the Jew Simon to the apostle Peter, and with the crude sexuality of the Arcadian woods. Even though the image of the touch remains central to his image, the restitution of human sexuality to its higher Christian form is the subtext of the image. But through this the erotic had to be connected

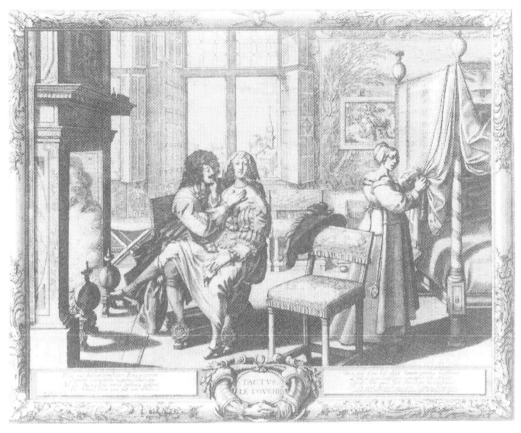

Fig. 62. The erotic touch in the bedchamber in a seventeenth-century line engraving by Abraham Bosse, *Tactus, le Touche*, an allegory of the sense of touch (Paris, n.d.).

with the religious. Thus the primary references of Touch in this image are sexual but ambiguous. For the male–male relationship of Christ and Peter is not exalted over the crude heterosexuality of Arcadia. The sign of the scorpion points towards the earthly nature of Christ's sexuality which is, however, on a far superior plane to that of the gross heterosexual act of Arcadia, with its hidden motif of the illness of the shepherd Syphilis.

By the close of the seventeenth century the image of touch seems to have become one with the heterosexual erotic; the contradictory subtext of van de Passe's image of the superiority of male–male bonding had been suppressed as the image became secularized. The feminine figure of touch in C. Drebbel's engraving becomes the object of seduction, and in a seventeenth-century French print by Abraham Bosse the act of touching is the prelude to seduction (fig. 62). The placing of the icon of touch, the woman, in the bedchamber, with the bedclothes being drawn back, points towards a Richardsonian view of the

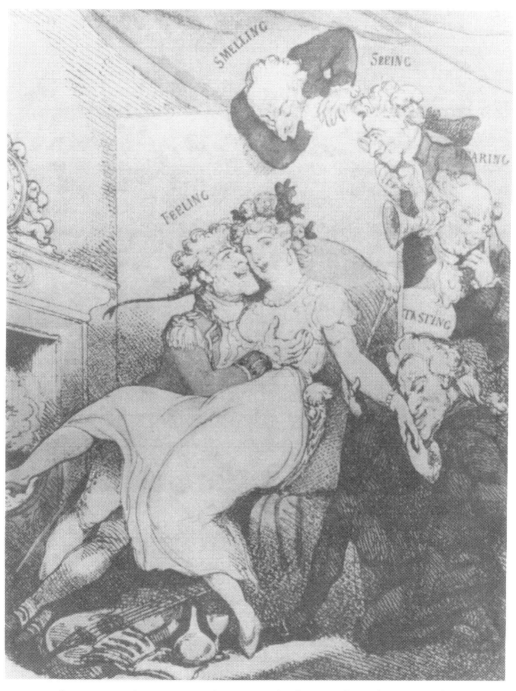

Fig. 63. The erotic touch as satire in Thomas Rowlandson's eighteenth-century *The Five Senses*, *c.* 1800.

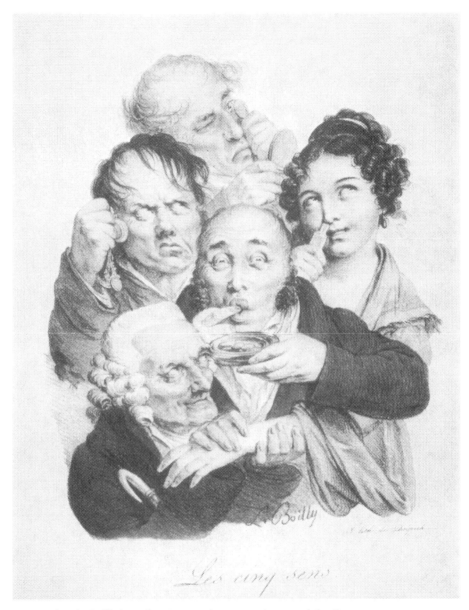

Fig. 64. Louis Boilly's early nineteenth-century image of the five senses.

role of the senses in the male's seduction of the female. It is the incorporation of the icon of coitus, the bed, with the act of seduction, exemplified by the touch. Indeed, the painting which adorns the back wall is of Amor and Psyche, a theme which becomes inherently entwined with the sexualization of the representation of touch in the following century. It is the image of the male's seduction (and penetration) of innocence. This fantasy is necessary to create a boundary between the pure (i.e., uninfected) object of desire and the sexually polluting female. The touch of the male, the sign of seduction, makes the female into the pure object; her seductive touch makes her into the diseased seductress, the succubus. Thomas Rowlandson, in the mid-eighteenth century (fig. 63), ironically recognizes this domestication of the sense of touch in his satiric print of the five senses, in which 'feeling', with all of the multiple associations of that term, is abetted in its seduction of the female by the other senses. All of the senses are subordinate to 'feeling', and all aim towards the seduction of the pure female. In Louis Boilly's image of the five senses, the object touched is the female and the touch itself is inherently erotic (fig. 64). The traditional feminization of Touch is thus made possible because of the implicit shift from the female touching to the female being touched. The touched female becomes the icon of the object of desire, a desire stimulated by and through the senses. And the male touching becomes the image of the touch which does not hurt, the touch without disease. The banishment of pain from these images is a banishment of both the projected pain of the male (the acquisition of sexually transmitted disease) and the banishment of the pain associated with defloration (the only heterosexual coital act in which the transmission of disease to the male was viewed as impossible). But hidden within the seduction of the pure female through the sense of touch is a further indicator of the association of touch with inferior femininity. For Touch is a sign of the inferior senses, of the non-rational aspects of sexuality. It is also the source, for the male observer, of both pleasure and pain, both coitus and disease. Touch becomes the exemplary means of representing the complexities of sexuality, a sexuality written on the skin. It evokes the potential of a disease which is exemplified by the state of the skin and is linked to the organ of seduction, the skin. The image of touch thus becomes part of the repertoire of images which deal with the body and illness in the seventeenth and early eighteenth centuries.

The touch of AIDS

The association of touch with sexuality and disease remains a constant through the eighteenth and nineteenth centuries. Its association with images of pollution and difference, specifically racial difference, is maintained. Lorenz Oken's view, which reflects an eighteenth-century understanding of embryological development (and it was Oken who first stated that 'A human fetus is a whole animal kingdom'), places the skin at the nadir of development, which accounts for the primitive basic nature of skin responses.[26] Oken used the senses as a means of differentiating among the various classes of his animal world.[27] While Oken believed that all of the human 'races' were related, he did see a hierarchy of human beings, the highest being the 'Eye-Man, the White, the European' and the lowest being the 'Skin-Man, the Black, the African'. The skin is the most primitive of all the sensory organs, its information the crudest. It is, indeed, the source of irrational empiricism. Again, Havelock Ellis later in the century speaks with great authority of touch as 'the least intellectual and the least aesthetic' of the senses.[28] Logically, if 'Eye-Men' live by sight, by the aesthetic, it means that their world, the world of images and words, is a world of heightened visual sensitivity; the corollary should be that the 'Skin-Man' should have a heightened physical response to tactile sensation. However, the Black, to whom Hegel denied any sense of the aesthetic, is denied even the status of the heightened sensibility of the skin. In this age of expanding colonies, the Black becomes the primitive *per se*, his primitivism mirrored in the stultifying quality of his dominant sense, touch. Thus Friedrich Nietzsche, writing in *The Genealogy of Morals* three-quarters of a century after Hegel, can comment (in line with the medical views of his age) that the history of the painful touch could be written through the examination of atavistic cases:

Perhaps in those days – the delicate may be comforted by this thought – pain did not hurt as much as it does now; at least that is the conclusion a doctor may arrive at who has treated Negroes (taken as representatives of prehistoric man –) for severe internal inflammations that would drive even the best constituted Europeans to distraction – in the case of Negroes they do *not* do so.[29]

Nietzsche's view places the Black, the 'Skin-Man' in a position of insensitivity, for sensitivity (at least the word in both German and English) is an aesthetic term, and the nineteenth century knew that Blacks had no aesthetic sensibility. But the Black was also viewed, as I have detailed elsewhere, as the primitive sexual being who marked the boundaries of the Western European 'civilized' sexuality.[30]

The image of the Black as the representation of the pathological touch reappears within the iconography of AIDS in the 1980s in a surprising unaltered form. It is as if the discovery of germ theory had never taken place. For the inherent fear of AIDS is the fear of the polluting touch, the sexualized touch, the touching of polluted products of the body as much as it is the fear of sexual or blood-borne transmission of the disease. And it is a sense of touch associated with race. Indeed as Nelkin and Hilgartner indicate in their study of the Queens School Board case, the central preoccupation of a community confronted with the presence of a child with AIDS in their school system seems to have been with the questions of 'body fluids – saliva, tears, sweat, vomit, stools'.[31] Children, the epitome of innocence, were portrayed as 'wallowing in their secretions, unsocialized in sanitary behavior and basically out of control'. It is the fear of the corrupting touch, associated with the extraordinary power of stigmatized sexual pollution, which lies at the centre of this anxiety about coming into contact with infected and infecting bodily fluids.

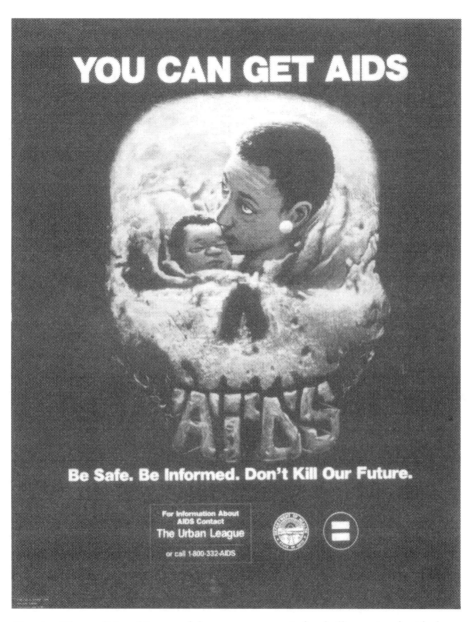

Fig. 65. The traditional image of the *memento mori*, the skull associated with the image of the female, is here expanded to include the image of the black child.

If the dying child, the epitome of sympathy in American culture (from Little Eva to the television fund-raising marathons of the present), can become a 'danger' to society, how much truer of those images traditionally associated with representations of pathology. The African-American child infected with AIDS comes to represent the movement of the centre of anxiety about the corrupting touch from the world of homosexuality to the world of the Black. While African-American children were at risk, as were all other children, the image of the black child came to signify the individual at risk (fig. 65). Initially the association of blackness and disease was not localized to the home community. In the United States AIDS was quickly labelled an 'African' or 'Haitian' disease. Whatever the reality of the origin of the disease, this is, of course, very much in line with the white American sense that blacks have a basically different relationship to disease, because of their inherent difference. This was true in the case of mental illness, where Blacks were assumed for over a century to have a much higher rate of illness because of their inability to cope with civilization.[32] Indeed, it was also assumed that African-Americans had a greater immunity to syphilis because of the 'African' origin of the disease. This led to the horrors of the Tuskegee syphilis experiment, in which black patients infected with syphilis were observed, without any medical intervention, until their death.[33] The irony, of course, is that African-Americans were at special risk from AIDS because of the nature of treatment for sickle-cell disease, through transfusions. It was the polluted blood supply that placed African-Americans, at least those suffering from such genetically transmitted diseases, in the forefront of those who were at risk.[34] But they were not understood as being in the same category as the haemophiliacs. Blacks were deemed to be at risk because of their perceived sexual difference, their sexual practices and their hypersexuality, as well as their sociopathic use of drugs. Black sexuality, associated with images of sexually transmitted disease, became a category of marginalization, as it had in the past.[35] And that image even entered into the sympathetic (even erotic) representation of the black person with AIDS. By the 1980s, after white America had been made aware of the intolerable state of African-Americans in the United States through the civil rights movement of the sixties and seventies, white America could no longer as easily localize the source of disease among African-Americans, as had been done in the Tuskegee experiment. Rather, the source of pollution was seen in foreign Blacks, in black Africans and Haitians, thus assuaging American 'liberal' sensibilities while still locating the origin of the disease within the paradigm of American racist ideology. Indeed, in the African-American community the very evocation of this paradigm generated older images of enslavement and powerlessness (fig. 66). It is as if the evocation of the diseased Black represented a return to an older well-known image of risk associated with the Black.

It is important to understand that the association of the image of those

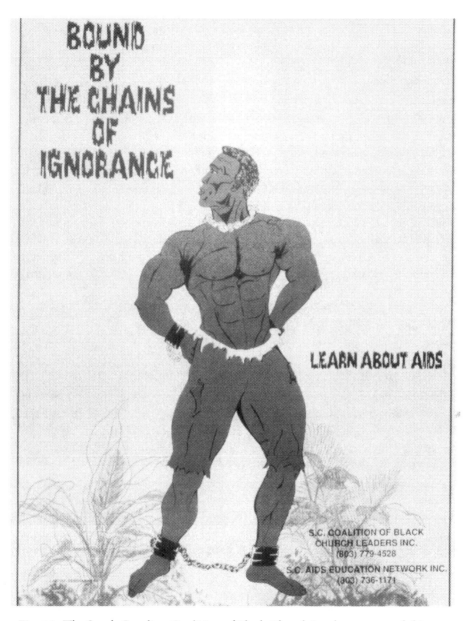

Fig. 66. The South Carolina Coalition of Black Church Leaders generated this poster in the late 1980s which evoked both the beautiful male body and the image of the African-American in chains.

individuals living with AIDS with the icons from the history of sexually transmitted diseases such as syphilis is not coincidental. It is clear that the initial
association rests on that population of those living with AIDS, homosexuals,
and their being perceived as having suffered from a sexually transmitted
disease. But it is also clear that the 'taming' of syphilis and other related sexually transmitted diseases with the introduction of antibiotics in the 1940s left
Western culture with a series of images of the mortally infected and infecting
patient suffering from a morally repugnant disease but without a disease sufficiently powerful with which to associate these images. During the 1970s there
was an attempt to associate these images with genital herpes, but even though
it was a sexually transmitted disease, its symptomatology was too trivial to
warrant this association in the long run. AIDS was the perfect disease for such
associations, even if it was not a typical sexually transmitted disease.

We turn to a vocabulary of images of an individual living with AIDS, who
then comes to represent the disease in itself, when we explore the official
public health images generated in the 1980s.[36] These images were created to
influence attitude and behaviour in the wider public. The images that follow
are all posters, that is they were all intended for public display and they were
all intended to communicate specific information directly to a mass audience.
The tracking of the public awareness of the disease, the images used to evoke
the disease, the visual and verbal language employed to characterize those who
have or are at risk of the disease, provide an index of how the disease was
understood over time and in various visual cultures both within and outside
the United States. These posters are the product of a complicated advertising
culture (whether or not they were designed and circulated by official 'advertising' agencies) which has a specific set of assumptions about its audience, their
capacity for the quick assimilation of information and the means by which to
communicate this information. Our assumption will be that these posters had
an overt 'intention'. We can explore what this intention was and whether or
not the visual and verbal vocabulary selected was appropriate for that overt
intention. Central to an analysis of this material is a close reading of the iconography, the visual vocabulary, of each poster. The tracing of specific visual
themes, the question of who and what is represented on the poster and how
they are portrayed will give us a vocabulary of images which is tied closely to
the public image of AIDS and HIV infection. The image which results (and
which shifts over time and from group to group) can provide us with a clear
understanding of how the person with AIDS or at risk of HIV infection is
presented ideologically.

In many of these public health representations, there is a sense of the need to
universalize the image of the patient, but in a way to avoid the powerful association of the disease with gay men. An AIDS poster created by the Urban
League, a conservative African-American political organization, stressed the

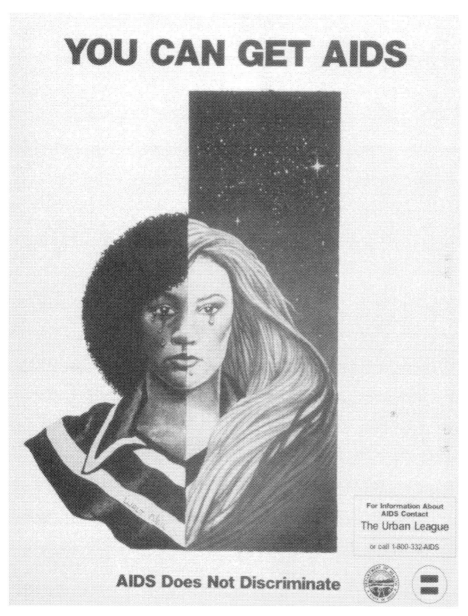

Fig. 67. The composite person with AIDS is black and white, rather than male and female, in this poster from the Urban League.

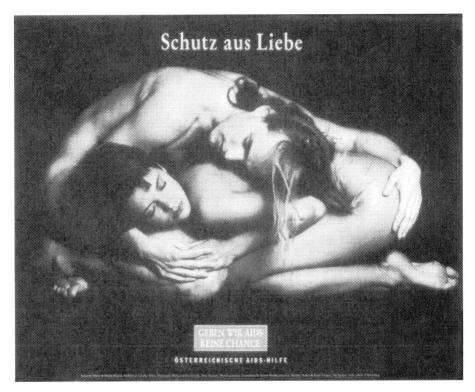

Fig. 68. The image of the protecting male restructures the meaning of the erotic touch in this poster from the Austrian AIDS Organization.

risk to black and white women alike (fig. 67). And it is in this image of the merging of the two groups within the discourse of gender that the powerful association in the United States of the person with AIDS and the homosexual male is sundered. The person with AIDS can be an African-American or a white woman (as well as a male, black or otherwise). But the person with AIDS is both the poor sufferer as well as the cause of his own suffering. The person with AIDS is both the 'male' victim and the 'female' source of infection.

And the sexualized touch which is present in these images becomes one with the older images of the *memento mori*. The sexualized touch, the erotic, is revealed to be but a mask for disease and death (fig. 68). In this image from the Austrian AIDS organization, there is a sense of the male protecting the female, rather than exposing her to risk. The sexualized touch here is a dangerous one. And this is evoked precisely in the piercing and painful touch in the use of the image of martyrdom in a poster from 1989 which incorporated a painting of the martyrdom of St Sebastian by the seventeenth-century Piedmontese artist Tanzio da Varallo (fig. 69). It is the sexualized touch which is painful that is

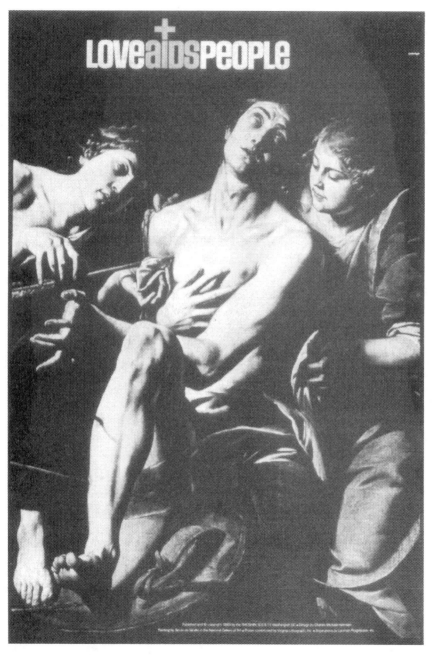

Fig. 69. This poster, designed by Charles Michael Helmken, incorporates a painting of the martyrdom of St Sebastian by Tanzio da Varallo and echoes the earlier implication of the dangerous, painful touch of sexually transmitted disease.

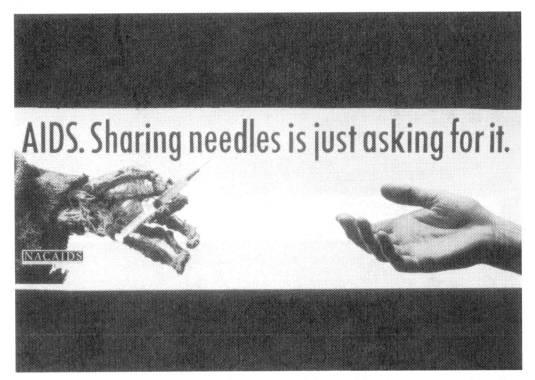

Fig. 70. The *memento mori* as the image of the painful, infectious touch of the dirty needle is evoked in this poster from the late 1980s.

evoked here using the image of St Sebastian, an image which has wide currency in the gay community.

The painful touch as the polluting touch is evoked in the images of AIDS associated with the dangers to intravenous drug users in sharing used needles. The bounds of the polluting touch, even within the context of medical treatment, echo the general cultural association of AIDS and touch. Death, represented by the classic image of the 'grim reaper', comes to represent the touch of the dirty needle (fig. 70). Over and over again, the hand, which is the icon of touch, comes to stand for the potentially deadly touch, just as the erotic touch has hidden within it the potential for pain. We have not come very far from the Renaissance in associating the sense of touch and the image of blackness with the sense of disease. This powerful cultural tradition continues even into our iconography of AIDS.

12

Sense and sensibility in late nineteenth-century surgery in America

GERT BRIEGER

'Therapeutic surgery', Samuel D. Gross wrote in the preface to the 1882 edition of his widely used textbook, 'was never in so healthful condition as it is at the present moment.'[1] Science combined with skill, he enthused, had led to astonishing progress in the decade since 1872. This was not merely the idle rhetoric of a promoter, but was the felt reality for many of his contemporaries as well. It was the increasingly consistent results of surgical therapy in the late nineteenth century that helped once again to elevate the image of the physician, and of the medical profession as a whole, in the eyes of the public.

It is the implicit tensions of the public image and the private doubts and sensibilities of the surgeons of a hundred years ago that one of America's great artists, Thomas Eakins of Philadelphia, portrayed in two of his best known paintings. What follows, then, is hardly a conventional view of surgery in the United States. It is, rather, an attempt to view surgery as the surgeons viewed it, and as they wished to be seen. It will be an attempt to trace an increasing sensibility of surgeons towards their own work, and in doing so I will use sources common to the work of the art historian, as well as those of the medical historian. Neither a visual portrait, such as a photograph or a painting, nor a verbal picture, such as a conventional historical account, can hope to do more than evoke a series of images for further contemplation by the viewer or reader.

For this portrait of surgery, I have chosen to focus upon a decade and a half between 1875 and 1889, a time about a century ago, when, in the words of J. Collins Warren, 'no other generation of physicians in the history of medicine

This chapter is a modified and shortened form of 'A portrait of surgery: surgery in America', *Surgical Clinics of North America*, 67 (1987), 1181.

has seen such extraordinary changes in the practice of medicine and surgery'.[2]

Our focus in this essay will be on the fourteen-year period between the two magnificent paintings by Eakins, *The Gross Clinic* of 1875 and *The Agnew Clinic* of 1889. Here the attempt will be to understand something of the science of surgery as well as its place in American medicine during these eventful years. This was a time when contemporaries themselves noted a shift from the old to the new. Stephen Smith, using the period between the two editions of his own textbook *The Principles and Practice of Operative Surgery* was explicit: 'Within the period 1879–1886 the principles and practice of operative surgery have undergone so complete a revolution that the term "the new surgery", applied to the present practice, is not inappropriate.'[3] The principles of wound treatment so modified practices that diseases and injuries previously regarded as untreatable or incurable were now yielding to surgery. This new surgery, then, imposed new obligations upon the surgeon. Diligent attention to the details of antisepsis before and after surgery was the hallmark of the new approach.

Medicine in America, in the last quarter of the nineteenth century was just emerging from its heroic age. Heroic medicine was so called because the vigorous application of therapies such as blistering, bleeding and purging produced a profound effect on most of their recipients. And it was a heroic medicine no less because as much fortitude was necessary on the part of the patient to withstand such treatments as for the physicians to prescribe it. It would not be many years into the twentieth century that the surgeon would be looked upon more as a healer than as a hero. Courage and optimism fused with an increasing understanding of pathophysiology and ever-better results came to differentiate the newer heroism of surgery from its earlier version.[4]

The older surgery was also invested with the spirit of exaggeration, even notoriety. A leading Boston surgeon, Henry J. Bigelow, noted in 1850 that in order to become known in his field so as to acquire a practice, the surgeon had often to become 'The hero of extraordinary operations'.[5] Bigelow also drew attention to what he called a spirit of exaggeration that invested surgery in 1850, just four years after he and his Boston colleagues had witnessed the marvels of anaesthesia:

Why is the amphitheater crowded to the roof, by adepts as well as students, on the occasion of some great operation, while the silent working of some well-directed drug excites comparatively little comment? Mark the hushed breath, the fearful intensity of silence, when the blade pierces the tissues, and the blood of the unhappy sufferer wells up to the surface. Animal sense is always fascinated by the presence of animal suffering.[6]

As Dr John Brown wrote earlier in the nineteenth century in his story about Rab and his friends, 'It is a natural, and not wicked interest that all boys and men have in witnessing intense energy in action.'[7] Nor should one think the young medical students as heartless when they run to the amphitheatre to secure a good place to see an operation, Brown claimed. They too need to overcome their natural professional horrors to prepare them for their proper work.

It is true, as Elizabeth Johns has pointed out in her fine study of Thomas Eakins, that surgery in the nineteenth century had become 'a major professional opportunity for heroism'.[8] But what weakens her argument for viewing Eakins's painting as a portrait of heroism is that precisely by the time of the Gross and Agnew paintings surgery was becoming more precise, increasingly grounded upon scientific principles. Thus as Gross, Agnew and their contemporary surgical writers were proclaiming that surgery was becoming more and more an integral part of the modern scientific medicine of their day, it was shedding its long historical cloak of heroic therapy. Furthermore, if we are to give any credence to Gross's words about the principles according to which he conducted his life, then the surgeon should *not* be viewed as a hero. Gross firmly believed that the most skilful and accomplished surgeons were also 'men of the keenest sensibilities and the warmest sympathies'.[9] He hated applause from his students as he entered the amphitheatre: 'I always said, Gentlemen, such a noise is more befitting the pit of a theatre or a circus than a temple dedicated to Aesculapius'.[10] Nor did he have more patience for the surgeon too ready to use the knife. Knivesmen, as he called them, were to be equated with knaves.[11] With the progress of American Surgery, Gross proclaimed in his centennial essay of 1876, 'Comparatively few knivesmen, properly so called, exist among us, and it is worthy of note that their career is usually as shortlived as it is inglorious.'[12]

Surgical writers of the later nineteenth-century frequently wrote about the dramatic changes they perceived, but it was Thomas Eakins, the friend of many surgeons, who set out to put them on canvas for all to see. The profound belief in the realization of a true surgical progress rested upon theory as well as practice, and upon some equally significant developments in the institutions of American surgery. I will confine the examples to a very few, only briefly explained.

For the theory of surgery, the new view of appendicitis, especially culminating in the epochal paper of Reginald Fitz in 1886, is perhaps the most graphic example. Fitz not only put the natural history of appendicitis into perspective, but he also urged surgeons to operate *before* perforation took place. With theory then leading the way, surgeons such as Charles McBurney of New York worked out the best surgical approach. The diagnostic criteria and the incision are still associated with his name.[13]

Among the changes in the practice of surgery during these latter decades of the nineteenth century, the slow acceptance and spreading use of the techniques of Listerism cannot be overlooked, though this is by now a well-known story and one that I have already told.[14] Beyond this, three important institutional changes, also well known, deserve to be noted in the context of the development of this new surgery. These are the establishment of the American Surgical Association in 1880, the founding in 1885 of a journal devoted exclusively to surgery, the *Annals of Surgery*, and the opening of the Johns Hopkins Hospital in 1889 which quickly led to the founding of a true school of surgery on the wards, in the clinics, and in the laboratories directed by William S. Halsted.

Ours has been called a visual age, as E. H. Gombrich has noted, though one must wonder how much do we really see?[15] A great deal has been written about ways of seeing. In reading a painting or a photograph we must constantly ask ourselves how well the picture portrays the character of a scene or of a person, how does it describe the culture of its time? How well, for instance, did the great surgical scenes of Thomas Eakins portray, or in the terms of the historian, describe, the culture of surgery, of a hospital, and of medical education? What do these paintings reveal about the general traits of the surgeon and of surgery, of the relationships between doctors and their assistants, doctors and their patients, and of teachers and their students?

Among art historians there has arisen a sizeable literature about the surgical paintings of Thomas Eakins.[16] Just as William Schupbach has recently suggested that the well-known *Anatomy Lesson of Dr. Tulp* does not merely reveal a morphological theme, but quite probably a religious one as well, so these Eakins paintings are much more than the portraits of two renowned surgeons at their work.[17] For the history of surgery, it is not so important to decide whether *The Gross Clinic* is best viewed as a portrait of Dr Gross or as a genre painting of a surgical scene, and whether it is a group portrait or meant as the study of a single individual. Whether these very large, one might almost say overpowering, paintings were meant by the artist to portray the surgeon as a hero or at least engaged in an heroic pursuit, does, however, speak directly to the question of the image of the surgeon in the eyes of the public, in those of his colleagues, and to an extent to how he perceived himself and his work.

To understand the art one must know something of the artist. For our purposes we must also know to what extent he understood surgery and the surgeons of his time. As we shall see, Eakins was an avid anatomist, and there is little doubt that he was quite familiar with the many activities of the Jefferson Medical College in Philadelphia. And he seems to have been nearly as keen a student of the surgical scene as he was of the anatomical. Since he was known for his teaching of art and of anatomy, it was perfectly natural for him not merely to depict the scene of an operation, but to turn that into one of surgical teaching as well.

Thomas Eakins spent his entire career in Philadelphia where he was born in 1844. He was the eldest of the children of Benjamin Eakins, a writing master, and his wife Caroline. Benjamin Eakins seems to have been a very supportive father, both financially and emotionally. As several art historians have pointed out, it is likely that it was the artistic nature of his father's work as well as the warm and important support that he received from him that influenced Tom Eakins to study art rather than medicine, though the inclination for the latter was there as well.

After attending Central High School, an unusually fine institution of its kind, where Eakins was exposed to good drawing courses, mathematics and languages, as well as the natural sciences, he began to study art at the Pennsylvania Academy of Fine Arts in 1862. As many young medical students in the 1860s recognized, their studies would be immeasurably enhanced if they could travel to the leading medical centres in Europe. The same was true for the young artists of the time. Like the physicians, those whose families could afford to send them headed for France or Düsseldorf and Munich. Eakins chose Paris, where he remained for over three years.[18]

It is probable that while Eakins was studying in Paris during the years 1866–9 he became well aware of French medicine and the legacy of the Paris School of the early nineteenth century in which surgery had played such a significant role. It is probable, however, that in planning *The Gross Clinic* in 1875 he wished to reveal to the world the importance of medical Philadelphia while simultaneously showing the grand nature of his own work and ability.

After leaving Paris, Eakins spent about six months in Spain, where the seventeenth-century painter Diego Velázquez had been one of the first artists who had fully understood the idea and the importance of painting directly from life. And as would also be unfortunately true of Eakins, Velázquez had been largely unnoticed in his own day. The work of both Velázquez and his countryman José de Ribera made a lasting impression on the young American.

Eakins returned home to Philadelphia in 1870. There, with his father's continuing support and encouragement, he began his career. He produced some justly famous rowing scenes as well as a quite sophisticated portrait of Professor Benjamin Howard Rand in 1874. Rand had taught at Central High School when Eakins was a student there, and was now nearing the end of his tenure as Professor of Chemistry at the Jefferson Medical College.

Sometime before Eakins left for his four-year European period in 1866, he had begun the serious study of anatomy with Joseph Pancoast and his son William at Jefferson. There remains a ticket to William Pancoast's lectures in 1864–5.[19] Eakins did not confine himself to lectures and books, for he dissected avidly. Nor did he confine himself only to human anatomy.

After his return from Europe in 1870, he renewed his Jefferson ties. He became a prosector for another Jefferson surgeon, Dr William W. Keen, who taught the course for art students at the Pennsylvania Academy. By 1879 Eakins himself directed his drawing students in human and animal dissections.

Many of Eakins's contemporaries were well aware of his interest in anatomy. 'Anatomy is his passion', the critic Mariana van Rensselaer wrote in 1881.[20] Eakins himself was quoted at length in 1879 about his views on dissection and on the importance of anatomy for the artist. He said: 'To draw the human figure it is necessary to know as much as possible about it, about its structure and its movements, its bones and muscles, how they are made, and how they act.'[21] Asked if he did not find the students' interest becoming too scientific, with dissection becoming an end in itself, Eakins is quoted as saying, 'we turn out no physicians and surgeons . . . but we are considerably concerned about learning how to paint'.[22] Thus one dissects, as Eakins stressed, to know how beautiful things are put together, so as to be able to imitate them.

After 1879 Eakins assumed increasing teaching and administrative duties at the Academy. It is unfortunate that what seems to be best known about Eakins as a teacher is that he was fired from all his duties there in 1886.[23] The final straw seems to have been complaints about the use of nude male models in the women's painting class, but there were far deeper differences and some petty jealousies among faculty and directors that need not detain us here. They have been well described by Lloyd Goodrich and other Eakins scholars.

Despite this blow to his pride and to his teaching career, Eakins continued active teaching in Philadelphia, New York and Brooklyn for many years after he lost the Academy position. Thus his intense, almost career-long involvement with students and with teaching can readily explain why the two surgical scenes are not merely pictures of surgeons performing an operation. There are also scenes of Gross and of Agnew teaching, and of their students learning. Eakins was not only a teacher but also an avid student. Once again, it is not chance that finds him as one of the onlookers in both of these major paintings, while at the same time he is urging us to look at the scene with him.

Eakins's main teaching, of course, was devoted to the principles of art, of drawing, composition, perspective and the like. In his large surgical paintings, I believe, he also wished to teach the viewer something about the surgeon's work. As he disrobed his models, and himself was photographed on several occasions in the nude, so too in his paintings he wished to remove the mystique from surgery.

A final word about Eakins the man and his work: some claim that he had considered a career in surgery, but the evidence for this is lacking. That he was a man of active pursuits and of a muscular, athletic build there is no doubt. He frequently painted the scenes of his own active pursuits, such as rowing, swimming, sailing and hunting. He was also interested in other sports such as wrestling, boxing, baseball and running, all reflected in his paintings and photographs. Many of his pictures involve motion. Thus the surgical scenes were in character for a painter with such interests and inclinations. The surgeons portrayed in both *The Gross Clinic* and *The Agnew Clinic* reveal controlled motion and much power.

The motion implicit in the surgical scenes includes retraction and incision of tissues, the holding of limbs and the administration of anaesthesia. Teaching too is filled with the motions of gesture, of speech and of eye contact with an audience. All are manifest in the manner in which Eakins executed these scenes. The actual or implied movement of the rower in his shell, the artist in his studio, as much as the surgeon in the amphitheatre, is what lent emphasis to the drama inherent in so many of Eakins's major works.

With the use of motion as well as the element of drama, Eakins conveyed a sense of optimism about the progress of surgery. He was not merely celebrating the career of a great man, but wished to communicate to his viewers that the drama had a purpose, a useful outcome that resulted from the vast learning and experience that the venerable teachers were communicating through their work. It was optimistic also because Eakins chose to show the next generation learning from its elders so that they would be prepared to continue the work and to contribute to the progress of healing.

This chapter is not the place to discuss at any length the role of realism in the work of Thomas Eakins, or indeed his place in the history of art in America. Suffice it to say that it was very definitely in the realist tradition to portray the dignity, and even the heroism, of daily work and of manual labour. Thus we may view Eakins as depicting the daily work of the surgeon while simultaneously showing him in the service of humanity.[24]

Eakins did write long letters to his family while he was studying in Europe, and occasionally in his later career either he or his students preserved a few pieces of his philosophy of art. Since *The Gross Clinic*, at least, was the product of a young artist barely thirty years old, his thoughts from his student days are pertinent. In 1868, for instance, he wrote to his father that 'The big artist does not sit down and copy monkey-like . . . but he keeps a sharp eye on Nature and steals her tools. He learns what she does with light, the big tool, and then color, then form, and appropriates them to his own use.'[25] In the same letter Eakins maintained that 'In a big picture you can see what o'clock it is, afternoon or morning, if it's hot or cold, winter or summer, and what kind of people are there, and what they are doing and why they are doing it.'[26]

One of Eakins's contemporaries, the lawyer and social critic Clarence Darrow, captured, I believe, the feelings that are so well portrayed in much of Eakins's art. 'The greatest artists of the world today', Darrow wrote in 1893, 'are telling facts and painting scenes that cause humanity to stop and think, and ask why one shall be a master and another a serf'. As if to answer those critics who objected to the graphic details of these surgical scenes, Darrow also noted that 'Not all the world is beautiful, and not all of life is good. The true artist has no right to choose only the lovely spots, and make us think this is life.[27]

If the creative spirit of Thomas Eakins had not manifested itself in his paintings, he could quite probably have become a fine writer. His paintings frequently have rich implications for story-telling, and indeed each of the surgical scenes contains several separate stories, to which I now turn.

In the Eakins surgical portraits one can readily feel the artist's desire to have the viewer see more of the surgical scenes than is normally available to laymen. This was an age, one must remember, long prior to the time when medical and surgical events could be viewed on a cinema screen or at home in a television drama. Nor had photo-journalism, except for the occasional picture of war or an accident, yet emerged. A line drawing or a reproduced woodcut was a relatively new feature in popular magazines such as *Harper's* or *Scribner's*. Only after 1880 did the camera become available for a wider public. The question for us is whether paintings of surgical scenes such as the clinics of Gross, Agnew and Billroth helped to shape, in their time, the public's image of the new ways of surgery? In these paintings it was not merely the surgeons who should be seen in nearly heroic proportions, but their teaching and their craft should also take on a grand scale. Eakins thereby celebrated both the surgeon's art and that of the painter, even as the surgeons themselves were insisting that their art was no longer heroic but rather progressive and scientific.

To return then to the first of the large Eakins surgical scenes, the painting originally known as *The Portrait of Dr. Gross*, now generally called *The Gross Clinic*, was finished in 1875. This is a painting that measures 96″ by 78″, or 8 by 6 ½ feet, and it must be viewed first hand at the Jefferson Medical College in Philadelphia to experience its full impact. After completing the *Portrait of Professor Rand*, Eakins decided upon his first large medical scene. It is probable that he had the forthcoming Centennial Exhibition to be held in Philadelphia in the summer of 1876 in mind, but whatever motivated the thirty-year-old artist to paint the renowned seventy-year-old surgeon, it was a private decision. The painting was not commissioned by Gross nor by the medical school.[28]

Samuel D. Gross, by virtue of his many books, active participation in medical affairs, and a teaching career that began in Cincinnati, continued in Louisville, and since 1856 had been in Philadelphia, was by any measure one of the country's leading men of medicine. Many of his contemporaries remarked on his great skill as a teacher. Part of his success, no doubt, lay in the fact that by deed as well as by an imposing appearance he possessed real charisma.[29]

Eakins increased the dramatic effect of his painting because he chose not only to present the idea of a surgeon and his team about to operate, but also to

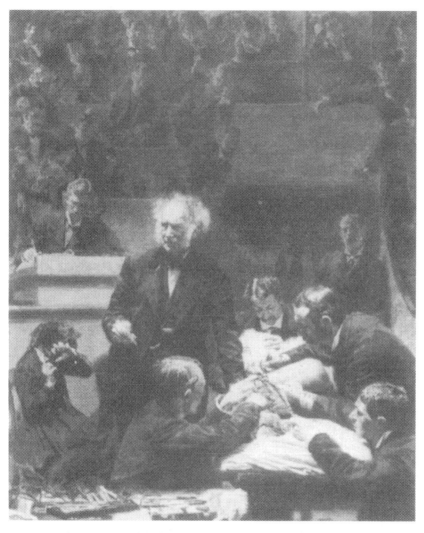

Fig. 71. Thomas Eakins, *The Gross Clinic.*

show the surgical procedure actually in process with retractors holding the wound open, probes probing and blood flowing. There were precedents for this in the great dissection scenes of Vesalius and of Rembrandt's Dr Tulpius, in both of which the forearm was actively being dissected. But for the history of surgical scenes, this was a most unusually vivid depiction because the object of the dissection was not a dead body.

It is also important to remember that surgery, until the later decades of the nineteenth century was still a dramatic and often a quite public event. As had been true throughout the long history of surgery, an operation was a capital occasion, much like public dissections in the Renaissance or executions in the centuries that followed. Surgery too, unless carried out on the privacy of the kitchen table, was often still open to public view. The anatomical theatre and its descendant, the operating theatre, provided the stage for public spectacles. These events are now private and sterile occasions. In an earlier time neither the painter nor later the photographer was necessary to publicize the event or to open it to public view. By the time of Thomas Eakins, however, usually only physicians and medical students were found in attendance at a surgical clinic. It was his aim both to celebrate the work of the surgeon and once again to open it to wider, public view. And it was on this latter point that the critics of the time were most negative in their reviews.

Eakins received relatively little attention and even less praise during his lifetime. Nor was he ever able to sell many paintings. That the Jefferson Medical College has refused offers of several million dollars for *The Gross Clinic* would have astounded as well as pleased Eakins. That subsequently his surgical scenes have been called masterworks and among the most important works by any American artist would have pleased him even more.

Only one contemporary critic of *The Gross Clinic* was consistently favourable in his reviews of the painting. The Philadelphian William Clark, Jr, of the *Evening Telegraph* regarded it as a work of great learning and of great dramatic power. He went so far as to say, 'we know of nothing greater that has ever been executed in America'.[30] This was fairly heady praise for a young artist who wished to establish himself with such a major work. But, alas, Clark's fellow reviewers had quite a different reaction.

The first blow to Eakins's pride came when the committee that chose the American art for the Centennial Exhibition did not include *The Gross Clinic*. Instead, the painting was hung in a government building that housed a medical exhibit. This slight must have been a serious blow to Eakins, lessened only by the fact that five of his other paintings were chosen. In 1878 the painting was bought by the Jefferson Medical College for $200. When the painting was exhibited in New York in 1879, the reaction was swift. The *Herald* called it strong and startlingly lifelike, but 'decidedly unpleasant and sickenly real in all its gory details'.[31] The critic for the *Tribune* went so far as to wonder why it was ever painted in the first place and exhibited in the second. The *Times* asserted that the showing of a bare thigh was indecent. Calling it a violent and bloody scene, the *Times* critic chided Eakins for confusing the beauty of the nude and the indecency of the naked, but admitted that power it had, if little art.[32]

There were other aspects of the painting which were the subject of criticism and discussion that also deserve our attention. The *Tribune* critic made a condescending remark about the young man who was recording the scene: 'A mile or so away, at a high-raised desk another impassive assistant records with a swift pen the Professor's remarks'.[33] What this critic apparently failed to realize was that the reports of the clinics of many professors of surgery were regular features of the medical journals of the day. Gross's operations, for instance, appeared about monthly in the *Philadelphia Medical Times*. These clinics, then, were important surgical teaching exercises that discussed the criteria for operating, the natural history of the diseases in question, the types of surgical approach used, the types of dressings and post-operative care that seemed to work best, and the complications that might arise. By thus appearing in print, the teacher of surgery was able to reach an audience far beyond the walls of the operating theatre.

Art historians have discussed the enigmatic elements of *The Gross Clinic*. At first glance it is difficult for the viewer to orient the body of the patient properly. That the bare thigh belongs to a person lying on his right side and is indeed attached to a body with a head at one end and feet with socks at the other takes a bit of study. Beyond the enigmatic elements, the surgical scene presents as a contemporary statement of surgical history. I would also suggest that Eakins was sufficiently familiar with the art and the science of surgery in 1875 that he left little or nothing to chance.

We may even postulate that Eakins, in his attempt to portray the intense drama inherent in such an operation, also signified for us an aspect of medicine of great and enduring importance – the element of uncertainty.

Still another aspect of the painting that poses an interesting puzzle for the historian of surgery is the presence of the cringing woman to the right and rear of the surgeon. She adds great drama to the scene; an unfriendly New York critic called it melodrama. The woman has been variously called a relative or the mother of the patient. Common wisdom among art historians is that in charity cases a relative of the patient was required to be present. For this assertion we should examine the evidence, for if it is true, it would be a very important comment upon the sociology of nineteenth-century medical care.

I will begin by stating that I am sceptical about this requirement. What is perhaps most difficult for the historian who knows anything about the work of Thomas Eakins is simply to dismiss this cringing woman in her dark dress as a bit of dramatic licence on the part of the artist. Eakins was justifiably known for his painstaking study of shape, form, perspective and grouping. His was a realism that permitted no such casual intrusion, I believe. As I have said, he left little or nothing to chance.

I have also, so far in my own search, been unable to find any discussion of such a requirement of a relative's presence. The critic for the *New York Tribune* in 1879, previously cited, chided Eakins for painting the woman out of proportion, with an effect that she was perceived to be a great distance from the operating table. This writer also asked the crucial question: '. . . is it usual for the relatives of a patient who is undergoing a serious operation to be admitted to the room?'.[34] Whether or not it was, this writer believed that her presence in the painting introduced a wholly unnecessary melodramatic effect. Unfortunately, he continued, 'neither the recording scribe or the old woman has any right at all to be in the picture. They are only here for the sake of effect.'[35]

I say 'unfortunately' because a scribe was probably frequently present in the surgical amphitheatre. Can we then simply dismiss the woman's presence as done for effect? Possible, but I believe not likely. If, as has also been the claim of art historians, the patient was a young boy (and there really is no very firm evidence for this either, I believe), then one possible interpretation is that Eakins here tried to suggest parental consent. This would be somewhat more understandable than the stipulation of a relative's presence.

In the absence of any good evidence, I will, for the time being, still maintain the position that Eakins must have observed such a scene, for he was not a frivolous reporter, nor was he in the habit, as the *Tribune* critic asserted, of taking much artistic licence. Melodrama was not his stock-in-trade either. So, for the moment we are left without a full interpretation of the meaning of this part of the painting.

The drama of the scene is heightened for the viewer because we must confront the emotional response of this woman whose gnarled and claw-like fingers serve to evoke sensations of horror, disgust and the like. It is of interest that none of the art historians I have so far read has commented on a major anatomical abnormality of the woman's hand – the one raised in front of her face has six fingers. Eakins did not have to become an expert on human anatomy to avoid such a glaring mistake. The only plausible explanation, I believe, is that the hand of the almost invisible assistant sitting at the table behind Dr Gross is comforting the distraught woman. So the extra finger belongs to his hand, partly resting upon hers. I am indebted to Dr Frederick Wagner of the Jefferson Medical College for this astute observation.

About the surgical procedure itself, there is much less doubt. Contemporary sources claimed that Gross was about to remove a sequestrum of the femur from his patient. This was an operation he much favoured over amputation, and it was the hallmark of what his contemporaries called conservative surgery.

The important procedure of removal of a sequestrum could only come into general use after the advent of anaesthesia. As Theodor Billroth notes, 'the operation is a very violent one, and the chiselling, sawing, and hammering about the bony case appear horrible to a looker on, especially as the operation may require a great deal of time. An amputation is a trifle in comparison with it.'[36] Perhaps it was just this horror that Eakins was trying to convey in the image of the cringing woman sitting behind Gross, unable to watch. With the advent of the newer surgery such horror was relegated to the past. Viewed in

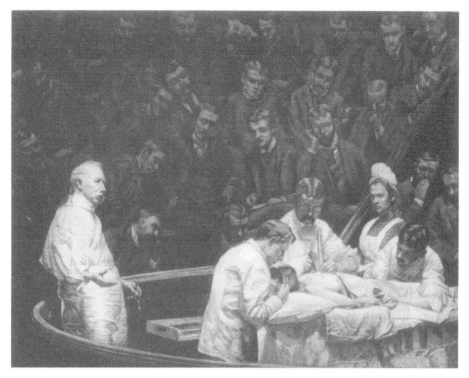

Fig. 72. Thomas Eakins, *The Agnew Clinic*.

this way, the painting itself was a historical lesson as well as a contemporary statement.

Very early in 1889, the students of the three classes at the University of Pennsylvania School of Medicine decided to pool their funds and commission a painting of their retiring Professor of Surgery, Dr D. Hayes Agnew. They approached Eakins and offered him $750 to paint the portrait. It was his largest commission, and with it he set out to paint his largest canvas. Since the students wished to have it finished so they could present it on graduation day, 1 May, Eakins literally had to work day and night for three months. That he finished the task in time is proof not only of his great skill and concentration, but of his physical stamina as well.

A painting is fundamentally, of course, the creation of the artist, but it does, nevertheless, invite us to historical appreciation and speculation about what is portrayed. The fourteen years since *The Gross Clinic* of 1875 witnessed the evolution of a new surgery, as already discussed. All this is very evident in *The Agnew Clinic*, a painting quite different from its large predecessor. The sterile appearance of the scene, better lighting and a horizontal grouping are the most obvious changes.[37] Agnew, in a regal pose, is definitely off to the side of the scene. It is possible that Eakins wanted to convey him as an Olympian figure, while Dr Gross was more involved as a man of the people with whom he worked.

It is sad, if not surprising, that the public reaction to *The Agnew Clinic* was not a great deal more positive than had been the case fourteen years before. Eakins is reported to have told a friend, with tears in his eyes, 'They call me a butcher, and all I was trying to do was to picture the soul of a great surgeon.'[38]

David Hayes Agnew, like his older Philadelphia surgical contemporary Samuel D. Gross, was born in Pennsylvania. In contrast to Gross, who came from sturdy but humble stock, Agnew's father was a physician and his family had business assets. Eakins, who admired Agnew as a surgeon and teacher but probably identified far more readily with the less patrician Gross, captured the difference in social origins of these two surgeons in a striking manner in the two paintings.[39]

Agnew received his medical degree from the University of Pennsylvania in 1838, and for a few years joined his father in a country practice. Like Gross and Eakins, he was also an avid anatomist, taught in the Philadelphia School of Anatomy. He became Professor of Surgery at his Alma Mater in 1871, and on its founding in 1878 was the first to hold the distinguished John Rhea Barton chair in surgery. Once again Eakins chose to portray his subject in a teaching role.[40] Although both Gross and Agnew were renowned for their teaching, it is important to remember that they belonged to those generations of surgeons who were largely self-taught.

Agnew was known to be an ambidextrous surgeon, a circumstance of necessity because of an early injury he suffered to a finger of his right hand. Eakins portrayed him with scalpel in the left hand. Agnew also was widely involved in surgical consultations, his most famous case being President Garfield in 1881. It was at this time, as his biographer noted, that the eyes of the world were on that scalpel.[41]

Coming just at the midway point between our two paintings, the shooting of Garfield in July 1881, and his daily care until his death two months later, was the first medical case to be so consistently and publicly reported in the press and in the medical literature. For the historian of surgery it provides elements of both the new and the old surgery, and thus good evidence for a transition period. Viewed in this light the case deserves further historical study.

As one great physician's career was winding to a close with the gift of his portrait that would ensure his lasting fame, another's career was about to take a remarkable turn on its path to fame. As Agnew Day was being celebrated at the University of Pennsylvania, the students' much beloved Professor of Clinical Medicine was giving his farewell address before he departed from

Philadelphia to head ninety miles farther south to take up a post in a brand-new hospital whose fame along with his own would soon take on almost legendary proportions. The title of the talk the graduates heard on that day in Philadelphia was 'Aequanimitas', and the name of its author was William Osler. The subject matter of Osler's talk, equanimity, was incidentally an ideal one for Agnew Day. Though Osler did not so acknowledge it, the retiring surgeon was well known both for his stamina and for his equanimity.

Since one of the main themes of this chapter is a focus upon the fifteen-year period that separated the Gross and the Agnew paintings, it is time to compare them, at least briefly. How did the characterization of Gross differ from that which Eakins ascribed to Agnew? Can we detect any differences in the surgical settings themselves? Do the students and assistants vary in their places of their roles? Did the artist's choice of disease reflect a changing pattern or a change in the surgical approach to disease? Do we see in these paintings an evolution from conservative to radical surgery? These, and many more, questions come readily to mind. Answers, unfortunately, are more problematic, but the paintings serve as convenient a focus for a series of discussions about the evolution of surgery a hundred years ago, as do any historical documents.

Both paintings are very large, *The Gross Clinic* is 6½ × 8 feet, and *Agnew* 6½ × 11 feet, and thus quite overpowering just because of their scale. There is an immediate perception of a dark, sombre and dramatic scene in the Gross painting, compared to the more open, better-lit, sanitized scene that greets the viewer in the Agnew one. Part of the effect was no doubt intentional on the part of Eakins. It has been said that Agnew wished no visible evidence of blood on his hands: both he and Eakins were well aware of the intense reaction which had been aroused by *The Gross Clinic*. But there was also an important technical advance in the operating theatre by 1889: Agnew worked with the help of artificial light. In Gross's time, surgery was still usually done during the midday hours when daylight shining through a skylight was its maximum intensity. Thus once again the artist was faithfully recording the scene before him. The more even light in the Pennsylvania amphitheatre allowed him to paint the onlookers with recognizable detail. That some of the students appear a bit distracted, and that one of them is reclining and possibly asleep, all give the painting a still more realistic feeling.

That the artist himself appeared in both paintings, as indeed he did in rowing, swimming and hunting scenes as well, seems evidence enough that he wished to be as closely identified with the surgical activities as he was with the sporting ones.

There is no doubt that Eakins had great admiration for both Gross and Agnew, but because of his closer relationship to Jefferson he doubtless was more intimate with Gross. In any event, Eakins did indeed choose to characterize them differently. Whether the difference arose from a greater or lesser familiarity, or whether it was a result of his own choice of Gross as a subject, while the Agnew painting was done on commission by request of the graduating class at Penn, need not detain us, for it is a difficult question to decide.

What we see in the Gross Clinic is an imposing figure, deeply involved in the surgery at hand, appearing knowledgeable and about to share that knowledge with his class. There is also little doubt that the figure of Gross is that of a surgeon fully in command. The surgeons are all intent on their tasks, a feature common to both scenes. But the most noticeable difference between them is the type of clothing they wear to the operating room, a point to which I will return.

Another major difference between the two paintings is the presence of the nurse in the later one. Stolid, ready to assist, but not actively involved, she is one of two women in the painting; the other is the patient. The nurse contrasts with the only woman in *The Gross Clinic*, who has the role of an unwilling bystander. In neither painting are there any women students or assistants. Agnew was a known opponent of women in medicine, and for a time left his position at the Pennsylvania Hospital rather than teach a mixed class of students.

Agnew, as well as Gross, was known for his teaching. His massive three-volume textbook is certainly evidence of that. Since Eakins too was a dedicated teacher, as I have already noted, it is not surprising that in both of his large surgical canvases he chose to portray a teaching scene. Agnew's students, of course, wished to commemorate their revered professor on his retirement from his chair. Both of the paintings clearly reveal the stages of a surgical career – from eager student, to junior assistant, then to active senior assistant and, finally, to the pinnacle reached by Gross and Agnew.

Both Eakins's surgical scenes show teaching in an amphitheatre setting. There are scores of photographs and some additional paintings as well as countless descriptions of this method of teaching. Only rarely did anyone question how much the onlookers could see and learn. The artist of an 1889 picture of a surgical scene at the Massachusetts General Hospital hints to his viewers that both seeing and hearing were probably difficult. One of the onlookers in the very first row is using binoculars, another is cupping his ear. One man in the back row also has binoculars. What the others who are looking without such aid actually see is, of course, the question.

Abraham Flexner, in his usual pungent style, was very critical of such learning at a distance:

Its pedagogical value is relatively slight; for operations are performed in large amphitheaters in which the surgeon and his assistants surround the patient, to whom they give their whole mind, in practical disregard of the students, who loll in their seats without an inkling of what is happening below. Most of the students see only the patient's feet and the surgeon's head.[42]

To convey to us the remarkable changes that had occurred in surgery during the years between his two paintings, Eakins may well have used the setting of the operative scene itself, and also the striking difference in the garments of the surgeons. He may have used the light of the room to reveal the onlookers in far greater detail in the Agnew painting for two reasons. In the first place, since they all have been identified, we may assume that they were those who paid the artist's commission. Eakins thus acknowledged their contribution to both art and medicine. But he was a far more subtle painter than such a simple interpretation would indicate. I believe the symbolic change between the 'enlightened' students in the Agnew painting and their confreres, who were literally in the dark in the Gross painting, should not be lost upon us – improvements in mechanical lighting notwithstanding. It was an improved understanding and the optimism of the new surgery that he wished to convey.

We come, then, to the most noticeable difference between the two scenes. Agnew and his assistants are robed in white gowns and the table and patient are draped in far more elaborate fashion than in the 1875 painting. By 1889 the antiseptic principles of Lister had achieved far more understanding and acceptance than had been the case fourteen years earlier. In terms of art history, we are now iconographically in the age of Lister.

The last of the institutional developments in our fourteen-year period that was to be of profound significance for surgery was the organization of the Johns Hopkins Hospital. Its planning began in 1875, and the first patients were admitted in May 1889, thus corresponding almost precisely to the years between the two Eakins paintings. This story, too, is sufficiently well known that it does not need repetition here.

What is of importance for the theme I have been trying to develop is that with the organization of the Johns Hopkins Hospital and its close relationship to the University and its Medical School (which for financial reasons did not admit its first students until 1893), we now see the early culmination of the 'new surgery' in the work of William S. Halsted. Both in the laboratory approach to the problems of the surgeon, such as wound healing, and in the organization of a formal training programme of which the aim was to turn out not merely competent surgeons but, rather, surgical leaders, Halsted was guiding American surgery along a new path. Of course he was not alone, nor was the Johns Hopkins Hospital the only place to carry out such a systematic training program; but in its early years after 1889, physicians from around the country and abroad acknowledged its leadership role.

The Trustees of the Johns Hopkins Hospital, not immediately confident that Halsted had fully regained his health after his severe cocaine addiction just a few years before, appointed him as director of the surgical clinic when the hospital opened in May 1889. His quiet and methodical ways in both the laboratory and the operating room soon convinced them that he had recovered, and he was appointed Surgeon-in-Chief in 1890. By the time of his death thirty-two years later, his former residents were spread throughout the country, many of them heading their own departments of surgery. The hallmark of Halsted's surgical technique was an exquisite sensitivity in handling tissues and a very careful control of even the smallest bleeding vessels.

Halsted's close friend, the French surgeon René Leriche, summed it up most concisely. Leriche noted in his obituary of Halsted that he was the father of a school of surgery

which may be described as the surgery of safety; of a technique which sacrificed everything to the immediate and future success of the operation and the welfare of the patient. He put in force the most rigorous asepsis and the most uncompromising discipline in guarding the tissues from insult by neglecting no details, no matter how small . . .[43]

Thus in the work of Halsted we see the culmination of the early phase of the new surgery, a surgery based as much on physiology as upon anatomy, and a surgery that moved from the theatricality of the operating theatre to the privacy and relative sterility of the operating room. With the careful and methodical approach, indeed because of it, Halsted and other surgeons of this time were able to bring to surgery true therapeutic power. More and more in the literature of the 1880s, and certainly in the work of Halsted in the following decade, do we find the radical approach, meaning a decisively curative means of hernia repair, breast surgery for malignancy, and appendectomy prior to abscess formation.

While the juxtaposition of radical surgery with conservative surgery may at first sight seem contradictory, it was not so in the least. Radical surgery was the logical outgrowth of the conservative approach, and radical 'cures' could make little sense in the conditions under which surgeons operated prior to the 'school of safety', as Leriche called it. Thus the decade and a half that separated the two Eakins paintings was indeed an epoch in the history of surgery, as those who participated in it were well aware.

Surgeons have long been concerned with their image – in the eyes of their fellow medical practitioners, as well as in those of their patients. A sympathetic portrayal of surgery is not what one always finds, but surely in Eakins's hands, especially from a century's distance, one cannot but be impressed favourably. That the surgeons continue to be concerned about their image was evident in the opening paragraph of a recent brief history of surgery in America by an eminent surgeon. Acknowledging surgery as a part of the science of medicine, Allen O. Whipple stressed not only the healing that may result from the use of the knife, but claimed for his colleagues an important measure of sympathy as well. That he should feel the need to say that a sympathetic, understanding, tactful and courteous surgeon will achieve greater success, underlines the need to counter the still lingering image of the cut-and-slash type of surgery.[44]

In 1923, at the memorial meeting in honour of William Halsted, his friend Rudolph Matas clearly indicated how the surgeons wished to be viewed:

It is the harmonious unison of mind and the senses, the hand and the head, science and craft, exhibited in the supermen who have exalted the fine arts, from antiquity to the present time, that we find the ideal, difficult to attain it is true, that should be in the mind of those who aspire to the mastery of our profession.[45]

Of interest to our present theme of the relationship of the history of surgery to art is that Matas viewed the surgeon as a sculptor of the human form who needed sensitive fingers as does the sculptor and painter. 'But even more,' Matas waxed enthusiastically, 'he needs the broad vision, the cultivated imagination, the catholicity of artistic taste and human sentiment, that give to his manual accomplishments the attributes and qualities that glorify the hand in the higher arts.'[46]

And it was the marked successes registered by surgeons in the decade and a half between 1875 and 1890 that gave a significant impetus to the many medical developments that followed in the succeeding decades. While it is a theme I cannot elaborate further at the moment, it is important to stress, nevertheless, how much of the characteristic hospital-based medicine of the first eight decades of this century we owe to the sense and the sensibility of surgeons.

13

Training the senses, training the mind

MERRILEY BORELL

The introduction of instrumentation into medicine in the second half of the nineteenth century markedly altered the face of medicine and the place of physicians within it. New diagnostic apparatus derived from laboratory research instruments such as the recording drum kymograph transformed both the perceptions and expectations of medical practitioners.[1] Between 1870 and 1900 these new perceptions and expectations were increasingly built into medical education through the development of practical preclinical courses. Physiology was particularly influential in shaping this intellectual revolution. It led the way in developing an explicitly experimental approach to replace didactic training.[2]

The new practical courses developed in physiology and other preclinical sciences illustrate the changing values and new emphases associated with the use of precision instrumentation in the late nineteenth century. Exact measurement initially supplemented and ultimately supplanted the qualitative distinctions emphasized by preceding generations of practitioners. Diagnostic and research instruments, used at first to train the senses of medical students, soon became an important means for ensuring that students internalized the basic tenets of the scientific method. Practical courses, explicitly oriented towards laboratory analysis of physiological function, served to adapt these same students to the increasingly complex and specialized diagnostic techniques that

The Wellcome Trust generously supported this research. This chapter developed out of a paper prepared for the conference 'Twentieth-century health sciences: problems and interpretations', organized by Guenter Risse and Jack Pressman at the University of California, San Francisco, 23–4 May 1988. I would especially like to thank Bill Bynum, Ghislaine Lawrence, Alan Morton and Brian Bracegirdle for their many courtesies during my visit to London and Adele Clarke for kindly allowing me to prepare the manuscript on her personal computer. I am also grateful to Stella Butler, John Pickstone and Mike Cattermole who helped me to discover many intriguing resources in Manchester and Cambridge.

were to burgeon in the twentieth century. Indeed, instruments integral to the laboratory-based sciences both trained the senses and trained the mind in well-defined patterns of perception and reasoning that were to ensure the pre-eminence of laboratory medicine in the twentieth century.

This chapter explores aspects of the introduction and utilization of recording instruments in medical education in the latter half of the nineteenth century and the early decades of the twentieth. Important perceptual and cognitive changes resulted from researchers' increasing ability to record and evaluate dynamic physiological processes. The use of related diagnostic instruments supplemented and finally challenged the primacy of anatomical reasoning and with it numerous observational techniques that had been so successfully exploited in previous decades through the introduction of the achromatic microscope and the subsequent rise of pathology and bacteriology. In contrast to these optical instruments, recording apparatus accentuated process. It focused attention on the succession of individual events occurring in the body over time. The use of such registration techniques, and later electrical instruments which extended them, bound medicine more firmly to the physical sciences, linking medical research to a variety of commercial opportunities associated with chemical and electrical technology.

Provision of teaching apparatus and the furnishing of magnificent new laboratories for research extended the material foundations of medicine, attracting much attention and, in some countries, significant resources from the state.[3] The contemporary rationale for adoption of such analytical apparatus within medicine is thus of great historical interest. It helps us to understand how the physician's senses gradually came to be replaced by machine-based technologies in the twentieth century.

The late nineteenth-century context

Historians of medicine have recently explored the historical origins of twentieth-century diagnostic technology in the instrumentation of the nineteenth century. However, merely examining inventions, tests and devices introduced in the late nineteenth century gives us little insight into the important transitions, then well underway, that were shaping the technology-dominated medicine of the twentieth century. By looking instead at the context of instrument justification and use in this period, we can see clearly the consolidation of a new investigative rationale and a powerful organizational infrastructure that fostered later dependence on machines.

Stanley Reiser, Audrey Davis, Christopher Lawrence, Joel Howell and Robert Frank, among others, have examined in detail the introduction and use of new instruments in laboratory medicine and their reception among practitioners in the closing decades of the nineteenth century and the opening years of the twentieth.[4] Their accounts focus on analysis of contemporary debates as to whether instruments of precision actually provided the practitioner with new and useful data as advocates claimed, as well as on the extent to which diagnostic instruments intruded upon the doctor–patient relationship, shifting the focus from the patient to the disease. I shall extend their analyses by reconsidering this set of concerns from the point of view of late nineteenth-century pedagogy.

Late nineteenth-century instruments were for the most part investigative tools transformed for clinical purposes. Devices like the clinical polygraph, for example, represented the strong emphasis on measurement and quantification that permeated the sciences in the nineteenth century and transformed traditionally descriptive areas of investigation into quantitative, experimentally oriented new sciences. Recording apparatus like the polygraph derived from the revolving drum kymograph introduced at mid-century. Related instrumentation – in fact, a whole family of adaptations of these recording machines – spread from physiology to botony, zoology and psychology, as well as to clinical medicine, in the latter decades of the nineteenth century. In the early twentieth century, scientific medicine and experimental biology emerged together. These new terms were watchwords representing new emphases. Within each research arena, be it medicine or biology, new investigative tools and standards of exactness transformed the workspace, habits and professional ethos of practitioners.[5]

Late nineteenth-century researchers developed and adapted recording techniques, precision instruments and chemical diagnostic tests to make medicine more quantitative and exact. Most important among the procedures then being investigated were spirometry, sphygmography, cardiography and plethysmography. These analytical techniques supplemented the stethoscope, microscope, ophthalmoscope and thermometer as central tools in medicine. These precision instruments recorded changes in function. They yielded either actual numerical data or graphic records that could be measured to determine precise levels of function. Advocates presumed that measurements of lung volume or pulse patterns, for example, would permit more accurate diagnosis of disease. The temperature fluctuations portrayed graphically in temperature charts from the late 1860 had indeed given a precision and typology to the diagnosis of fevers. During these same years, research-oriented investigators argued that sphygmograph and polygraph records would be able to accomplish the same for pulse-correlated phenomena. The debates over the clinical usefulness of these new research tools, particularly the sphygmograph, mechanical cardiograph and electrocardiograph have been thoroughly documented by Christopher Lawrence, Joel Howell and Robert Frank.[6]

Despite the intensity of these debates and the limited clinical value of some of these techniques, such machine-based procedures did acquire stature in medicine by the turn of the century. This fact must be explained. By that time, recording instruments represented, indeed symbolized, the exactness of laboratory techniques and the ideal of a precise scientific medicine. Medical schools introduced laboratory training into their curricula through practical work in physiology, bacteriology, pharmacology and biochemistry, all laboratory-based sciences. Such work supplemented the traditional observational sciences of anatomy and pathology. Students practised new procedures and techniques in order to learn to measure as well as to observe, to portray function graphically and to incorporate scientific method into their diagnoses of disease. Educators argued that the laboratory experiences then being formalized not only trained the senses, thereby developing student facility in the art of medicine, but also trained the mind, introducing students to the scientific method, and bringing to medicine the rigour and critical thought representative of the sciences in general.

The graphic method

The use of recording instrumentation grew out of recognition of the limitation of the human senses in detecting and measuring physiological processes. Investigators could not analyse events which occurred very rapidly, nor could they measure the transitions which occurred. In the winter of 1846–7, the German physiologist Carl Ludwig invented the recording drum kymograph or 'wave writer' by placing a float atop a mercury manometer and attaching a pen to the float. The pen traced the changing height of the mercury onto a paper wound around a revolving drum. The height of the mercury, which previously could only be estimated by eye and which wobbled as the experimental animal's blood pressure varied, could now be measured precisely from the kymograph tracing. Ludwig used the kymograph to study blood pressure changes and their relationship to respiration.[7]

In the 1850s and 1860s, other investigators adapted this recording technique for study of the activities of nerve and muscle, as well as local circulatory changes in organs. In the 1860s and 1870s, the French physiologist Etienne-Jules Marey popularized these procedures, as well as the use of the term 'the graphic method'. In his classic work *La méthode graphique*, he displayed the simplicity and power of registration and graphic techniques for examining change over time. During the second half of the nineteenth century, physiologists around the world created other sensing devices and specialized recording drums to monitor a wide range of physiological events which had not previously been amenable to quantitative study.[8]

In 1873, in his discussion of the sphygmograph or 'pulse writer' in the *Handbook for the Physiological Laboratory*, John Burdon-Sanderson, then

Professor of Practical Physiology at University College, London, summarized the outstanding features of registration devices:

The purpose of the sphygmograph is to measure the complicated succession of alternative enlargements and diminutions which an artery undergoes whenever blood is forced into it by the contracting heart, to magnify those movements, and to write them on a surface, progressing at a uniform rate by watch-work.[9]

Like many of his contemporaries, Burdon-Sanderson understood the advantages of this instrument to be the magnification and measurement of internal phenomena which could not be analysed by the human eye. The pulse was already detectable by touch, but through use of the sphygmograph, main features of this physiological event could be 'seen' through the registration process. None the less, Burdon-Sanderson cautiously compared this method for evaluating the pulse to the physician's tactile sense. He referred to the 'supposed' value of instrumental measurement over the subjective and variable assessments of individual observers:

In man, no artery can be directly measured either as regards pressure or expansion. In feeling the pulse, we attempt to measure both by the sense of touch, and obtain results which, although incapable of numerical expression, are sufficiently exact to be of great value. In the sphygmograph, an attempt has been made to obtain the same kind of information by a mechanical contrivance, which the physician obtains by the *tactus eruditus*; the supposed advantage of the instrumental results over the others being, that they can be estimated by measurement and weighing, and that they are unaffected by variation in the skill and tactile sensibility of the observer.[10]

Twenty-five years later Charles Sherrington, opening the new Thompson-Yates Laboratories for Physiology and Pathology at University College, Liverpool, would express much more emphatically and directly the limitations of the human senses. Sherrington stressed the desirability of apprising students of these limitations. In reviewing the apparatus provided for each student in the new laboratory, Sherrington noted:

Experiments in examination of the senses are also conducted in this room, and the student is taught to test the delicacy and the deficiencies of his vision, hearing, touch, sense of temperature, tune, and space, &c. Few guess the possibilities, fewer still the limitations and deceptions of their own senses until they are systematically introduced to them.[11]

During the two-and-a-half decades between Burdon-Sanderson's and Sherrington's remarks, practical teaching in physiology became systematic and formalized. Throughout Britain, and in the United States as well, entrepreneurial physiologists created new practical courses, as well as the texts to accompany them. These courses surveyed the principal insights and discoveries of the new experimental instrument-oriented physiology that had been created since mid-century.[12] By the 1890s, experimental physiology was strongly linked to the

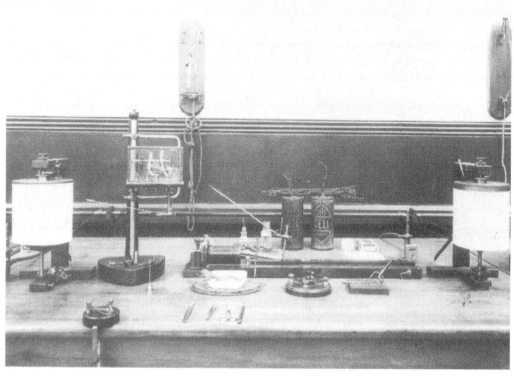

Fig. 73. Examination apparatus for physiology, University of London, 1890s.

graphic method and to exact measurement (fig. 73). A refined vivisectional technique exposed hidden processes to view. Sherrington noted that:

Each student's place is provided with electric light, water, gas, electric wire for supply of current, induction coil, electric battery, recording drum driven by fixed pulleys from the shafting running above the table, electric keys, heliostat apparatus for examining contraction of muscle, the beat of the heart, the measurements of respiration, &c.[13]

He stressed: 'In this room there is accommodation for a class of more than thirty students to carry out exercises on muscle and nerve, and in doing so to allow of each student for himself making use of the "graphic" method of study.'[14]

The experimental method

While William Sharpey had merely demonstrated the principles of the kymograph to his students with a cylinder hat,[15] by the turn of the century the centrality and necessity of such apparatus was assumed by medical educators. Physiology was seen as absolutely fundamental to training students in the new scientific medicine. In 1902, M. S. Pembrey argued in the preface to the first edition of *Practical Physiology*:

Physiology is the basis of medicine, and the further advance of these sciences depends mainly upon the 'experimental method'. The medical student, the future physician, should undergo a training in practical physiology, for thereby he learns the most important of all lessons; he learns to observe, to draw conclusions from his observations, and to unravel the causes of his failures.[16]

Although these educators assumed the primacy of physiology teaching in medical education, there emerged considerable debate as to which aspects of physiology deserved most emphasis. Muscle and nerve physiology had been particularly amenable to the graphic method and had assumed a central role in most physiology courses on both sides of the Atlantic. Pembrey observed:

The importance of practical physiology is undoubted, but as to the nature and scope of the experimental work which is most suitable for the medical student, there is considerable difference of opinion among teachers of physiology. In this country, perhaps, too much stress has been laid upon the physiology of muscle and nerve; for the hope that a study of the properties of these tissues will unfold the enigma of life is likely ever to remain without consummation.[17]

In the previous year, on the other side of the Atlantic, Edward T. Reichert, Professor of Physiology at the University of Pennsylvania, had summarized the main pedagogical issues relating to the teaching of practical physiology:

The general characters of the equipment must depend, apart from the matter of the cost, largely upon the main objects sought – whether the chief aims are, the illustration of the didactic course, the exhibition of physiologic apparatus and methods, etc. (which can satisfactorily be done in the lecture and demonstration rooms); or whether they are, the training in the use of instruments of precision with especial reference to clinical and experimental medicine, the cultivation of the individual powers of observation and deduction, the encouragement of and insistence upon accuracy of method and expression, the prosecution of collateral work with the view of the co-ordination of facts and their broad application, etc. If the latter, they cannot satisfactorily be attained with crude instruments, which at best are unscientific makeshifts and very often merely toys, and generally so regarded by the student. Aside from any other consideration the moral effects attending the use of instruments of precision and the pursuit of broad objects are far more salutary than the inexperienced, as a rule, are apt to believe, and it is perhaps needless to state that this course in the University has been based upon such views, and that time, labor and expense have not been spared to secure the highest results. It must not be supposed, however, that thoroughly satisfactory apparatus and expensive apparatus are necessarily synonymous terms.[18]

Reichert noted here that, in principle, teaching equipment could be adapted for demonstration or for actual use by students. As educators refined their goals, they demanded new instruments to secure these ends. Furthermore, suppliers emerged to satisfy the needs and requirements of large practical courses. Reichert, emphasizing the desirability of developing in students powers of observation and deduction, noted the necessity for good-quality instruments that were simple, compact, strong, easily manipulated, adapted to a variety of uses, compatible with one another, precise and reasonably priced. The main elements of Reichert's system for teaching practical physiology were the laboratory table, the recording apparatus and the stimulating apparatus. All of the instruments for his laboratory, over 2,000 pieces, had been made in laboratories at the University of Pennsylvania.[19]

Each university in Britain also provided extensive apparatus for its teaching laboratories. Between the late 1880s and 1910s, in fact, the manufacture and supply of instruments, as well as of laboratory fittings, had emerged as important support industries for science and medicine. This growth is particularly evident in the quality and quantity of recording instrumentation made available for student use during this period. In the mid-1880s, for example, the newly established Cambridge Scientific Instrument Company equipped laboratories at Manchester and Cambridge with driving pulley systems to provide power to turn recording drums in newly fitted lecture rooms and teaching laboratories.[20]

In 1895, William Stirling, Brackenbury Professor of Physiology and Histology at Owens College, Manchester, added an appendix on recording apparatus to the third edition of his *Outlines of Practical Physiology*. At the time, motors drove drums for student work; clockwork and weight drive were frequently used in research, although they could be adapted to motor drive by the use of small cogwheels. Motors were driven variously by gas, water or electricity. They were connected to the drums either by a driving pulley or by shafting with coned pulleys that allowed a range of speeds. At the Experimental Laboratory of the New Medical School buildings of Yorkshire College, Professor de B. Birch utilized a fifty-four-inch bicycle wheel as part of the gearing mechanism. At Owens College, Stirling used a gas-engine pulley drive system. Cambridge, Oxford and University College, London each had different drive systems in operation, constructed by their own physiological departments or local craftsmen. By the early 1900s, such shafting was provided commercially.[21]

The Sherrington physiological recording drum constructed in brass by C. F. Palmer (of 5 Kellet Road, Brixton) could be obtained in 1895 at the cost of five pounds, twelve shillings and six pence. Kymograph drums varied as to the mechanism for achieving different speeds. Stirling noted that Hawksley's form of the drum used different axles, while Ludwig's drum had an adjustable wheel. Non-drum recording mechanisms were also used, especially for studies of muscle, where the standard rotatory form was replaced by other types, i.e. a specially designed stationary, swinging pendulum, or horizontally displaced

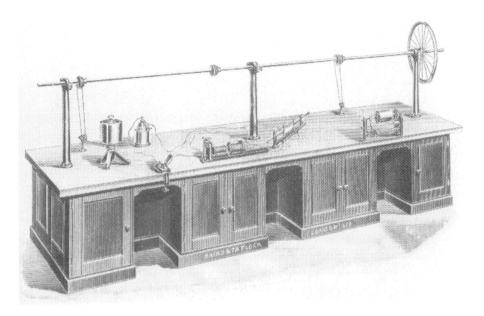

Fig. 74. Bench for physiological work for six students showing shafting and grooved pulley wheels. The large pulley on the right is fitted for coupling with a motor. Note the drum kymograph, battery, electric key, inductorium and spring myograph arranged from left to right across the bench.

plates. By the early 1900s, there was considerable variation in instruments and the data they produced. A body to review standardization issues was set up by a resolution made at the meeting of the International Physiological Congress held in Cambridge in 1898.[22]   The scientific supply company Baird & Tatlock supplied benches and shafting for physiological work at least by 1910. The then standard arrangement of shafting, flanked by standard physiological equipment may be seen in fig. 74. In their 1910 catalogue, Baird & Tatlock noted that laboratory fittings 'ha[ve] now become a very important branch of our business, and we have fitted up many of the principal new laboratories both in this country and abroad'. Indeed, at this time, Baird & Tatlock published a separate list for physiological apparatus. It covered blood testing and urine testing apparatus, as well as microtomes and dissecting sets for histological work. The widening industrial base of Baird & Tatlock's sales is evident in their identification at this time as 'manufacturers of assay, bacteriological, chemical, physical, and physiological apparatus, &c. &c. Laboratory benches, apparatus, and fume cupboards, &c.'. From the early 1890s, the signs on the front of their building at 14 Cross Street, Hatton Garden, London had advertised them as 'laboratory furnishers', 'pure chemical and scientific instrument makers' and 'dealers in chemical & physical apparatus'. At that time, their Glasgow office bore the signs: 'scientific instrument makers', 'educational and laboratory apparatus' and 'chemical warehouse'. By 1910, Baird & Tatlock, London, had become contractors to His Majesty's Government, India and Colonial Offices etc. While the majority of laboratories listed in the 1910 catalogue as fitted by them were chemical, bacteriological or pathological, they had also fitted the Physiological Institute, the Pharmacological Laboratory and the Chemical-Physiological Laboratory at University College, London, and physiological laboratories at St Bartholomew's Hospital, London and Queen's College, Belfast. Baird & Tatlock, 'makers of simple physical apparatus, suppliers of general laboratory apparatus and importers of German and Bohemian glassware', had been founded in 1881 in Sauchiehall Street, Glasgow by Hugh Harper Baird. The London company was set up in 1889. Baird & Tatlock were to acquire the kymograph manufacturer C. F. Palmer in 1964.[23]

When the new Physiological Laboratory opened at Cambridge University in 1914 it, too, had been fitted in part by Baird & Tatlock. There the Experimental Room for elementary classes was equipped for forty-six students, each operating his own recording drum; the nearby Histology Laboratory held 150 students working simultaneously. In the Experimental Room, the shafting was driven by an electric motor with pulley and cord. There were sixteen drums from the old physiological laboratory, some of which had been in use since 1884 when the Cambridge Scientific Instrument Company constructed the pulley drive mechanism. In 1914, by means of shafting and clutch, drums could be driven at six different speeds from one revolution per second to one revolution per thirty-five minutes. This allowed study of a very wide range of physiological phenomena. Indeed, the Experimental and Histological Room for advanced classes provided apparatus for measuring one ten-thousandth of a second.[24]

New laboratory facilities such as these in medical schools throughout Britain and North America reflect the growing material prosperity of experimental science before the First World War. Journals from this period proudly display the new spaces designed for teaching and research, as well as the fine precision equipment which these rooms housed. By the early 1900s, the Cambridge Scientific Instrument Company, C. F. Palmer and Baird & Tatlock all supplied recording apparatus to the burgeoning university and school trade in Britain. Both the Cambridge Scientific Instrument Company and C. F. Palmer worked closely with individual physiologists to perfect recording apparatus. Baird & Tatlock, on the other hand, like several other scientific supply houses of this period, served primarily as suppliers and fitters for the larger-scale needs of education and industry. The contents of the catalogues of these several companies reveal an important but unexplored interface between industrial and scientific enterprises in this period. These catalogues suggest that support industries and services for chemical and bacteriological laboratories in industry and medicine opened the way for development of parallel enterprises utilizing mechanical and electrical devices.

Promotion of the laboratory method

Stanley Reiser in *Medicine and the Reign of Technology* gives attention to the rise of bacteriological, serological and chemical tests, as well as to the increasing use of hardware, that is, instruments *per se*, in twentieth-century medicine. The close ties between the establishment of the teaching laboratory and acceptance and utilization of diagnostic tests and instruments has not been fully explored by historians. The promotion of quantitative techniques over qualitative methods was achieved by this important means in the late nineteenth century. Students were urged to utilize tools which not only extended the senses and made invisible processes visible but also promoted observation and detailed study of precisely those phenomena which could be measured. The rise and decline of the sphygmograph and polygraph illustrate this process well. Investigators sought to define graphic states that signposted disease. The pulse-tracing thus became the subject of intensive scrutiny until it was determined that blood pressure and electrical activity (also quantifiable events) could provide the deterministic signs physicians sought.[25] As practical handbooks from the 1890s and early 1900s stressed the importance of learning these evaluative techniques, the reading of graphic data came to surpass the value of ascertaining clinical signs directly from the patient (figs. 75 and 76).

In another project, Deborah Coon, Hughes Evans, Gail Hornstein and I examined the importation of the 'exact method' espoused in Germany and its transformation into the 'laboratory method' in the United States. In this work, we showed the large extent to which philosophical issues of the validity of exact measurement as a route to progress in natural science dropped out during the importation process. In the United States, methods, techniques and procedures were accepted with limited reflection or criticism of the assumptions inherent in them. Instead, American scientists seized upon, applied and utilized this approach in the scurry to establish laboratory-based science in American universities. For example, William James, unlike most American investigators, had serious reservations about the brass-instrument psychologists who tried to measure all phenomena of mind.[26] I suspect that this same attention to tools, techniques and methods in practical courses both in the United States and Great Britain explains in part the ready entry of new diagnostic procedures and instruments into early twentieth-century medicine. The rush to establish well-equipped laboratories and well-designed buildings presumed the validity of the exact method and quantitative, machine-based technologies for economic, intellectual and social progress generally.

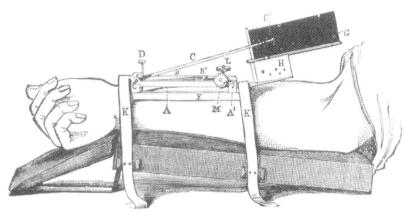

Fig. 75. Marey's sphygmograph arranged for student work.

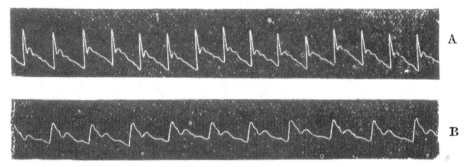

Fig. 76. Tracings from Marey's sphygmograph showing a 'hard pulse' and a 'softer pulse'.

The supply and advocacy of instruments

The use of instrumentation in the routine work of biology and medicine began in the nineteenth century and has continued without abatement to the present day. Diagnostic and monitoring devices now dominate laboratory, clinical and hospital settings. Most of these large and intricate machines derive from the proliferation of electronic apparatus after the Second World War. However, their roots lie deep within the changing ethos of medicine in the late nineteenth century – that is, in the transition from clinically oriented to laboratory-oriented medicine. Such instruments are the material expression of the new experimentalism observed in the everyday work, procedures and habits of both biologists and physicians from the turn of the century.

Looking at the tools being explored by investigators in the period 1900–30, noticeably lacking are the therapeutic emphases of the late nineteenth century, as they were expressed especially in electrotherapeutic devices. Lisa Rosner characterized the shift in her paper, 'The professional context of electrother-apeutics', where she commented explicitly on the differing goals of electrother-apeutists as opposed to surgeons and advocates of laboratory medicine. Rosner also noted how the significance of X-rays, extensions in a sense of the electrotherapeutic instrumentation of the late nineteenth century, was rapidly perceived as scientific and investigative rather than therapeutic. Joel Howell has begun to document the appearance of X-ray machines in hospitals, noting how their original role as curiosities changed as technicians were supplied and fees generated for the use of these instruments. The electrocardiograph machine gained acceptance in hospitals in a similar manner in the 1920s. Routine incorporation of data generated by these instruments into patient records correlates well with the curricular reforms that promoted the laboratory-based preclinical sciences.[27]

As already noted, it is during the period of transition at the end of the nineteenth century that scientific supply companies emerged. These companies were distinct from medical and surgical supply houses. For the most part they dealt in the new mechanical and electrical apparatus invented and popularized in the late nineteenth century. Elsewhere I have documented how, at the turn of the century, Associate Professor William Townsend Porter created one such company, the Harvard Apparatus Company. His goal was to supply cheap, high-quality, reliable and durable precision apparatus for the use of medical students in his newly restructured experimental physiology course at the Harvard Medical School. Porter's course, like those of many of his com-patriots at other medical schools across the United States, emphasized hands-on experience in the laboratory. Porter's innovation, the quantity pro-duction of teaching apparatus for physiology, was but one aspect of a major pedagogical revolution sweeping that country, as laboratory experience replaced didactic lectures and the culture of science gained prominence in American universities.[28]

The basic sciences claimed an increasing role in medical education in the United States, especially from the 1890s. Their successful move to positions of power and influence is evident in curricular reorganization during this period and in the Flexner Report of 1910. Educators argued that training the senses, developing coordination and training critical faculties were integral to the establishment of scientific medicine. Every medical student exposed to these newly established laboratory courses gained experience at the laboratory bench. Clinical correlation was a theoretical presumption but not necessarily an essential part of these laboratory exercises. Students on Porter's course at Harvard or Stirling's course at Manchester, for example, often used models or schema to simulate physiological phenomena like the circulation rather than relying on human subjects or clinical tools *per se*.

In one critique of the new laboratory medicine, Richard Cabot – physician at Massachusetts General Hospital and later Professor of Clinical Medicine at Harvard – in his 1907 address to the Congress of Physicians and Surgeons identified a developing paradox. He noted: 'There are methods in use to-day quite uselessly exact, and others in which a greater exactness is very desirable.' He argued that a dangerous dichotomy between the clinic and the laboratory has been created. Cabot stressed scientific medicine, not laboratory medicine *per se*. He emphasized the skills of analysis and deduction rather than the techniques and tools of experimental science. Cabot perceived two different choices for medicine, both modelled on the scientific tradition. He chose the route that stressed analytical rigour specifically. In the period 1910–30, Western medicine took the second route, the one rejected by Cabot, borrowing tools explicitly without the philosophical safeguards underlying the scientific method. The allocation of space, resources and personnel within medicine in this period increasingly went to the development of new laboratories and research institutes that represented the more narrowly defined pragmatic domain of laboratory-based medicine, which was linked explicitly to the use of diagnostic tests and precision instrumentation.[29]

While it took two or three decades before machine-based procedures were fully integrated into hospital practice and utilized to any large extent by practitioners, they none the less moved readily from the research laboratory to the hospital setting where they were used to a greater or lesser extent.[30] This transmission occurred because these instruments could be manufactured and sold even before their clinical value had been demonstrated. As noted above, numerous support for industries for laboratory research had emerged between 1870 and 1900, and instrument supply companies grew and multiplied. Supply is, of course, an important organizational factor that facilitates the acceptance of a new technology. The rapid transformation of cumbersome research devices into compact, often portable bedside tools meant that the usefulness of new devices could be readily explored by practitioners. The market was created, so to speak, as the instrument was utilized and its value reinterpreted in a new context, in this case at the bedside or in the hospital rather than at the laboratory bench.

Describing the development of biomedical instrumentation in recent decades, the authors of *Biomedical Instrumentation and Measurements* observed that 'the medical profession and hospital staffs [in the 1960s] were suspicious of new equipment and often uncooperative'.[31] These reactions certainly extend back to the turn of the century. They accompanied the appearance of new instrument-based techniques, which required the development of new technical skills not usually associated with professional training.[32] One common strategy of advocates was to create very simplified compact machines. Such black-box instruments entered medicine throughout the twentieth century through training in the preclinical sciences. Sturdy, simplified investigative devices adapted for teaching accustomed new generations of medical students to precision instrumentation and awakened them to the potential of quantitative techniques for understanding internal processes and detecting disease. Such strategies appeared prior to demonstration of the actual value of such quantitative techniques in medical practice. They represent the new values and scientific ethos being inculcated in students in practical preclincial courses from the turn of the century.

Conclusions

The entry of a variety of instruments and measuring devices into the everyday experience of practitioners is thus only one facet of the manifold intellectual and social transformations that marked late nineteenth and early twentieth-century medicine. By the period 1900–30, instrumentation in biology and medicine served four main purposes: diagnostic, therapeutic, investigative and pedagogical. Diagnostic devices were as yet fairly limited. The microscope and chemical and serological tests were utilized for diagnostic purposes. Electric diagnostic techniques like the electrocardiograph and electroencephalograph were introduced in this period and not fully accepted until compact models were made available in the 1930s. Therapeutic devices were also fairly limited; electrotherapy was then in evident decline. Investigative uses, however, were numerous. Recording apparatus generated a wide variety of graphs that extended the senses, vividly portraying functional change in graphic form. The fourth and most important use was pedagogical, i.e. to teach the attitude of scientific medicine by using these investigative techniques in newly standardized formats or exercises. It is through this latter process, I contend, that instruments became emblematic of the diagnostic and therapeutic potential of laboratory medicine. I am not arguing that these instruments had yet produced great changes in the physician's ability either to diagnose or treat disease. Rather, they were indicative of the faith and optimism that underlay the rise of scientific medicine. Like the large electrotherapeutic machines of the late nineteenth century with flashing lights and buzzing noises, they represented to new generations of physicians and patients alike the progress yet to be achieved by applying the scientific method to complex medical problems.

In the twentieth century, biomedical researchers have been exceedingly successful in designing increasingly precise investigative and diagnostic machinery. The use of these larger, more intricate machines has furthered the compartmentalization, specialization and fragmentation apparent in medicine from the turn of the century. Registration and monitoring techniques, in particular, have been refined and popularized through the development and marketing of portable units that, like the early laboratory instruments designed for student use, are sturdy, not delicate, and convincing in their visualization and simplification of complex body processes.

The persuasive power of machines and of laboratory evidence more generally was promoted in the early twentieth century in debates over the reform of medicine. Once these values were accepted and new laboratories built, new objectives followed: specifically, emphasizing investigation rather than reflection, and science rather than art (and clinical judgement) in medicine. This ethos is a persistent theme in twentieth-century medicine. It explains in part the ready entry of unproven technology into our health care system. Paul Torrens has observed quite accurately:

A still more profound effect of technology is its ability to insinuate itself into the values of not just the system but also of the people who work in the system. The student entering a health profession rapidly learns that academic success and, later, professional success, comes from mastery of the scientific technology. Increasingly, the student views excellence as being reached through technical achievements and gives decreasing importance to the more personal, nontechnical aspects of disease. By the time the student becomes a fully accepted member of the profession, a value system has been established that views illness as a series of technical problems to be solved by the application of specific technical solutions. This value system is then reinforced in practice by the expectations of the public and by the requirements of the regulators, both of whom have come to view quality in terms of technical excellence. The result frequently is a professional performance that is excellent in technical terms and rather poor in human terms.[33]

The set of values inherent in laboratory-based medicine became apparent only as this style of medicine grew in the twentieth century. Late nineteenth-century advocates of experimentally oriented medicine did not appreciate the full import of the promotion of laboratory-based medicine. What we see in this period is not so much technology-driven change as the creation of an intellectual climate and institutional context in which only numerical data mattered. Cabot contrasted the '*laboratory* methods of examination' ('the most *exact* instrumental methods') with the '*rougher* and more approximate processes used at the *bedside*'. He cautioned that '*clearness of statement*' was often more desirable than 'the use of figures and quantitative terms which mislead those who hear or read our statements'. 'What we want to know from every man is – "Just what did you observe, and just what inference can be legitimately deduced therefrom?"' 'We may easily have too much as well as too little exactness', he argued.[34]

As machines provided that precision and new tests proliferated, data rather than the patient claimed the physician's attention. Diagnosis rather than treatment became the focus of interest in this newly emergent milieu. Cabot's fuller vision of a truly scientific medicine was lost as methods, techniques, procedures and new instruments created research-oriented goals for those generations of practitioners newly trained in the ideology of the laboratory.

Practical manuals from the turn of the century attest to the hopeful aspirations of reformers. The display of tools and techniques laid before medical students asserted the limitations of the human senses and the ability of machines and chemical tests to go beyond them.[35] Practical experience in the laboratory taught the student to see and to think in a new way, accustoming him or her to data and insights which the human senses alone could not provide; that is, it taught the student to think as a scientist would, to remove intuition and quality and replace it with exact reasoning.

Such training at the laboratory bench was presumed to be ultimately applicable to the bedside. Russell Burton-Opitz, Associate Professor of Physiology at Columbia University, implicitly assumed this goal in 1920 in his introduction to *Advanced Lessons in Practical Physiology for Students of Medicine*:

Obviously, the acquisition of knowledge by the laboratory method consumes a longer period of time and requires a definite experimental attitude on the part of the student. Furthermore, this method of teaching entails the expenditure of large sums of money for apparatus and the salaries of additional teachers. These difficulties, however, have been overcome in recent years in all the schools of higher grade, and practical courses in physiology are now an accomplished fact and rightly so, because the benefits which the students derive from this kind of work cannot be overestimated. It cultivates the faculty of close observation and accurate rating of facts. It develops the power of logical thought and expression and impresses upon them facts and principles otherwise scarcely noted and comprehended. Indeed, many students must see things in order to obtain a clear mental picture of them, but when once seen, the impression is lasting. Where else than in medicine could this manner of teaching be of greater service?[36]

In the early twentieth century, the increasing preference for reason over the senses was evident even within clinical medicine. Cabot, in the introduction to his book *Case Teaching in Medicine*, argued that the data of physical diagnosis 'do not crystallize spontaneously into conclusions'. They need to be interpreted. Students ought to be trained in interpretive skills:

For this secondary and relatively easy step in the development of medical knowledge, one does not need the actual presence of a patient. With a book and a teacher it can be learned anywhere and at any time as well as in the clinic. Indeed it is easier to concentrate attention upon the processes of memory, comparison, and exclusion, which form the essence of diagnostic reasoning, if the senses are not distracted by the presence of the patient. *After the student has learned to open his eyes and see, he must learn to shut them and think*, and when he is thinking the less he has to distract him the better.[37]

Emphasis on scientific reasoning and the use of quantitative, often machine-derived, data permeated the elite medical culture of the early twentieth century. Students' senses were not simply extended or trained by experience in practical preclinical courses. Rather, medical students were taught to distrust their senses, even as they were trained to use them. As a result, the precise numbers generated by laboratory instruments came to signify the power of machines to go beyond the human senses and to define the domain of data on which the new scientific medicine would be based.

14

Technology and the use of the senses in twentieth-century medicine

STANLEY J. REISER

This chapter explores how the growing use of technology in medical practice of the twentieth century has influenced the application of the senses in patient care. It examines the nineteenth-century background that led to a new practice pattern in the twentieth century, focused around technology. It explores how particular technologies, such as electrocardiography, imaging technologies, laboratory examinations and computers, have replaced the senses in the acquisition of the evidence of illness directly from the patient. This has produced important consequences for medicine, including changes in the ways in which illness is perceived and understood by the doctor; in the ability of patients to present and have analysed the full range of problems and requests they may have; and in the future standing of the physician and medicine. In the discussion of these events, particular attention will be paid to the nature of the interaction between people and machines, and the problems that develop when technological relationships compete with and replace human relationships.

When in 1816 René Laënnec, in an inspired act of scientific creation, rolled into a tube a sheath of paper lying next to the bedside of his patient, placed one end to his ear and the other to the patient's chest, and heard the sounds of the motions of the organs within, he appreciated the potential of this discovery for improving diagnoses of chest diseases. But he could not foresee the even more significant outcome it would have of altering the diagnostic habits of all of medicine.

When Laënnec approached his patients, armed with this new technology, he was flaunting deeply held medical convictions that encountering patients with technology was inappropriate – that tools were reserved for action in the common trades and the specialities in medicine of lower station such as surgery. The physician was to observe and question patients to gain diagnostic knowledge, not to poke and probe their bodies.

But gradually the saliency of physical examination of the body using the doctor's senses, aided and extended by simple tools, overcame the resistance of custom to such an engagement. By the middle of the nineteenth century use of the stethoscope, as Laënnec's tube became called, was commonplace, and acceptable to doctor and patient. Moreover, the ideology of physical examination was, by now, a part of the mainstream of medical thinking. This ideology emphasized illness as a physical event, to be detected by tools placed physically on and within the body, but always connected at one end with a particular sense of the doctor.

The anatomic view of illness had by this time been accepted. Beginning with the interest in anatomy stimulated by Vesalius's 1543 treatise *On the Structure of the Human Body*, which depicted normal anatomy, continuing to Morgagni's 1761 work *The Seats and Causes of Diseases Investigated by Anatomy*, and ending with Virchow's *Cellular Pathology* of 1858, a clear perspective had developed on what diseases were. Diseases had, to use Morgagni's term, 'seats', loci in the body whose places were denoted by the fingerprints of structural disruption. Each of these prints was specific and thus characteristic of a particular disorder and, when discovered by the anatomist's scalpel or the microscopist's lens, gave to the beholder dependable signs of illness.

The use of tools and the doctor's senses to probe the body of the living patient for evidence of these signs was the hallmark of nineteenth-century diagnostic medicine, and the basis of its accomplishments. The doctor became a detective, seeking physical evidence of particular disorders. The patient's body became the field of investigation and the doctor's senses the media. When, towards the end of the century, Dr Arthur Conan Doyle created Sherlock Holmes, the arch-criminologist whose essential quality was detecting physical clues and deducing causes from them, it followed rather naturally that this fictional character was based on the qualities of one of Conan Doyle's professors in medical school, Joseph Bell.

We can argue fairly, then, that the nineteenth-century doctor had become a skilful diagnostician, whose highly developed senses and simple extending technologies provided the basis for acquiring the evidence for diagnosis. Doctors probed, listened and looked into the body – like explorers, self-reliant, seeking treasures. This self-reliance replaced a dependence on the patient's views to gain the facts about an illness, which was the hallmark of pre-nineteenth-century medicine. The patient's story, a medical biography, was a tapestry woven of events subjectively experienced. It contained the patient's feelings produced in the body by an illness, and the patient's suppositions about events of life implicated in their cause. It told of the patient's wants and hopes. But it was for doctors often a biography of truths and half-truths, exaggeration and belittlement. It was for them evidence they could not usually verify. From such dependence on the reportorial skill, memory and veracity of patients, it was an exhilarating liberation to rely on their own senses to detect the symptoms of illness. The result was a diminution in the doctor's attention to the subjective, experience-centred account of illness by the patient, and a turning to the evidence of illness the doctor could acquire directly through the senses.

Surely, the strides taken within nineteenth-century medicine to make the physician the analyst of physical signs, the detective armed with educated senses, had elevated the accuracy of diagnoses, and thereby the doctor's self-esteem and the patient's confidence in the medical enterprise. All of this was of decided significance, a large step forward for medicine – but was it enough for the doctor as the nineteenth century ended? Was something yet missing? Yes. The advances in chemical and physiological instrumentation and monitoring emerging from the scientific laboratory were making doctors feel that, in their understanding of disease, there still remained large gaps that only a new technology had a chance to close. A new technology emerged depending not on the senses of the doctor for their effect but on self-registering processes that 'saw' and 'felt', unaided by human perception. Such technologies would take the doctor into the twentieth century, and into a new realm of activity in which the significance of the doctor's senses in the actions of diagnosis would be challenged.

While physicians of the nineteenth century were grooming themselves as physical diagnosticians, developments were occurring in the laboratories of Europe and the United States that would change medical practice and custom in the succeeding century. Scientists of this time developed rudimentary tools to characterize and analyse the chemistry and motions of the body's organs and tissues. Simple chemical tests were developed by mid-century to detect in the human body the presence of uric acid, implicated in gout, and of albumin, implicated in kidney diseases. At this time, efforts to depict internal body motions such as the movements of muscles and the flow of blood also met with success through the development of the sphygmograph. This device required the placing of a needle in the body part to be monitored; the needle was connected to a mobile arm, which in turn was linked by a pen at its tip to a rotating drum banded with paper. The device then recorded the movements as a wave pattern. Such graphic and quantitative depiction of body events became an important ingredient in an effort to make medicine into a scientific discipline.

This development continued in the second half of the nineteenth century, from which emerged an innovation that serves to illustrate the competition of technology with the application of the senses in medicine that would emerge in the twentieth century. Like the stethoscope it was simple, small and portable,

an unlikely device to challenge the developments of a century. Unlike the stethoscope its origins went back hundreds of years to the end of the sixteenth
century – it was a technology in waiting, destined to linger unused until refined
to fit the needs of ordinary practice. This instrument was the thermometer.
The person principally responsible for developing it as a significant clinical
instrument was the German physician Carl Wunderlich in his 1868 treatise *On
the Temperature in Diseases*. Its use caused one of the quintessential sensory
examinations – touching the body to estimate its heat – to fall into disuse. It
had the virtue, typical of this new class of instruments being developed, of
seeming uninfluenced not only by the patient's subjective views, but also by the
doctor's. Wrote one enthusiast: 'While the doctor is chatting with his patient,
or interrogating the friends, the thermometer may be silently recording its
truthful tale in the patient's axilla.'[1] This 'truthful tale' was not a story of
words but a narrative of numbers.

Pictorial representation was a second important mode through which the
evidence of disease was depicted in this new vanguard of technology. The
principal device through which this became possible was the X-ray. X-
radiation, discovered by the physicist Wilhelm Röntgen at the end of 1895, was
a mode of energy capable of penetrating solid objects and recording their
image on a fluorescent screen or photographic plate. At first, the
announcement of this phenomenon left the world incredulous, even suspecting
a hoax. But when the first X-ray portrait of Madame Röntgen's hand was
published, incredulity became belief, and a new era was inaugurated. The
medical profession and the public marvelled at this new-found power to see
through structures opaque to the eye. Fears even developed that walls could no
longer shield inhabitants from the piercing power of the X-ray held in inquisitive hands, and thus that the era of privacy was at an end. Such fancies eventually gave way to more sober appraisals of the X-ray's benefits and burdens. But
even considered appraisal produced a view among physicians that X-ray
images provided unparalleled evidence about pathologies in all parts of the
body. Doctors of the day became enthralled 'in devising endless applications of
this wonderful process'.[2]

A third device captured another form of evidence that would become a
significant way of representing disease in the twentieth century – the device
was the electrocardiograph, which allowed the electrical activity generated
within the heart to be detected and depicted graphically. It was developed into
a clinically usable form principally by the Dutch physiologist Willem
Einthoven, who in 1901 first described his string galvanometer type of electrocardiograph. Its origins were the mid-nineteenth century device described
earlier, the sphygmograph. This electrical record of the physiological activity
of the heart provided an innovative view of its normal and abnormal conditions. It detected changes which could not at all be appreciated in typical

examinations of the heart through the senses – neither the hand which felt its beat, nor the eye which observed it through the skin, nor the ear which detected its sounds through the stethoscope could provide clinicians with the view its electrical activity could, when engraved graphically on a moving paper strip.

These technologies, prototypes of those that would dominate diagnosis in twentieth-century medicine, shared characteristics that produced their transcendence. Four have been selected for discussion.

The first is objectivity. One of the features that made the laboratory experiment an important feature in the advancement of scientific learning in medicine in the nineteenth century was the view that its procedures could be controlled in such a way that evidence produced through it would not be tainted by human subjectivity and bias. A characteristic of that which was called scientific was this freedom from such bias, or objectivity.

By the nineteenth century's end, as biological medical research was achieving the status of being scientific, it was natural for bedside clinicians to seek a similar achievement. If scientific medicine at the bedside were possible, its methods of gathering evidence must share the same hallmark as their laboratory brethren – the hallmark of objectivity.

As early twentieth-century clinicians soberly reviewed the means that formed the foundation of medical diagnosis, it became painfully apparent that, of its many excellent characteristics, objectivity in the sense it was now used was not among them. The techniques of physical examination were all dependent on the doctor's natural sensory apparatus to gather information. The eye would probe the body through simple tubes with devices for illumination – the opthalmoscope, laryngoscope and gastroscope for example. The ear would listen for sounds brought to it through myriad forms of stethoscopes. And touch was used increasingly to feel and palpate the body and the organs within it. These sensory signals, generally apparent only to the physician and hidden from other observers and the patient, were appraised by the doctor. Often they were translated by physicians into a written form and entered into the medical record for colleagues to see.

From the very start of this process, bias could creep in. Who knew what the doctor heard, saw or felt; or how events of the previous day, the nature of previous medical training or even the mark of heredity influenced the perception? The shadow cast by subjectivity over the accuracy of these perceptions was deepened by reflection about the interpretation given them. By what yardstick did the doctor's mind measure what was heard, seen or felt on the way to reaching a decision about their meaning? If observers could not themselves unambiguously discern the nature of the sensory signal perceived by the doctor, how could they judge whether its interpretation was appropriate?

When physicians who introduced the technology and ethos of physical diagnosis argued for its dominance, they presented the contrast as being between observations made by the doctors themselves through the use of their own trained senses, and the memories and descriptions of patients of the feelings and events that accompanied their illness. When given this choice, doctors selected as superior evidence they themselves gathered. Thus the views of the doctor about the illness replaced those of the patient, and the cast of nineteenth-century medicine was set.

The self-registering, numerical, pictorial and graphic evidence generated by the new technology, as in turn it was compared with the sensory impressions of doctors by the yardstick of objectivity, found doctors and their senses wanting.

A second critical variable in the diagnostic reorientation of twentieth-century medicine was one always in scarce supply in the life of a busy physician – time. To elicit the biography of the illness from the patient and observe the effects of disease as they were written on the body's external surfaces – the key pre-nineteenth-century techniques of diagnosis – or to physically examine the patient with the simple technologies of physical diagnosis, like the stethoscope, to enquire of the state of the body organs within – the principal diagnostic technique of the nineteenth century – both required the physician to spend time with the patient. The more meticulous the questioning or the examination, the greater the time spent together by doctor and patient. The diagnostic linkage between them that seemed so fundamental and unchangeable for pre-twentieth-century generations began to break down in our century.

The technology of self-registration made it possible to separate the act of receiving medical data from the act of interpreting it. A nurse, for example, could be given a thermometer, instructed in its use, and then could take the temperature of a patient and record its daily movement on the chart. All the physician need do was to come to the ward to read the chart. As Wunderlich put it, the doctor's job was 'not merely taking observations, but the superintendence, control, and right interpretation of them. The mere reading of thermometer degrees helps diagnosis no more than dispensing does therapeusis.'[3] Thus the acquisition of medical data with such instruments could be delegated to persons having less training and skill than those whose task it was to interpret them.

These events changed the face of medicine and the doctor's work in the twentieth century. The ability to develop a host of different self-registering technologies that focused on particular aspects of the body and its functions, and to train personnel to apply and record their results without the need for an extensive education, created a new and large cadre of technically focused personnel divided into specialities. For example, by the mid-1970s the allied health profession, which encompasses many of these less highly trained specialists such as the cytotechnologist and the X-ray technician, numbered within its ranks in the United States 152 different specialities and 1.8 million people.[4] Stated in another way: as the twentieth century began, one person in three in American health care was a physician; by 1980, this ratio was one in thirteen.[5]

This expansion of personnel in health care by technological advances has had an enormous influence on its organization and costs, events that must be noted but – in the context of this chapter – not discussed. However, the ability to become divorced from the gathering of data did mean a considerable saving of time was possible for the modern doctor. No more would it be necessary to spend time at the bedside meticulously percussing the chest to outline the heart, or moving the stethoscope slowly from place to place over the chest and back listening for sounds that would indicate a lesion. Instead, a swiftly written order to the X-ray department would produce the evidence needed. Moreover, as the twentieth century progressed, departments such as X-ray also routinely provided doctors with an interpretation, further diminishing the time they had to spend on case analysis.

So, the substitution of technological examinations by machines and technicians for sensory examinations made personally by the physician was encouraged not only by a belief in the technologies' greater objectivity and accuracy, but also by their time-saving and labour-saving qualities.

A third cause of the reduction in attention to the senses in twentieth-century medicine has been the advantage conferred by the new technology in terms of standardization and ease of communication. When it was time for physicians to convey to colleagues the evidence gathered through their senses by eye, ear or touch, problems of transmission generally materialized. Even doctors who used one of the earliest sense-driven procedures of diagnosis – pulse-feeling – reported on this difficulty. One nineteenth-century physician noted that a physician could pursue 'the habit of discriminating pulses instinctively (and learn) valuable truths from it, which he can apply to practice. Yet how difficult – how impossible – is it for the skilled physician to impart his knowledge to his less experienced junior.'[6]

The fundamental reasons why this and other sensory-derived evidence travelled so poorly from teacher to student or doctor to doctor was the problem of being sure each person was feeling, hearing or seeing the same phenomenon, and transforming what was sensed into words. The phenomenon in question was fleeting – a pulse beat or heart sound. One could not be sure that the second or third person who felt or listened experienced the same effect as the first – either because of a temporal change in the biological character of the phenomenon or because observers slightly but imperceptibly varied their examining technique, e.g., pressing on the pulse more strongly than their colleagues, or placing the stethoscope on a slightly different portion of the chest in listening for breath sounds.

In addition to variations imposed on sensory analysis by these factors, there was the problem of using language as the medium of exchange: how to know if one person calling a heart sound a 'grade two murmur' interpreted what was heard in the same way as colleagues. The dilemma demonstrated a major problem of sensory evidence – the difficulty of standardizing terms through which it is described.

Alvan Feinstein, Professor of Medicine at Yale University, studied this issue with his medical staff in the 1960s by having each physician specify the characteristics of a given physical sign that led them to call it normal or abnormal. He found that different physicians used different criteria to interpret what they experienced through their senses. In evaluating heart sounds, for example, one physician might focus upon pitch to determine its character, while another would add duration or change with posture. Only when Feinstein and his staff developed standards to use in eliciting or sensing physical signs, and in identifying them did their disagreements decline.[7]

The problem of developing standards for the acquisition of sensory evidence and its transmission to observers present at the bedside, or to those distant from it via medical records or journal articles, remained troublesome to clinicians during the twentieth century. Despite the great effort by Feinstein to address the problem, few medical staffs joined him in pursuing the arduous task of standardization. Moreover, an alternative form of evidence was before them that seemed free of the standardization and communication problems of sensory data – the numerical, graphic and pictorial evidence of technology. Such data had the advantages of being observable simultaneously by all members of a group. A machine which generated a picture, like an X-ray, or a graph, like an electrocardiograph, produced evidence on which all viewing it could agree. Further, this type of evidence could be compared, more readily than sensory data, with subsequently generated data. Moreover, the same evidence could be transmitted readily to others at a distance through medical records, correspondence or journals without loss of content.

From the earliest stages, inventors and users of diagnostic technology providing data in such forms recognized the advantages over sensory-based evidence for interpersonal communication. For example, Julius Herisson, the inventor in 1835 of a machine, called by him the sphygmometer, to make a column of mercury rise and fall synchronously with the beat of the pulse, promoted it as allowing doctors to observe the pulse simultaneously as a group. He noted that doctors in different cities distrusted sensory-based accounts of the pulse they had to accept when being consulted through the mails, but that 'a far greater degree of accuracy may now be introduced into such correspondence . . . the measure obtained at St Petersburgh will be perfectly understood at Paris'.[8] Writing in the early twentieth century about his newly developed electrocardiograph, its inventor, Willem Einthoven, conveyed the same measure of confidence as did Herisson: 'Every EKG, when and where it may have been recorded, is immediately comparable with every other EKG.'[9]

The greater dependability of machines than humans to detect and characterize the biologic data of illness has imprinted upon medicine of the twentieth century one of its most significant features – that secondary depictions of patients by technologic means can be more valuable than primary sensory-based portraits of patients themselves. Thus, the image of the patient developed through X-ray, ultrasound or magnetic resonance imaging technologies can be in this view more revealing of pathology than the patient herself.

This view is shared by the public. As the twentieth century has progressed, people have increasingly requested technological testing from physicians and hospitals to detect disease. They have been impressed by popular accounts of the scientific power of the new technology, which began, essentially, in media coverage of the discovery of X-rays.

The fascination of patients with diagnostic technology and the conviction that the power of the machines is greater than the power of the senses has led them increasingly to demand technological procedures, and to distrust examinations without them. The learned and well-known American physician Walter Alvarez commented in 1943 that when people 'go to see a physician they hardly think it necessary to give a history or to have a physical examination'.[10] Rather, they sought technological answers to questions about illness: 'All the average patient wants in a consultant's office today is tests and plenty of them; he wants to "be given the works".'[11]

This behaviour has continued to the present, fuelled by the belief of both doctor and patient in the new technology. By 1987, there were almost 1400 technologically based diagnostic tests, from blood chemistries to CAT-scans. In the United States that year approximately 19 billion were done, which amounts to 80 for each person in the country. The cost of doing these diagnostic tests was over $100 billion, or about 20 per cent of the total cost of health care in the United States in 1987.[12]

Thus, we have an interesting prospect to consider. If numerical, graphical and pictorial evidence with its qualities of dependability, objectivity and ready transmission among medical observers, is superior to the data gained through bedside examination using the senses, why should the doctor require the physical presence of the patient to conduct diagnosis? It might be done quite well in the hospital, office, or even in the doctor's study at home without the patient, using computer print-outs of laboratory test data, graphic depictions of physiologic function and evidence from imaging technologies sent in from imaging departments via a telephone line to a facsimile machine. Even the patient's story of illness could be taken by an interactive computerized history program and transmitted to the physician. Imagine the convenience to all concerned – physicians not becoming involved with the complex personalities of patients – and patients not having to struggle to gain the attention of busy physicians, whom studies show devote around six minutes in the United Kingdom (consultation with a general practitioner) and about twelve minutes in the United States (the average office visit) to the ordinary medical encounter.[13] I overstate such a future possibility (which I believe would be harmful) to sharply delineate the pernicious consequences of overvaluing the diagnostic saliency of technologic information and undervaluing evidence provided by the patient.

A similar extension of other technologic developments makes even a more simplified, odd and decidedly troublesome medical future possible – diagnostic medicine in the physical absence not only of the patient but of the doctor as well. This possibility, feared by some, and most undesirable, was created by the development of clinically useful computing power. From its introduction into clinical medicine in 1959, the computer has been embraced by physicians as an answer to handling the overwhelming load of clinical data being generated by technology, but also feared by them as the first technology to analyse evidence. All previous technology had either assisted the senses or replaced them, but in both cases the physicians were left the critical function of interpretation. The computer, with its power through programs to array, compare and portray the significance of data, now provided the interpretive function.

Programs were developed in the 1960s and 1970s to scan and analyse X-rays, electrocardiograms and microscopic finds, and also to diagnose diseases in limited fields like ophthalmology; these often performed as well as or better than clinicians. New computer programs for general diagnosis are being developed, such as one by the expert diagnostician Jack Myers and his colleagues at the University of Pittsburgh.[14]

This new analytic technology of computers challenges the decision-making capacity of doctors, just as earlier technology challenged their sensory abilities. Where then does this new situation leave the doctor and the patient of the present and future?

The application of the senses in the diagnosis of illness in the United States, where technology has been in the vanguard of practice more than in any other country, has declined during the twentieth century. Thus in 1931 James B. Herrick, an American physician and teacher, noted that medical schools were leading students 'to place the emphasis on the instrument of precision rather than on the eye, ear, hand of the physical examiner'.[15] This trend has continued as technology has been introduced that probes, using its own sensing system, the innermost reaches of the cellular structure, physiology and chemistry of the body.

Predictably, instruction in physical examination in the United States has declined, as techniques to detect illness which reach further than is possible with the senses are developed.[16] As diminished instruction creates diminished ability to use the senses, they will be applied less and less in cases where critical judgements are needed. Such diminished confidence in the senses points to their selective and limited use in the future.

This situation leaves the patient's biography of illness – the story the patient has to tell about experiences, needs and sensations – as the principal way doctors will have of connecting with the persona of the patient. The necessity of this dialogue and personal meeting is great. For the increasing range of data that it is possible to acquire through machines does not include insight into how the lives of the patient are interwoven with their illnesses. Further, the interaction through dialogue allows a crucial merging of the doctor's and the patient's views of the illness to occur. What doctors bring to this encounter is a knowledge acquired through experiences with people in like circumstances to the patient, whom they have met in the course of clinical learning and practice and whom they have read of and studied in the pages of medical texts and journals.

To this knowledge of the past, this distillation of how people with illness similar to the patient's experienced it, is added the thoughts of the patient in the present. The patient brings to this encounter a unique set of requests, hopes, fears and needs; a singular group of physical and mental reactions to the presence of illness. Both physician and patient must hear the other's story and combine the perspectives on the events of illness that each possesses in order to achieve a common view of what matters and what should be done. The physician's view of the past and the patient's view of the present merge in the ideal situation to form a common perspective on appropriate therapeutic actions in the future.

The necessity for such interaction precludes diagnosis wholly through technologic means. It precludes the two scenarios of medicine I described earlier in which doctors replace their own interactions with the patient with those with machines, or in which a computerized analysis replaces doctors themselves (an outcome that developers of such techniques, generally, have not intended).

The decline in physical examination and the use of the senses in diagnosis, as technologic substitutes are invented, seems to me inevitable, and as long as these techniques provide more dependable evidence, justifiable. However, there is a dimension of diagnostic medicine whose maintenance remains significant – direct connection with the patient. In order for a traditional stethoscopic examination to occur both doctor and patient must be together. Such personal communication must be maintained: for the doctor to know the patient and the patient the doctor is an important understanding for each to achieve. But as long as this interpersonal dimension of medical care is achieved through dialogue, I do not view with trepidation this aspect of the declining application in diagnosis of the human senses.

It is not possible to maintain skill in all techniques. This is one of the losses of progress in medicine. As new techniques and their accompanying theories are introduced, a decline occurs in the use of older ones. This decline is produced by the limit on the time available for learning and maintaining skill in a number of techniques. For example, the art of diagnosis through pulse-feeling could take a medieval physician a lifetime of hard study and practice to apply at its highest level. How then were nineteenth-century doctors to acquire and maintain pulse-feeling skills, while at the same time learning and applying the large number of new techniques of physical examination? They could not. The decline also is the result of the inevitable criticism launched by advocates of new techniques of those which are older, in order to encourage adoption of the newer ones.

While generally there have been developing reasonable technologic substitutions for sensory data, there is none for dialogue between doctor and patient. This keeps the presence of the patient in person essential in medicine, and is the best means of preserving its humanistic orientation in the technologic future.

Notes

Introduction

1 Saint Augustine, *Confessions*, trans. by R. S. Pine-Coffin (Harmondsworth, 1961), pp. 213–14.
2 Although a good deal of work has been done on the history of vision and hearing, sensory physiology more generally has been rather neglected, except as it relates to the history of the reflex. Probably the best way to approach the earlier history of the special senses is through the relevant sections of E. A. Schäfer (Sir Edward Sharpey-Schafer) (ed.), *Textbook of Physiology*, 2 vols. (Edinburgh, 1898–1900).
3 Diderot's *Lettre sur les aveugles* (1749) is a shrewd commentary on the interdependency of the senses.
4 A point stressed by Erwin H. Ackerknecht, *Medicine at the Paris Hospital, 1794–1848* (Baltimore, 1967).
5 Harris L. Coulter, *Divided Legacy: A History of the Schism in Medical Thought*, 3 vols. (Washington, D.C., 1973–7).
6 Cf. Erwin H. Ackerknecht, 'Elisha Bartlett and the philosophy of the Paris clinical school', *Bulletin of the History of Medicine*, 24 (1960), 43–60.
7 The phrase is from the title of Foucault's book: Michel Foucault, *The Birth of the Clinic*, trans. A. M. Sheridan Smith (London, 1971).
8 David M. Vess, *Medical Revolution in France, 1789–1794* (Gainesville, Fl., 1975).
9 John Harley Warner, 'Science, healing, and the physician's identity: a problem of professional character in nineteenth-century America', *Clio Medica*, 22 (1991), 65–88; John Harley Warner, 'The medical migrant's baggage unpacked: Anglo-American constructions of the Paris clinical school', in Ronald L. Numbers and John V. Pickstone (eds.), *British Society for the History of Science and History of Science Society. Programs, Papers and Abstracts for the Joint Conference* (Madison, Wis., 1988), pp. 213–20.
10 Martin Kemp (ed.), *Dr William Hunter at the Royal Academy* (Glasgow, 1975); Martin Kemp, *Leonardo da Vinci: The Marvellous Works of Nature and Man*, (London, 1981).
11 W. F. Bynum and Roy Porter (eds.), *William Hunter and the Eighteenth-Century Medical World* (Cambridge, 1985).

1 Galen at the bedside

1 Ernst Künzl, *Medizinische Instrumente aus Sepulkralfunden der römischen Kaiserzeit* (Bonn, 1983); G. M. Longfield-Jones, 'A Graeco-Roman speculum in the Wellcome Museum', *Medical History*, 30 (1986), 81–9.

2 L. Edelstein, *Ancient Medicine* (Baltimore, 1967), pp. 184–9; Michael Frede, 'The method of the Methodical school', in Jonathan Barnes, Jacques Brunschwig, Myles Burnyeat and Malcolm Schofield (eds.), *Science and Speculation* (Cambridge, 1982), pp. 1–23.

3 Paul Potter, 'Epidemien I/III: Form und Absicht der zweiundzwanzig Fallbeschreibungen', *Proceedings of the 5th Colloque Hippocratique*, Berlin, 1984 (Wiesbaden, 1989), pp. 9–19; V. Langholf, *Medical Theories in Hippocrates* (Berlin, 1990); J. Jouanna, *Hippocrate* (Paris, 1992).

4 Edelstein, *Ancient Medicine*, pp. 65–85.

5 W. D. Smith, 'Implicit fever theory in *Epidemics* 5 and 7', in W. F. Bynum and V. Nutton (eds.), *Theories of Fever from Antiquity to the Enlightenment* (London, 1981), pp. 1–10.

6 G. E. R. Lloyd, 'The Hippocratic question', *Classical Quarterly*, new series, 25 (1975), 184–7.

7 Hypochondrium: *Epid.* I.2; 3; 4; 8; 10; 11; 12; III.2; 3; 4; 8; 13; 16; spleen: *Epid.* I.3; III.3; 6.

8 Edelstein, *Ancient Medicine*, pp. 14, 17, 18 and 24.

9 *Prognostic* 7; 11; 12; 13.

10 Compare Edelstein, *Ancient Medicine*, pp. 71–81; Antoine Thivel, *Cnide et Cos?* (Paris, 1981), pp. 189–203; and Renate Wittern, 'Diagnostics in Classical Greek medicine', in Yosio Kawakita (ed.), *History of Diagnostics* (Osaka, 1987), pp. 69–89.

11 Edelstein, *Ancient Medicine*; Frede, 'The method'; G. Rubinstein, 'The riddle of the Methodist method' (University of Cambridge, Ph.D. thesis, 1986).

12 Frede, 'The method', offers interesting speculations about the philosophical rationale behind the Methodist claim to derive treatment securely from appearances.

13 The key text is Plato, *Philebus* 56B; cf. also Celsus, *De medicina*, Pr. 48ff., for the role of 'coniectura' (which may or may not be based on rational principles) in medicine.

14 The most relevant study of diagnostics in Galen (who is cited here by the volume and page in the edition of C. G. Kühn, 20 vols. in 22 (Leipzig, 1821–33) is Luis Garcia Ballester, 'Galen as a medical practitioner: problems in diagnosis', in V. Nutton (ed.), *Galen: problems and prospects* (London, 1981) pp. 13–46.

15 Galen, x.29; 629; XIII.116. The rewording of this conceit in XVI.81 is a Renaissance forgery. M. Frede, 'On Galen's epistemology', in Nutton (ed.), *Galen*, pp. 65–86.

16 Galen, XVIII B.632–57, summarized by Ibn Ridwan, *Compendium of Galen's Commentary of Hippocrates'* ΚΑΤ᾽ΙΗΤΡΕΙΟΝ, ed. and trans. M. C. Lyons. Corpus medicorum graecorum, Suppl. Orient. 1 (Berlin, 1963), p. 103.

17 Hippocrates, *On the surgery* 1; the discussions of the senses in two Galenic commentaries, XVII A. 336–41 and, especially, XVI.212–19, are both Renaissance forgeries (by G. B. Rasario?).

18 Galen, XVIII B. 652–3.

19 It is interesting that Garcia Ballester in his survey of Galenic diagnosis does not say anything about the sense of smell. At XI.700 Galen expresses doubts about the certainty of distinctions made purely from smell.

20 Justinian, Digest 21.1.12.4, a reference I owe to Ralph Jackson.

21 Martial, *Epigr.* x.3; XI.30; XII.85; cf. also the reverse of this joke at II.12, where Martial attacks the clean-smelling Postumus, because: 'non bene olet qui bene semper olet'.

22 Galen, XI.445, cf. VIII.87; XVIII B. 653.

23 Galen, VII.105. The reference at XVI.217 to the importance of tasting the sweat before making a diagnosis is a Renaissance fabrication.

24 Wittern, 'Diagnostics', pp. 85–6: cg. Galen, VIII.390; 951.

25 Galen, VIII.951.

26 Galen, XVIII B. 653. Others thought that the senses were those of the patient, the judgement that of the doctor.

27 Rufus of Ephesus, *Medical Questions*, ch. 1; for Rufus as a Hippocratic, see Wesley D. Smith, *The Hippocratic Tradition* (Ithaca, 1979), pp. 240–6.

28 In particular, Galen, XIV.640.

29 There is a good photograph of Dr Jason in J. Scarborough, *Roman Medicine* (London, 1969), pl. 37.

30 M. Michler, 'Die Palpation im Corpus Hippocraticum', *Janus* 57 (1970), 261–92; Wittern, 'Diagnostics', pp. 83–5.

31 C. R. S. Harris, *The Heart and the Vascular System in Ancient Greek Medicine* (Oxford, 1973), pp. 111–12 and 184–94.

32 Although no ancient text specifically attributes these names to Herophilus, they resemble in their fancifulness the anatomical terms he coined.

33 Harris, *The Heart*, pp. 397–402.

34 His major treatise on pulses consists of four interdependent sets of four books, which he later summarized in a single tract of double book length. He also wrote a treatise, one book long, on pulse doctrine for beginners.

35 Galen, XIV.661.

36 *Ibid.* Cf. VIII.616–7, for further examples of what Garcia Ballester terms his 'baroque conceits' of sphygmology.

37 Galen, VIII.504–6.

38 Harris, *The heart*, pp. 396–431.

39 Cf. W. H. Broadbent, 'The Croonian lectures on the pulses', *British Medical Journal* (1887), 655–60.

40 Harris, *The Heart*, pp. 187–92.

41 Wittern, 'Diagnostics', p. 77.

42 Galen, III.110–11.

43 Wittern, 'Diagnostics', pp. 87–8.

44 The quotation is from Plato, *Phaedrus* 270 c 2; the alternative explanation is that 'the whole' refers to the whole of the patient's body and not just to the affected part. Despite vigorous debate, the precise interpretation of this phrase still seems to me to be elusive.

45 For the latter, see the quotation preserved by al-Masudi, trans. B. de Meynard, *Les prairies d'or*, vol. II (Paris, 1863), p. 33.

46 Especially in his commentary on *Epidemics* VI, trans. F. Pfaff, Corpus medicorum graecorum, V 10,2,2 (Berlin, 1956), pp. 483–95.

47 His whole tract *On Prognosis* is designed as an exemplary series of cases, and many of his other treatises, for example, the *Method of Healing*, have case histories as the climax to individual books.

48 Galen, *On Affected Parts*, v.8 (VIII.362–6.).

49 This is the overall message of *On Prognosis*. Cf. Garcia Ballester, 'Galen as a medical practitioner', *passim*.

50 Galen, *On Prognosis*, 7 (XIV.635–41).

51 Garcia Ballester, 'Galen as a medical practitioner', p. 20.

2 Sensory perception and its metaphors

1 Paris, Bibliotheque Nationale, fr. 412, fol. 228r. A virtually identical image appears in this manuscript on fol. 237v, at the opening of the accompanying *Response* (a reply in a woman's voice to the contents of Richard's text). The texts are edited by C. Segre in *Li bestiaires d'amours di Maistre Richart de Fornival e li response du*

bestiaire (Milan, 1957); translated by J. Beer in *Master Richard's Bestiary of Love and Response* (Berkeley, 1986). These two works are cited hereafter as Segre and Beer, respectively. On MS fr. 412, see Segre, pp. xxxvii f.; C. Hippeau, *Le bestiaire d'amour* (Paris, 1860) – a transcription of the manuscript with forty-eight line-drawn reproductions. On the image, see C. Nordenfalk, 'Les cinq sens dans l'art du moyen âge', *Revue de l'art*, 34 (1976), 17–28, esp. pp. 22–3 and fig. 9.

2 In the Latin 'Omnes homines natura scire desiderant' (G. Vuillemin-Diem (ed.) *Aristoteles Latinus*, vol. xxv (2) [Leiden, 1976], p. 7). On the widespread employ of this *sententia* see Segre, p. vii.

3 Segre, p. 4; Beer, p. 1.

4 'Ceste memoire si a .ij. portes, veïr et oïr, et a cascune de ces .ij. portes si a un cemin par ou on i puet alet, che sont painture et parole. Painture sert a l'oel et parole a l'oreille. Et comment on puist repairier a le maison de memoire et par painture et par parole, si est apparant par chu ke memoire, ki est la garde des tresors ke sens d'omme conquiert par bonté d'engien, fait chu ki est trespassé ausi comme present' (Segre, pp. 4–5; Beer, p. 1). Richard's revealing statements about speaking and writing, hearing and reading, and text and image have been analysed by S. Huot in *From Song to Book: The Poetics of Writing in Old French Lyric and Lyrical Narrative Poetry* (Ithaca, 1987), pp. 135–73.

5 More normally illustrators would show the poet writing or reading aloud, sometimes in the presence of his lady. Segre, p. clvii; Huot, *From Song to Book*, pp. 164–73.

6 Paris, Bibliothèque Ste-Geneviève, MS 2200, fol. 173r. A. Boinet, *Les manuscrits à peintures de la Bibliothèque de Ste-Geneviève de Paris*, Bulletin de la Société Française de Reproductions de Manuscrits à Peintures, vol. v (Paris, 1921), pp. 47–59; Segre, pp. xlv–xlvii.

7 Boinet, *Manuscrits à peintures*, p. 57.

8 Paris, Bibliothèque Nationale, MS fr. 1951, fol. 1r. Described by V. A. Kolve within a discussion of medieval theories of memory and mental images in *Chaucer and the Imagery of Narrative* (Stanford, 1984), pp. 25–6. The verse redaction, anonymous, is edited by A. Thordstein in *Le bestiaire d'amour rimé* (Lund, 1941).

9 While a disembodied ear is most easily recognized straight on, the eye could have been rendered intelligibly either frontally or from the side. An eye in profile may have been preferred because it would not engage the viewer, but seem active and mobile and unaware of scrutiny. The artists may, too, have been fighting the mind's tendency to animate an entity bearing a frontal eye.

10 Huot wonders if the figure might be Richard's lady none the less, since the opening lines of the *Bestiaire rimé* address her and since it is her memory that Richard is seeking to reach (*From Song to Book*, p. 159). Rubrics for miniatures never executed in an early fourteenth-century manuscript (Paris, Bibliothèque Nationale, MS fr. 12786), to which Huot calls attention (p. 164), reveal that Memory was to be represented in the opening miniature ('ceste damoisele est memoire' (Segre, p. xxxix)). The personified Memory appears in a fourteenth-century copy of the *Bestiaire* (Paris, Bibliothèque Nationale, MS fr. 12469, fol. 1r): the female figure who stands before a castle with two bright orange gates holds two banners – unlikely attributes for Richard's lady to bear. Kolve, *Chaucer*, p. 381 n.27.

11 *Metaphysics*, 1013a40: 'ut finis; hoc autem est quod est cuius causa' (Vuillemin-Diem (ed.), p. 85).

12 Current efforts on the part of philosophers and biologists to defend teleological thinking against criticisms levelled at it since the early modern period encourage sympathetic reappraisal of medieval positions. 'What we now have in the natural sciences is teleology without mystery', says T. L. Short in 'Teleology in nature', *American Philosophical Quarterly*, 20 (1983), 311–20, at p. 311. Other recent defences of teleological thinking include L. Wright, *Teleological Explanations: An*

Etiological Analysis of Goals and Functions (Berkeley, 1976); A. Woodfield, *Teleology* (Cambridge, 1976). See also N. Rescher (ed.), *Current Issues in Teleology* (Lanham, Md, 1986).

13 The *Biblionomia* survives in a single manuscript, Sorbonne MS 636. L. Delisle's edition of the text in *Le cabinet des manuscrits de la Bibliothèque Impériale*, 3 vols. (Paris, 1868–81), vol. II, pp. 518–35, has remained standard. The manuscript is reproduced by H. J. de Vleeschauwer in Mousaion, vol. LXII (Pretoria, 1965).

14 'Fuit ergo sua intentio in ea plantare ortulum in quo sue civitatis alumpni fructus multimodos invenirent, quibus degustatis, summo desiderio hanelarent in secretum phylosophie cubiculum introduci' (Delisle, *Le cabinet des manuscrits*, vol. II, pp. 520–1.

15 Seminal work was undertaken by A. Birkenmajer, 'La bibliothèque de Richard de Fournival' (1924), rpt. in *Etudes d'histoire des sciences et de la philosophie du moyen âge*, Studia Copernicana, vol. I (Cracow, 1970), pp. 117–210. See also P. Glorieux, 'Etudes sur la "Biblionomia" de Richard de Fournival', *Recherches de théologie ancienne et médiévale*, 30 (1963), 205–31; R. H. Rouse, 'Manuscripts belonging to Richard de Fournival', *Revue d'histoire des textes*, 3 (1973), 253–69 (with bibl.); P. Zambelli, 'Da Aristotele a Abû Ma'shar, da Richard de Fournival a Guglielmo da Pastrengo', *Physis*, 15 (1973), 375–400 esp. pp. 377–81; D. Pingree, 'The diffusion of Arabic magical texts in Western Europe', in B. Scarcia Amoretti (ed.), *La diffusione delle scienze islamiche nel medio evo europeo* (Rome, 1987), esp. pp. 80–7. I owe the last two references to the kindness of Charles Burnett.

16 For Richard's biography see P. Paris, 'Richard de Fournival', in *Histoire littéraire de la France*, vol. XXIII (Paris, 1856), pp. 708–33, at pp. 708–17; P. Zarifopol (ed.), *Kritischer Text der Lieder Richards de Fournival* (Halle, 1904), pp. 1–3; Y. G. Lepage (ed.), *L'œuvre lyrique de Richard de Fournival* (Ottawa, 1981), pp. 9–12.

17 A. Birkenmajer, 'Pierre de Limoges commentateur de Richard de Fournival', *Isis*, 40 (1949), 18–31; rpt. in *Etudes d'histoire*, vol. I, pp. 222–35.

18 E. Langlois, 'Un document relatif à Richard de Fournival', *Mélanges d'archéologie et d'histoire*, 10 (1890), 123–5; E. Wickersheimer, *Dictionnaire biographique des médecins en France au moyen âge* (Paris, 1936), p. 700, and *Supplément* by D. Jacquart (Geneva, 1979), p. 258.

19 On Richard's vernacular writing, authentic and spurious, see Paris, 'Richard de Fournival', pp. 717–33; A. Långfors, 'Le bestiaire d'amour en vers par Richard de Fournival', *Mémoires de la Société néo-philologique de Helsingfors*, 7 (1924), 291–317; A. Saly, 'Li commens d'amours de Richard de Fournival (?)', *Travaux de linguistique et de littérature*, 10, no. 2 (1972), 21–55; G. B. Speroni, 'Il "Consaus d'amours" di Richard de Fournival', *Medioevo romanzo*, 1 (1974), 217–78; Lepage (ed.), *L'œuvre lyrique*, pp. 12–15 (with bibl.).

20 On Richard's scientific writing see Birkenmajer, 'La bibliothèque', at pp. 117–19. Both of the recent editors of *De vetula*, P. Klopsch (Leiden, 1967) and D. M. Robathan (Amsterdam, 1968), hesitate to attribute the work to Richard. Lepage (ed.), *L'œuvre lyrique*, would keep the question open (p. 10 n.12). That the Amiens-based Latin scholar and the vernacular poet were one and the same figure – not merely relations sharing a name – is substantiated by the explicit reference to the *Bestiaire* in a late thirteenth-century manuscript in Dijon (Bibliothèque Municipale, MS 526, fol. 31r): 'Ichi defenist li bestiaires damours ke maistres Richars de furnial canceliers damiens fist' (ed. Segre, p. lii).

21 For analysis of the literary genre see Segre, pp. vii–xxviii; G. Bianciotto, 'Sur le *Bestiaire d'amour* de Richart de Fournival', in G. Bianciotto and M. Salvat (eds.), *Epopée animale, fable, fabliau*, Actes du IVe Colloque de la Société Internationale Renardienne, Evreux, 7–11 septembre 1981 (Paris, 1984), pp. 107–19; Huot, *From Song to Book*, pp. 135–8.

22 Segre, p. 23; Beer, p. 8.

23 Segre, p. 45; Beer, p. 16. L. Vinge, *The Five Senses: Studies in a Literary Tradition*

(Lund, 1975), pp. 53–8; Huot, *From Song to Book*, p. 140 (who notes that the discourse on the senses appears at the midpoint of the tract).

24 Segre, pp. 33–4; Beer, p. 12.

25 Segre, p. 35; Beer, p. 12.

26 For sight it is the line (*li liens*), a white worm; for hearing the mole (*la taupe*); for smell the vulture (*li voltoirs*); for taste the monkey (*li singes*); and for touch the spider (*il araingne*) (Segre, p. 36; Beer, pp. 12–13). The five animals are represented in a North Italian manuscript of the first half of the fourteenth century in the Pierpont Morgan Library, New York (M.459, fol. 9v). For a survey of literary and pictorial treatments of the theme see Vinge, *Five Senses*, pp. 47–58; Nordenfalk, 'Les cinq sens', pp. 21–7; G. Casagrande and C. Kleinhenz, 'Literary and philosophical perspectives on the Wheel of the Five Senses in Longthorpe Tower', *Traditio*, 41 (1985), 311–27.

27 Segre, p. 42; Beer, pp. 14–15.

28 The visit of one distinguished thirteenth-century figure – Albertus Magnus – has been postulated. David Pingree, 'Arabic magical texts', observing that the magical books cited by Albertus Magnus in his *Speculum astronomie* were virtually all present in Richard's library, many of them in a miscellany identified as having belonged to Richard on palaeographical grounds (Paris, Bibliothèque Nationale, MS lat. 16204), suggests that Albertus had access to Richard's manuscripts, including his 'secret books' (pp. 80–7).

29 *Biblionomia*, nos. 61, 62, 71, 72 (Delisle, *Le cabinet des manuscrits*, vol. II, pp. 528–9).

30 Richard's manuscript of the *libri naturales*, necessarily a copy of the 'corpus vetustius', would have contained *De anima* in the translation of James of Venice (mid-twelfth century) and an anonymous translation of *De sensu*. William of Moerbeke's revised versions of these translations (*c.* 1260–80) subsequently became standard. B. G. Dod, 'Aristoteles latinus', in N. Kretzmann, A. Kenny and J. Pinborg (eds.), *The Cambridge History of Later Medieval Philosophy* (Cambridge, 1982), pp. 46, 50 and 55. The translations available to Richard have never been printed. I follow the readings in Oxford, Corpus Christi College, MS 114 (thirteenth century).

31 *De anima* 415b (CCC, MS 114, fol. 149v): 'Est autem anima corporis viventis causa et principium ... Manifestum autem est quod et propter quid anima est causa. Sicut enim intellectus propter hoc intelligit, eodem modo et natura, et hoc est ipsius finis. Hoc autem in animalibus anima est, et secundum naturam. Omnia enim phisica corpora anime instrumenta sunt.' I have consulted J. A. Smith's translation of the Greek text in the series, The Works of Aristotle translated into English, vol. III (Oxford, 1931).

32 *De anima* 418a; *De sensu* 439a–442b. On Aristotle's theories of perception see J. I. Beare, *Greek Theories of Elementary Cognition from Alcmaeon to Aristotle* (Oxford, 1906); Vinge, *Five Senses*, pp. 15–21; R. Sorabji, 'Aristotle on demarcating the five senses', *Philosophical Review*, 80 (1971), 55–79.

33 *De anima* 422b.

34 *Ibid.* 434a–435b; *De sensu* 436b–437a (CCC, MS 114, fol. 169r).

35 *De sensu* 437a. Information on the soul and sensory perception could be found in other volumes in Richard's library, among them Avicenna's *De anima* and Alexander of Aphrodisias' *De sensu secundum intensionem Aristotelis* (*Biblionomia*, nos. 64, 70; Delisle, *La cabinet des manuscrits*, vol. II, p. 528). Richard's own copies of the texts survive in the Bibliothèque Nationale – MSS lat. 16603 and 16602. Birkenmajer, 'La bibliothèque', pp. 176 and 179–80.

36 Birkenmajer ('La bibliothèque, p. 175) and Rouse, *Manuscripts*, pp. 263–4) have tentatively identified Paris, Bibliothèque Nationale, MS lat. 16162 as Richard's own. Michael Scot's translation of the *Historia animalium* in ten books, *De partibus animalium* in four books, and *De generatione animalium* in five books,

completed before 1220, would long hold its own against William of Moerbeke's translations from the Greek. Dod, 'Aristoteles latinus', and 48 and 52. I make reference to the text of a late thirteenth-century copy of Michael Scot's translation, Oxford, Balliol College, MS 252.

37 *Historia animalium* 489a, 492a–b and 532b–535a.

38 On the role of teleology in Aristotle's thought see A. Capecci, *Struttura e fine: la logica della teleologia aristotelica* (L'Aquila, 1978), esp. pp. 133–60.

39 *De partibus animalium* 639b–640a (= *De animalibus* XI, 1; Balliol, MS 252, fols. 71v–72r). I have consulted W. Ogle's translation of the Greek text in The Works of Aristotle translated into English, vol. v (Oxford, 1912).

40 *De partibus animalium* 656a–b (= *De animalibus* XII, 13). E. Clarke, 'Aristotelian concepts of the form and function of the brain', *Bulletin of the History of Medicine*, 37 (1963), 1–14.

41 *De partibus animalium* 658b (= *De animalibus* XII, 15; Balliol, MS 252, fol. 83v).

42 *Biblionomia*, nos. 133–62 (Delisle, *Le cabinet des manuscrits*, vol. II, pp. 532–5). Discussed by E. Seidler, 'Die Medizin in der "Biblionomia" des Richard de Fournival', *Sudhoffs Archiv*, 51 (1967), 44–54 (who counts 125 titles by 36 authors). Gerard d'Abbeville stipulated in his will that all medical manuscripts in his possession be sold at his death; thus it happened that this section of Richard's library did not enter the Sorbonne.

43 *Biblionomia*, no. 137 (Delisle, *La cabinet des manuscrits*, vol. II, p. 533). The text is printed in Galen's *Opera*, ed. D. Bonardus (Venice, 1490), vol. I, fols. 16r–32r. (hereafter cited as Bonardus). R. J. Durling, 'A chronological census of Renaissance editions and translations of Galen', *Journal of the Warburg and Courtauld Institutes*, 24 (1961), 230–305, at pp. 279 and 292. In 1317 Niccolò da Reggio made a full translation of the Greek text in seventeen books and, in his prologue, criticized the earlier translation. L. Thorndike, 'Translations of works of Galen from the Greek by Niccolò da Reggio (*c.* 1308–1345)', *Byzantina metabyzantina*, 1 (1946), 213–35, at pp. 214 and 232; Durling, 'Editions of Galen' pp. 233 and 292.

44 *De iuvamento membrorum* I, (Bonardus, fol. 16r): 'Corpora animalium sunt instrumenta animarum que sunt in eis ut per ea et per diuersitates membrorum compleatur illud quo indiget anima.' On Galenic teleology see the introduction to M. T. May's translation of the Greek text, *Galen, On the Usefulness of the Parts of the Body* (Ithaca, 1968); K. Gross, 'Galens teleologische Betrachtung der menschlichen Hand in *De usu partium*', *Sudhoffs Archiv*, 58 (1974), 13–24; P. Moraux, 'Galien et Aristote', in F. Bossier *et al.* (eds.), *Images of Man in Ancient and Medieval Thought: Studia Gerardo Verbeke ab amicis et collegis dicata* (Louvain, 1976), pp. 127–46. Of this aspect of Galen's thought G. W. Corner wrote: 'In his other large anatomico-physiological work, "The functions of the organs" ("De usu partium"), the many-sided Galen becomes a religious philosopher, using the marvels of the body to demonstrate the wisdom and power of the Creator. Such an attitude is dangerous to science, for if a man would glorify God by this means (rather than in the true way of patient and critical investigation) he must prepare an immediate explanation for every phenomenon, and thus he falls headlong into conjecture and dogmatism' (*Anatomy* (New York, 1930), pp. 8–9).

45 *De iuvamento membrorum* I, 1–6 (Bonardus, fols. 16r–17r).

46 *Ibid.* IV, 1 (Bonardus, fol. 18v).

47 *Ibid.* IX, 1 (Bonardus, fol. 28v): 'Et caput est fons sensus: et ex eo est motus voluntarius: et ex eo est origo nervorum mollium et durorum . . .'.

48 *Ibid.* IX, 2 (Bonardus, fol. 28v).

49 *Ibid.* IX, 4 (Bonardus, fols. 29r–29v).

50 Galen notes that the beneficent creator was often able to make single instruments serve multiple functions. *Ibid.* IX, 4 (Bonardus, fol. 29r): 'Et in hoc fuit solicitudo creatoris benedicti, quoniam multotiens ponit unum instrumentum utile ad operationes multas.'

51 *Biblionomia*, no. 73 (Delisle, *Le cabinet des manuscrits*, vol. II, p. 529).

52 Balbus observes that if you saw a great and beautiful house (*domus*), you could scarcely be led to believe, even if you did not see its master, that it was built by mice and weasels. *De natura deorum* II, 17 (ed. and trans. H. Rackham, (London, 1933), pp. 138–41; hereafter cited as Rackham).

53 *Ibid.* II, 140–6 (Rackham, pp. 256–65). Vinge, *Five Senses*, pp. 31–3.

54 *De natura deorum* II, 140 (Rackham, pp. 258–9): 'Sensus autem interpretes ac nuntii rerum in capite tamquam in arce mirifice ad usus necessarios et facti et conlocati sunt.'

55 *Biblionomia*, no. 80 (Delisle, *Le cabinet des manuscrits*, vol. II, p. 529): 'Ejusdem Tullii liber Tusculanarum questionum'.

56 *Tusculanae disputationes* I. 20, 46–7 (ed. and trans. J. E. King, (London, 1945, pp. 54–7). Vinge, *Five Senses*, pp. 33–4.

57 *Biblionomia*, no. 85 (Delisle, *Le cabinet des manuscrits*, vol. II, p. 530). Richard's copy was bound with the Hermetic *Asclepius*, Apuleius' *De deo Socratis* and *De Platone et eius dogmate*, and an epitome of the Platonic dialogues. Rouse identifies MS Reg. lat. 1572 in the Vatican Library as Richard's own (*Manuscripts*, p. 266). R. Klibansky suggests that Richard had the text copied from a Carolingian codex in the Abbey of Corbie, near Amiens. *The Continuity of the Platonic Tradition* (1939; rev. edn, Millwood, New York, 1982), pp. 6–7.

58 *Timaeus* 29D ff. (ed. J. H. Waszink (London, 1962), pp. 22ff.; hereafter cited as Waszink). F. M. Cornford, *Plato's Cosmology: The Timaeus of Plato Translated with a Running Commentary* (London, 1937), pp. 33ff.; G. R. Morrow, 'Necessity and persuasion in Plato's *Timaeus*' (1950), rpt. in R. E. Allen (ed.), *Studies in Plato's Metaphysics* (London, 1965), pp. 421–37. On Platonic teleology see H. J. Easterling, 'Causation in the *Timaeus* and *Laws* x', *Eranos*, 65 (1967), 25–38; Capecci, *Struttura e fine*, pp. 42–46.

59 *Timaeus* 32C–34A (Waszink, pp. 25–6).

60 *Ibid.* 44D–45B (Waszink, pp. 40–1).

61 *Ibid.* 45B–46C (Waszink, pp. 41–3).

62 *Ibid.* 46C–47E (Waszink, pp. 43–5). Cornford, *Plato's Cosmology*, pp. 156–9. Further on, in sections of the dialogue which Calcidius did not translate, Plato discusses the objects of the senses (61C–68D) at the beginning of a teleological account of the parts of the human body.

63 *Biblionomia*, no. 87 (Delisle, *Le cabinet des manuscrits*, vol. II, p. 530).

64 *Commentarii in Somnium Scipionis* I. 14, 9 (ed. J. Willis (Leipzig, 1963), pp. 56–7; trans. W. H. Stahl (New York, 1952), p. 144; hereafter cited as Willis and Stahl, respectively).

65 *Ibid.* I. 6, 77–81 (Willis, p. 33; Stahl, pp. 115–17).

66 *Ibid.* I. 6, 81 (Willis, p. 33; Stahl, p. 116). The numerological section in Martianus Capella's *De nuptiis Mercurii et Philologiae*, a two-volume manuscript shelved further on in Richard's library (*Biblionomia*, nos. 97, 98; Delisle, *Le cabinet des manuscrits*, vol. II, p. 530), would have yielded much the same information.

67 *Biblionomia*, nos. 107, 105 (Delisle, *Le cabinet des manuscrits*, vol. II, p. 531).

68 *Cosmographia* II. 3, 1 (ed. P. Dronke (Leiden, 1978), p. 123; trans. W. Wetherbee (New York, 1973), p. 94; hereafter cited as Dronke and Wetherbee, respectively).

69 *Ibid.* II. 13, 10–11 (Dronke, pp. 148–9; Wetherbee, p. 121).

70 *Ibid.* II. 13, 13; II. 14, 1–8 (Dronke, pp. 149–50; Wetherbee, pp. 122–3).

71 *Ibid.* II. 13, 13 (Dronke, pp. 149–50; Wetherbee, p. 122).

72 *Ibid.* II. 14, 13–108 (Dronke, pp. 150–3; Wetherbee, pp. 123–5).

73 *Ibid.* II. 14. 49–78 (Dronke, pp. 151–2; Wetherbee, p. 124): 'Auriculis quasi vestibulo suscepta priore, / Vox sonat et trahitur interiore domo: / Sermonis numeros extraque sonancia verba / Auris, sed ratio significata capit'.

74 *Anticlaudianus* I, 71–3 (ed. R. Bossuat (Paris, 1955), p. 59; trans. J. J. Sheridan (Toronto, 1973), p. 47; hereafter cited as Bossuat and Sheridan, respectively. On the

rhetorical tradition into which Alan's description fits, see S. Viarre, 'La description du Palais de la Nature dans l'Anticlaudianus d'Alain de Lille (i, 55–206)', in H. Roussel and F. Suard (eds.), *Alain de Lille, Gautier de Châtillon, Jakemart Giélée et leurs temps* (Lille, 1980), pp. 153–69.

75 *Anticlaudianus* IV, 95–212 (Boussuat, pp. 109–13; Sheridan, pp. 121–5).

76 Verona, Biblioteca Capitolare, MS CCLI, fols. 15r–16v. F. Mütherich, 'An illustration of the five senses in mediaeval art', *Journal of the Warburg and Courtauld Institutes*, 18 (1955), 140–1; Nordenfalk, 'Les cinq sens', p. 19; C. Meier, 'Die Rezeption des Anticlaudianus Alans von Lille in Textkommentierung und Illustration', in C. Meier and U. Ruberg (eds.), *Text und Bild* (Wiesbaden, 1980), pp. 408–549, esp. pp. 413–67 (on the Verona manuscript) and pp. 445–6 (on the illustrations of the senses).

77 Nordenfalk, who classifies devices for representing the senses, speaks of 'the depiction of the actual sensory organs, preferably by isolating each from the human body as a kind of physiological hieroglyph' ('The five senses in Late Medieval and Renaissance art', *Journal of the Warburg and Courtauld Institutes*, 48 (1985), 1–22, at p. 4).

78 Cf. S. L. Gilman, 'The uncontrollable steed: a study of the metamorphosis of a literary image', *Euphorion*, 66 (1972), 32–54.

79 Rouse, *Manuscripts*, pp. 254–7. To Rouse is owed the introduction of palaeographical and codicological considerations into the search for Richard's manuscripts.

80 Early representations are few. The names of the five senses were occasionally inscribed in diagrammatic images, but illustrations are to be found only on the Anglo-Saxon Fuller Brooch (ninth century), where five figures are depicted in the act of using their senses. See R. L. S. Bruce-Mitford, 'Late Saxon disc-brooches', in D. B. Harden (ed.), *Dark-Age Britain: Studies presented to E. T. Leeds* (London, 1956), esp. pp. 173–90. On the iconography of the senses see Nordenfalk, 'Les cinq sens', pp. 17–28; Nordenfalk, 'Five senses', pp. 1–22. For their suggestions on iconographical matters I am grateful to Adelaide Bennett Hagens and Nigel Morgan.

81 R. Branner, *Manuscript Painting in Paris during the Reign of Saint Louis* (Berkeley, 1977), p. 125 n.27; M. Camille, 'Illustrations in Harley MS 3487 and the perception of Aristotle's *Libri naturales* in thirteenth-century England', in W. M. Ormrod (ed.), *England in the Thirteenth Century*, Proceedings of the 1984 Harlaxton Symposium (Woodbridge, Suffolk, 1986), pp. 31–44.

82 Geneva, Bibliothèque Publique et Universitaire, MS lat. 76, fol. 327r (corpus vetustius). L. Minio-Paluello, *Aristoteles latinus codices: supplementa altera* (Bruges, 1961), pp. 121–2; B. Gagnebin, *L'enluminure de Charlemagne à François Ier* (Geneva, 1976), pp. 57–60 (no. 21); Nordenfalk, 'Les cinq sens', p. 21.

83 For descriptions of other initials to *De sensu* see Nordenfalk, 'Five senses', p. 2; Camille, 'Harley MS 3487', p. 38 n.29.

84 New Haven, Yale Medical Library, MS 12, fol. 180r. W. Cahn and J. Marrow, 'Medieval and Renaissance manuscripts at Yale: a selection', *Yale University Library Gazette*, 52 (1978), 196–7 (no. 24). For the later life of this motif see J. F. Kermode, 'The Banquet of Sense', *Bulletin of the John Rylands Library*, 44 (1961–2), 68–99.

85 Reims, Bibliothèque Municipale, MS 864, fol. 101v (corpus vetustius). *Catalogue général des manuscrits des bibliothèques publiques*, vol. XXXIX (Paris, 1904), pp. 173–5; G. Lacombe, *Aristoteles latinus*, 2 vols. (Rome, 1939–55), vol. I, p. 594 (no. 735); M. de Lemps, *Trésors de la Bibliothèque Municipale de Reims* (Reims, 1978), no. 35. Cited by Camille, 'Harley MS 3487', p. 38 n.29.

86 Munich, clm 527, fol. 64v. *Cat. codd. manu scriptorum Bibliothecae regiae monacensis*, vol. III (Munich, 1892), p. 149; Lacombe, *Aristoteles latinus*, vol. I, pp. 724–5 (no. 1023). In the first part of the codex, thirteenth-century in date, Aristotle's *De sensu* is transcribed. The diagram, inserted in the section dated 1347,

follows upon Avicenna's *De generatione embryonis*. E. Clarke and K. Dewhurst, *An Illustrated History of Brain Function* (Oxford, 1972), p. 30.

3 The manifest and the hidden in the Renaissance clinic

1 Theodor Puschmann, *A History of Medical Education*, trans. and ed. Evan H. Hare (London, 1891), p. 332; P. Lain Entralgo, *La historia clínica* (Madrid, 1950), p. 106; L. Münster, 'Die Anfänge eines klinischen Unterrichts an der Universität Padua im 16. Jahrhundert', *Medizinische Monatsschrift*, 23 (1969), 171–4; C. D. O'Malley, 'Medical education during the Renaissance', in C. D. O'Malley (ed.), *History of Medical Education* (Berkeley, 1970), pp. 95–6. For earlier literature on da Monte, see notes 24 and 25. It should be noted that the hospital had served as a teaching centre in Islam long before it did so in Western Europe; see Gary Leiser, 'Medical education in Islamic lands from the seventh to the fourteenth century', *Journal of the History of Medicine*, 38 (1983), 53–5 and 59–61. Furthermore, even in Europe students had routinely accompanied practising doctors on visits to patients since long before da Monte's time. Thus his (possible) priority has to do specifically with that form of bedside teaching in which a university professor gives formal presentations of hospital cases to an audience of students, i.e., gives clinical lectures.

2 I have discussed da Monte's clinical teaching in 'The School of Padua: humanistic medicine in the sixteenth century', in Charles Webster (ed.), *Health, Medicine and Mortality in the Sixteenth Century* (Cambridge, 1979), pp. 335–70, at pp. 346–52, and in 'Commentary', in Lloyd G. Stevenson (ed.), *A Celebration of Medical History* (Baltimore, 1982), pp. 200–11, at pp. 204–7. Da Monte's teaching of medical practice (including bedside teaching) is a major topic in a paper which I presented to the Second Galen symposium at Kiel in September 1982: J. Bylebyl, 'Teaching *Methodus medendi* in the Renaissance', in Fridolf Kudlien and Richard J. Durling (eds.), *Galen's Method of Healing* (Leiden, 1991), pp. 157–89.

3 Da Monte, *Consultationes medicae* ([Basle?], 1583), col. 938, my emphasis. Unless otherwise indicated, all subsequent references to da Monte's consultations and hospital discourses are to this edition, which is the reissue of the edition of 1572.

4 *Ibid.*, col. 939.

5 *Ibid.*

6 Galen, *Methodus medendi*, Bk III, chs. 7–8; Galen, *Opera omnia*, ed. C. G. Kühn, 20 vols. (Leipzig, 1821–33), vol. x, pp. 204–14.

7 Da Monte, *Consultationes*, col. 941.

8 *Ibid.*, col. 939.

9 *Ibid.*

10 Galen, *Methodus medendi*, Bk I, ch. 9, Bk II, ch. 1; ed. Kühn, vol. x, pp. 67–81; Galen, *De locis affectis*, Bk I, chs. 2–3; ed. Kühn, vol. VIII, pp. 20–34.

11 Da Monte, *Consultationes*, cols. 939–40.

12 *Ibid.*

13 *Ibid.*, col. 940.

14 *Ibid.*, e.g., cols. 630, 916, 954, 964 and 981. See also col. 943 regarding the second visit to this patient.

15 *Ibid.*, col. 940.

16 Da Monte, *De excrementis*, ed. Valentine Lublin (Venice, 1554); *De urinis*, ch. 5, p. 24.

17 *Ibid.*, p. 2v.

18 Da Monte, *Consultationes*, col. 940.

19 Da Monte, *In libros Galeni de arte curandi ad Glauconem Explanationes* (Venice, 1554), pp. 69v–70r.

20 Da Monte, *De excrementis*, Bk I, pp. 1v and 5. By the use of taste, however, he seems to have had in mind primarily the patient's tasting of his own sputum or tears.

21 Da Monte, *Consultationes*, col. 940.

22 *Ibid.*, col. 943.

23 Bylebyl, 'Commentary', pp. 201–2.

24 G. Rasori, *Opere complete* (Florence, 1837), pp. 293–6; G. Montesanto, *Dell' origine della Clinica Medica in Padova* (Padua, 1827).

25 Giuseppe Cervetto, *Di Giambattista da Monte e della medicina italiana nel secolo XVI* (Verona, 1839).

26 S. G. G. Bruté, *Essai sur l'histoire et les avantages des institutions cliniques* (Paris, 1803); Philippe Pinel, 'Clinique', in *Dictionaire des sciences médicales*, vol. v (Paris, 1813), pp. 364–71; L. P. Auguste Gauthier, 'Discours préliminaire surl'histoire des cliniques', in his trans. of J. V. von Hildebrand, *Médecine Pratique* (Lyons, 1824).

27 See especially Montesanto, *Dell' origine*, pp. 24–5, where he tries to find an alternative explanation for what clearly seem to be medical consultations. See also the article 'Consultation' by J. B. Nacquart, in *Dictionaire des sciences médicales*, vol. vi (Paris, 1813), pp. 33–9, esp. pp. 34–7, on 'les consultations cliniques' and their unfavourable reputation.

28 Cervetto, *Da Monte*, preface.

29 Bylebyl, 'The School of Padua', pp. 335–52; Bylebyl, 'Teaching *Methodus medendi*', *passim*.

30 J. Bylebyl, 'Medicine, philosophy, and humanism in Renaissance Italy', in J. W. Shirley and F. D. Hoeniger (eds.), *Science and the Arts in the Renaissance* (Washington, D.C., 1985), pp. 27–49, esp. 38–41.

31 Galen, *De anatomicis administrationibus*, Bk ii, ch. 2; ed. Kühn, vol. ii, pp. 286–7; *De locis affectis*, *passim*.

32 On this definition of disease, see note 10 above. In *De anatomicis administrationibus* (Bk i, ch. 4; ed. Kühn, vol. ii, p. 232), Galen refers to the typical vivisectional procedure as one which 'damages a function', using the same Greek terms as in his definition of disease. In *De locis affectis* he explicitly relates such vivisectionally induced functional damage to the diagnosis of human patients exhibiting similar functional impairment; see esp. Bk iii, ch. 14; ed. Kühn, vol. viii, pp. 208–14.

33 Luis Garcia Ballester, 'Galen as a medical practitioner: problems in diagnosis', in Vivian Nutton (ed.), *Galen: Problems and Prospects: a Collection of Papers Submitted at the 1979 Cambridge Conference* (London, 1979), pp. 13–46.

34 I have discussed these issues at some length in 'Teaching *Methodus medendi*'. Andrew Wear has discussed related themes in 'Explorations in Renaissance writings on the practice of medicine', in A. Wear, R. K. French and I. M. Lonie (eds.), *The Medical Renaissance of the Sixteenth Century* (Cambridge, 1985), pp. 118–45, esp. pp. 134–7 on da Monte.

35 Rhazes, *Nonus tractatus libri ad regem Almansorem*, ch. 14, in G. Kraut (ed.), *Opus medicinae saluberrimum* (Haganau, 1533), fols. 13v–14r.

36 Avicenna, *Canon medicinae*, Bk iii, fen. 5, tr. 1, ch. 11; (Venice, 1608), p. 586.

37 Da Monte, *In nonum librum Rhasis ad Mansorem … expositio*, ed. Valentine Lublin (Venice, 1554), pp. 242v–252v.

38 *Ibid.*, pp. 252v–257v.

39 *Ibid.*, pp. 270v–275r.

40 Da Monte, *In libros Galeni … Explanationes*, pp. 26v–27r. See also Andrew Wear, 'Galen in the Renaissance', in Nutton, (ed.), *Galen: Problems and Prospects*, pp. 242–5.

41 Da Monte, *Consultationes*, appendix, col. 104.

42 *Ibid.*, appendix, col. 83.

43 Da Monte, *Consilia medica omnia*, ed. Hieronymus Donzellini (Nuremberg, 1559), 'Consilia de curatione febrium', no. viii.

44 Da Monte, *Consultationes*, cols. 956–7.

45 *Ibid.*, col. 901.

46 *Ibid.*, col. 957.

47 *Ibid.*, col. 901.
48 *Ibid.*
49 *Ibid.*, cols. 185–6.
50 *Ibid.*, cols. 628–9.
51 *Ibid.*, col. 629.
52 *Ibid.*, cols. 629–30.
53 *Ibid.*, col. 630.
54 *Ibid.*, cols. 631–2.
55 *Ibid.*, cols. 619–20.
56 *Ibid.*, col. 629.
57 Alessandro Massaria, *Practica medica* (Venice, 1618), p. 487.
58 Da Monte, *Consultationes*, col. 939.
59 Donzellini, in the preface to his edition of da Monte, *Consilia medica omnia*, p. ix.
60 Da Monte, *Consultationes*, col. 489; see also col. 76.
61 Bylebyl, 'Commentary', pp. 205–7. However, I would now attribute to da Monte himself a clearer distinction between the hospital discourses, which he conducted on his own, and the consultations, which were inherently collaborative in nature. See below.
62 Da Monte, *Consultationes*, cols. 455–61, 619–26, 631–6, 901–7, 938–43 and 956–69.
63 *Ibid.*, cols. 938–9, my emphasis.
64 *Ibid.*, col. 939, my emphasis.
65 E.g., *ibid.*, cols. 61, 83, 85 and 89.
66 *Ibid.*, appendix, cols. 49 and 68.
67 *Ibid.*, col. 76, my emphasis.
68 *Ibid.*, col. 901.
69 *Ibid.*, col. 624.
70 *Ibid.*, col. 964.
71 *Ibid.*, col. 264.
72 *Ibid.*, col. 76.
73 *Ibid.*, cols. 61, 83 and 85; appendix, col. 88.
74 *Ibid.*, cols. 619 and 887.
75 *Ibid.*, col. 456.
76 *Ibid.*, col. 756.
77 *Ibid.*, appendix, col. 15; cf. main text, cols. 89–93.
78 *Ibid.*, col. 967.
79 *Ibid.*, cols. 80 and 631.

4 In bad odour

1 Useful discussions of these works are available in Gregory Vlastos, 'Plato's supposed theory of irregular atomic figures', *Isis*, 58 (1967), 204–9; A. J. Cappelletti, 'El sentido del olfato, segun Aristoteles', *Revista de la Sociedad Venezolana de Historia de la Medicina*, 27 (1978), 9–40; R. E. Siegel, *Galen on Sense Perception* (Basle, 1970); B. S. Eastwood, 'Galen on the elements of olfactory sensation', *Rheinisches Museum für Philologie*, new series, 124 (1981), 268–89.
2 Louise Vinge, *The Five Senses: Studies in a Literary Tradition* (Lund, 1975), esp. pp. 15–20.
3 The fragrant garden represents smell in the series of engravings of the five senses by Abraham Bosse dating from the 1630s (copy in the Wellcome Institute); the baby's bottom in a series of paintings of the five senses by Jan Miense Molenaer dating from 1637, illustration in *Mauritshuis. The Royal Cabinet of Paintings. Illustrated general catalogue* (The Hague, 1977), pp. 158–9; a man vomiting in P. Boone's representation of the sense of smell dated 1651 (original drawing in the Wellcome Institute). For earlier iconography, see Carl Nordenfalk, 'The five senses in late

Medieval and Renaissance art', *Journal of the Warburg and Courtauld Institutes*, 48 (1985), 1–22 and plates 1–9.

4 Charles Singer, *Vesalius on the Human Brain* (London, 1952), fig. 12, pp. 108–9.

5 C. V. Schneider, *Liber de osse cribriformi et sensu ac organo odoratus* (Wittenberg, 1655). On subsequent discussion in eighteenth-century Dutch medicine, see A. M. Luyendijk-Elshout, 'The cavity of the nose in Dutch baroque medicine', *Clio Medica*, 18 (1973), 295–303.

6 Avicenna, *Liber canonis* (Venice, 1507), liber 3, tract. 1, cap. 1, 'De anathomia nasi'. Ambroise Paré, *Oeuvres* (Paris, 1575), pp. 147–8.

7 The play is discussed in Vinge, *Five Senses*, pp. 98–103.

8 Bartholomeus Anglicus, *De genuinis rerum ... proprietatibus* (Frankfurt, 1609), pp. 68–9, 1162–8; book 3, chapter 19, 'De olfactu'; book 19, chapters 37–9, 'De odore', 'De effectu odorum', 'De foetore'. Theories of sense perception are usefully discussed in E. Ruth Harvey, *The Inward Wits: Psychological Theory in the Middle Ages and Renaissance* (London, 1975). Reisch's illustration is also reproduced in Singer, *Vesalius on the Human Brain*, p. 139.

9 Bartolomeo da Montagnana, *Consilia* (Venice, 1497), fol. 22v, 'De egritudinibus'.

10 Juan Bravo, *De saporum et odorum differentiis* (Salamanca, 1583), pp. 125–6, where the opinion of Vesalius is discussed.

11 Bartholomeus Anglicus, *De genuinis rerum*, p. 1162: 'Odor itaque est fumosus vapor a substantia rei resolutus, qui mediante aere ad cerebrum attractus est sensus olfactur immutativus'.

12 Bravo, *De saporum*, pp. 100–1. A similar view is presented in Gregorius Reisch, *Margarita philosophica* (Freiburg im Breisgau, 1503), ch. 18.

13 Petrarch, *Hülff, Trost und Rath* (Frankfurt, 1559), fol. xix r.

14 Marsilio Ficino, *The Book of Life*, trans. Charles Boer (Irving, Tex., 1980), pp. 52 and 76.

15 Bravo, *De saporum*, p. 116.

16 *Ibid.*, pp. 149–50.

17 Ficino, *Book of Life*, p. 19.

18 The engravings are amongst the iconographic collections of the Wellcome Institute. They are thought to derive from Laserre, *Le tombeau des délices* (Brussels, 1630).

19 Bartolomeo da Montagnana, *Consilia*, fols. 1r, 2r, 16r, 22r–25r, 44v, 50r, 74r, 77r, 113v.

20 Giovanni Battista da Monte (Montanus), *Consultationes medicae* (Basle, 1583), pp. 79 and 269–70.

21 Bravo, *De saporum*, p. 147.

22 *Ibid.*, pp. 114 and 151.

23 Harvey, *The Inward Wits*, p. 27.

24 Ficino, *Book of Life*, pp. 73–8.

25 Bravo, *De saporum*, p. 137.

26 Bartholomeus Anglicus, *De genuinis rerum*, p. 1168.

27 Ilza Veith, *Hysteria: The History of a Disease* (Chicago, 1965); Trotula, *The Diseases of Women*, trans. E. Mason-Hohl (Los Angeles, 1940), esp. pp. 10–13; Paré, *Oeuvres*, pp. 785–7.

28 John Sadler, *The Sick Woman's Private Looking-glasse* (London, 1636), pp. 61–9.

29 Simon Kellwaye, *A Defensative Against the Plague* (London, 1593), fol. 1v.

30 Galen, 'De febrium differentiis', in *Medicorum Graecorum opera quae exstant*, ed. C. G. Kühn, vol. vii (Leipzig, 1824), p. 279.

31 Bartholomeus Anglicus, *De genuinis rerum*, p. 1168.

32 Archivio di Stato, Venice, Provveditori alla Sanità, reg. 2 (a contemporary volume of laws and precedent-forming decisions of the Health Office of Venice), fol. 31.

33 Alberto Chiapelli, 'Gli ordinamenti sanitari del Comune di Pistoia contro la pestilenza del 1348', *Archivio Storico Italiano*, series 4, 20 (1887), 3–24.

34 Mario Brunetti, 'Venezia durante la peste del 1348', *Ateneo Veneto*, anno 32 (1909), vol. 1, pp. 289–311; vol. 2, pp. 5–42.

35 Archivio di Stato, Venice, Provveditori alla Sanità, reg. 725, fol. 63r.

36 This theme is discussed imaginatively in relation to the eighteenth and nineteenth centuries in Alain Corbin, *Le miasme et la jonquille: l'odorat et l'imaginaire social xviiie–xixe siècles* (Paris, 1982).

37 Bravo, *De saporum*, pp. 150–3 and 157.

38 Corbin, *Le miasme et la jonquille*, p. 32. This remark, made by Corbin in relation to the eighteenth century, is no less true of earlier periods.

39 Bartholomeus Anglicus, *De genuinis rerum*, p. 1165.

40 Bartolomeo da Montagnana, *Consilia*, fol. 1.

41 On the history of perfumes, see Frances Kennett, *History of Perfume* (London, 1975); Edwin T. Morris, *Fragrance: The Story of Perfume from Cleopatra to Chanel* (New York, 1984); Dan McKenzie, *Aromatics and the Soul: A Study of Smells* (London, 1923).

42 Thomas Dekker, *The Plague Pamphlets*, ed. F. P. Wilson (Oxford, 1925), p. 35.

43 G. G. Stewart, 'A history of the medicinal use of tobacco 1492–1860', *Medical History*, 11 (1967), 228–68, esp. p. 241.

44 Konrad Renger, *Adriaen Brouwer und das niederlandische Bauerngenre 1600–1660* (Munich, 1986), plate 4, 'Der Geruch'.

45 Eastwood, 'Galen on olfactory sensation' pp. 280–6; Siegel, *Galen on Sense Perception*, pp. 155–7.

46 Reisch, *Margarita philosophica*, ch. 17, 'Quid olfactus. Quid odor et que odoris species'.

47 Avicenna, *Liber canonis*, liber 1, fen. 2, doct. 3, cap. 4, 'De significationibus odoris urine'. Cf. Mazhar H. Shah, *General Principles of the Canon of Avicenna* (Karachi, 1966), pp. 213–14 and 256–66.

48 L. Münster, 'In tema di deontologia medica. Il "De cautelis medicorum" di Gabriele Zerbi', *Rivista di storia delle scienze mediche e naturali*, 46–7 (1976), 60–83, esp. p. 71.

49 Vinge, *Five senses*, pp. 68–70.

50 Nordenfalk, *Five senses*, plate 8.

51 On the *Speculum morale*, see Vinge, *Five senses*, pp. 66–7. Puget de la Serre, *An Alarum for Ladyes*, transl. Francis Hawkins (Paris, 1638), pp. 48–50.

52 Vinge, *Five senses*, pp. 71–2.

53 Ficino, *Book of Life*, pp. 64–8.

54 F. Mütherich, 'An illustration of the five senses in mediaeval art', *Journal of the Warburg and Courtauld Institutes*, 18 (1955), pp. 140–1 and plate 40.

5 Seeing and believing

1 In order to graduate as a doctor of medicine, French medical students had first to become bachelors and licentiates. Each degree was bestowed after a series of examinations which normally included the preparation of a dissertation and its defence in public in a three- to four-hour debate. The abstracts of these dissertations were usually printed and many have survived, forming one of the best sources for studying faculty teaching. The examination process is discussed in L. W. B. Brockliss, *French Higher Education in the Seventeenth and Eighteenth Centuries: A Cultural History* (Oxford, 1987), pp. 71–82.

2 Bibliothèque de la Faculté de Médecine de Paris, *Theses medicae Parisiensis* (hereafter Paris TMP), vi in-fol., no. 888. 'Experientia autem felices illorum [therapies] successus observat, ut rationis inventa et agitata confirmet: ita est utraque altera sine altera debilis; quamvis enim excolendis artibus principatum teneat ratio, numquam tamen experientiam tanquam ancillam et pedissequam ... Nihilominus

... sic versat sagacioris ingenii solertia, ut quamvis ex usu longo morbis medicinam quaesiverit: summo tamen, et unico ferme rationis consilio omnia impertita fuisse successus probet.' The dissertation record of the Paris faculty is particularly good thanks to the interest shown in the genre by the eighteenth-century physician H. T. Baron (1686–1758). The faculty library possesses two collections: 9 vols. in-fol. 1539–1724, and 16 vols. in-4 1599–1752. Their value is discussed in N. Legrand, *La collection des thèses de l'ancienne faculté de médecine depuis 1559 et son catalogue inédit jusqu'au 1793* (Paris, 1913).

3 This coterie used the *soutenance* to popularize its ideas. For another example from the 1640s, see the dissertation of J. B. Moreau, 'Estne Hippocratica medendi methodus omnium certissima, tutissima, praestantissima?' (1648), in Paris TMP, VI in-fol., no. 978. This abstract was also translated into French, evidence again of the coterie's anxiety to extend its influence: see British Library, Department of Printed Books, 1179 k 6(5). Moreau was the son of René, mentioned below.

4 The fullest list of the coterie is to be found in a letter written by Patin to the Lyons physician, Spon, on 18 January 1649, which contains twenty names. See G. Patin, *Lettres*, ed. J. H. Réveillé-Parise, 3 vols. (Paris, 1846), vol. I, p. 453. Patin, a well-known figure to both literary and medical historians is the only member of the group to have been seriously studied; see, for example, F. R. Packard, *Gui Patin and the Medical Profession in the Seventeenth Century* (London, 1924). The collection of Patin's letters edited by Réveillé-Parise is the fullest. An attempt by P. Triaire to publish a complete collection at the beginning of this century foundered after the first volume.

5 The standard biography is still Sir Charles Sherrington, *The Endeavour of Jean Fernel* (Cambridge, 1946).

6 Fernel's most famous textbook was his *Physiologia*, published for the first time under the title *De naturali parte medicinae* in 1542 (Colines: Paris). In 1554 Fernel published a complete *Medicina* (Wechsel: Paris), which contained his *Physiologia*, *Pathologia* and *Therapeutice*. Fernel's *Physiology* was reprinted thirty-one times after his death and was translated into French in 1655, an indication of its popularity as late as the mid-seventeenth century.

7 The first edition was published by Wechsel at Paris. The edition cited below is the second: *Joannis Fernelii Ambiani de abditis rerum causis Libri duo* (Jacques Dupuys: Paris, 1551).

8 *Ibid.*, pp. 2–3.

9 *Ibid.*, p. 181. 'Quamquam autem latent, naturae arcanis multaque obscuritate involutae, prae ignavia tamen sinendae non sunt, sed investigandae diligentius, non e primis tangendi secundisve qualitatibus, non e sapore, odore, sono vel colore, verum e solis effectis et operibus, quae tum longa usus observatione, tum optimorum authorum monimentis comparata confirmataque sint.'

10 *Ibid.*, p. 136. 'Haec causa est cur pestilentia non omnes regiones, nec omnes homines peraque efficiat et laedit.'

11 Thomist Aristotelians believed that only the rational soul, the substantial form of man, was specifically created and implanted in matter.

12 Fernel, *De abditis rerum causis*, pp. 127–9.

13 On the Galenic tradition, see Owsei Temkin, *Galenism: Rise and Decline of a Medical Philosophy* (Ithaca, N.Y., 1973).

14 France had sixteen universities by 1600 and all theoretically possessed a medical faculty except Orléans. Most, however, had a paper existence only and of the functioning faculties at this date Montpellier and Paris alone had a significant student body. See the general comments in Brockliss, *Higher Education*, pp. 13–19.

15 The Montpellier dissertation record is poor in comparison with the Parisian one (cf. note 2 above). Nevertheless, enough thesis abstracts survive to make this generalization sound. Most surviving Montpellier dissertations for this period are located in either the British Library, Department of Printed Books (hereafter BL) or

in the Bibliothèque Nationale, Département des imprimés (hereafter BN). Some of these are doctoral not student dissertations and are the abstracts of theses sustained as part of the contest for vacant chairs.

16 They drew the line at dysentery and quartan fevers. Apart from the plague, the malady that Fernelians most commonly attributed to occult causes was venereal disease; for example, Jacques Bellayus, 'An parentes lue venerea infecti possint generare liberos sanos?' (Montpellier, 1629) in BL, 1185 f 2(4), pp. 6–9; Pierre Haguenot, 'An lues venerea ab immoderato inter sanos amplexu suscitari possit?' (Montpellier, doctoral dissertation, 1639), pp. 9–10.

17 The commentary was first published in 1598. The edition cited below is the one printed in Riolan's *Opera omnia* (Paris, 1610). For a short account of Riolan's life and work, see J. A. Hazon, *Notice des hommes les plus célèbres de la faculté de médecine 1175–1750* (Paris, 1773), *sub nomine*. According to Riolan the elder, Fernel had been his model since graduation; see the preface to his 'Ad Fernelii Librum de Elementis Commentarium' also included in the 1610 *Opera omnia*.

18 Riolan the elder, 'Ad libros Fernelii de abditis rerum causis commentarium', in *Opera omnia*, pp. 149–50. The Fernelian position was sometimes sustained; see the thesis of Gabriel Biard, 'An in epilepsia quid occultum?' (1607), in Paris TMP, II in-fol., no. 387.

19 Riolan the elder, 'Ad libros Fernelii de abditis rerum causis', pp. 150–3. Riolan's explanation of the plague was idiosyncratic. Early seventeenth-century Fernelians preferred the views of their master; for example: Nicolas Lambert, 'An pestis a caelo?' (Paris, 1621); Nicolas Matthieu, 'An astronomis usui medico necessaria?', in Paris TMP, III in-fol., nos. 658 and 740. Riolan himself fell back on this view in his 'Generalis methodus bene medendi', in *Opera omnia*, pp. 382–3.

20 Riolan the elder, 'Ad libros Fernelii de abditis rerum causis', p. 166. 'Hoc si quis admiretur, meminierit totam fere medicinam esse empiricam, uti remediis experientia quam ratione, comprobatis.'

21 *Ibid.*, pp. 163–5. Among Pliny's *bêtises*, Riolan highlighted the Greek philosopher's belief that the chameleon survives on air.

22 Unfortunately, it is impossible to tell from the dissertation abstracts whether other early seventeenth-century Fernelians shared Riolan's realization of the need to treat the observations of others with caution. He himself, of course, had not even begun to grasp the difficulties inherent in evaluating sense experience: he was no Descartes *avant la lettre*.

23 B. Hachette, 'An in epilepsia θειον Τι, in Paris TMP, II in-fol., no. 281. 'Omnes [diseases] causam habere possunt obscuram, non tamen divinam.' Hachette believed all pestilential, contagious and poisonous fevers were the result of putrefaction.

24 *Lettres de Gui Patin 1630–1672*, ed. P. Triaire, one vol. only (Paris, 1907), p. 20, letter to Belin, no date [*c.* 1630]. See also Patin, *Lettres*, ed. Réveillé-Parise, vol. I, p. 13 (to Belin, 4 November 1631); II, p. 588 (to Falconet, 15 August 1651); III, pp. 59, 106, 199 and 648 (to Falconet, 29 March 1966, 27 December 1658, 27 April 1660, 29 April 1667). In the letter of 27 April 1660 Patin says that he often takes his sons to see Fernel's tomb in Saint-Jacques de la Boucherie, 'les exhortant de devenir comme lui'. In the case of this and other quotations in French in this chapter, the original orthography is followed.

25 J. B. Ferrand, 'An secta rationalis legitima?', in Paris TMP, VI in-fol., no. 711.

26 Patin has been incorrectly labelled a freethinker because he consorted with the Gassendi circle in the 1650s and held unorthodox views on monasticism and witchcraft. In fact, like Gassendi himself he was a strongly moralistic Christian and his unorthodoxy, as will be explained in the following section, was chiefly the product of his medical rationalism.

27 Triaire (ed.), *Lettres de Gui Patin*, p. 19.

28 Patin was particularly incensed by the misuse of the occult specific antimony. See

his remarks on the death of the *premier médecin du roi*, François Vautier, in 1652, who had been a great believer in the power of the drug. Vautier had himself deservedly died from taking antimony. If he had only died some seven years before (Vautier became the king's chief physician in 1646), then many more lives would have been saved. See Patin, *Lettres*, ed. Réveillé-Parise, vol. III, pp. 5–6 (letter to Falconet, 5 July 1652). The rationalists' objections to antimony are discussed below.

29 For example, Charles Bouvard, *Historicae hodiernae medicinae rationalis veritatis logos protreplikos ad rationales medicos* (Paris, 1655). Patin thought little of this particular defence of medical rationalism, dismissing it as 'bien chétif, embrouillé, force répétitions, mauvaises termes et pauvre latin': see Patin, *Lettres*, ed. Réveillé-Parise, vol. II, p. 242 (letter to Spon, 3 March 1656) and vol. III, pp. 427–8 (letter to Falconet, 23 March 1663). Bouvard (1572–1658) was *premier médecin du roi* in the 1630s: see the following section.

30 Hachette, 'An in Epilepsia'. According to Hachette the amulet would cure by a 'manifesta tractabilique facultate'. For occultist accounts of the treatment of epilepsy, see Fernel, *De abditis rerum causis*, p. 169, and Riolan the elder, 'Ad libros Fernelii de abditis rerum causis Commentarium', p. 159.

31 Account in A. Debus, *The Chemical Philosophy: Paracelsian Science and Medicine in the Sixteenth and Seventeenth Centuries*, 2 vols. (London, 1977), vol. I, ch. 3. See also H. Trevor-Roper, 'The Sieur de la Rivière, Paracelsian physician of Henri IV', in A. Debus (ed.), *Science, Medicine and Society in the Renaissance*, 2 vols. (London, 1972), vol. II, pp. 227–50.

32 Riolan and his son were the authors of numerous pamphlets in the 1600s attacking the court Paracelsians. For example, *Ad Libavimaniam Joan. Riolan [the elder] responsio pro censura Scholae parisiensis contra alchymiam lata* (Paris, 1606).

33 See L. W. B. Brockliss, 'Medical teaching at the University of Paris, 1600–1720', *Annals of Science*, 35 (1978), 221–51, at pp. 241–5. It must be emphasized that the neo-Paracelsians continued to call themselves Galenists and only accepted Paracelsian remedies. For a typical experiential defence of *metalla*, see J. de Bourges, 'An temeraria desperatis curatio?' (1619), in Paris TMP, III in-fol., no. 590.

34 Fernel, *De abditis rerum causis*, pp. 174–7.

35 P. Le Paulmier, *Lapis philosophicus dogmaticorum quo paracelsista Libavius restitutur, Scholae Medicae Parisienis iudicium de Chymiis declaratur, censura in adulteria et fraudes Parachymicorum deffenditur, asserto verae Alchemiae honore* (Paris, 1609). Le Paulmier's dates are unknown.

36 See especially chapter XI. Le Paulmier claimed that Galen, too, came to recognize the divine element in medicine.

37 See the remarks in Patin's letter to Belin, 4 November 1631: Patin *Lettres*, ed. Réveillé-Parise, vol. I, p. 13. The connection between Fernel and the neo-Paracelsians was strengthened by the fate of the great man's papers. These had been left to his valet who later became a Parisian physician and bequeathed them in turn to a nephew. The valet's nephew was none other than Pierre Le Paulmier; see Patin to Belin, 28 March 1643: *ibid*. vol. I, p. 280.

38 Patin became a doctor of medicine at Paris in 1627. His letters start from 1630.

39 Le Paulmier was ejected from the Paris faculty in 1610. By that date neo-Paracelsian theses were sustained at Montpellier without objection: for example, BL, 1180 b 1, Dissertations sustained by Charles de l'Orme in 1608, 'Assertiones', p. 34 (on the value of chemical medicine and the use of antimony). De l'Orme (1584–1678) is remembered for his promotion of the waters of Bourbon; see *Les Historiettes de Tallemant des Réaux*, 8 vols. (Paris, n.d.), vol. IV, pp. 180–2.

40 According to tradition, only graduates of the Paris faculty could legitimately practise in the capital. The sole exception were physicians officially attending the royal family. This right was legally confirmed in 1598. See Bibliothèque de la Faculté de Médecine de Paris, MS 9, fol. 55 (faculty minutes *sub* 1598).

41 J. Riolan the younger, *Curieuses recherches sur les escholes en médecine de Paris et de Montpelier* (Paris, 1651). For Riolan's defence of the rationalist position, see especially pp. 228–52. Courtaud's original pamphlet is referred to below, note 50. Riolan the younger's life and works are described in Hazon, *Notice des hommes, sub nomine*. On Courtaud, see the notice in J. Astruc, *Mémoires pour servir à l'histoire de la faculté de médecine de Montpellier* (Paris, 1767), pp. 261–2.

42 Much of Riolan the younger's book is a historical defence of the Paris faculty's monopoly, especially pp. 16–169.

43 In 1610 one Guillaume Desdames sustained a dissertation entitled 'An epilepsiae cranum humanum?' Unlike Hachette in 1598, Desdames castigated the use of the peony root and a host of other occult specifics: see Paris TMP, III in-fol., no. 436.

44 For a typical defence of theriac by a rationalist, see Philibert Morisset, 'An pestilenti febri theriaca?' (1626), in Paris TMP, IV in-fol., no. 676. The ingredients in theriac are described in Fr. Millepierres, *La vie quotidienne des médecins au temps de Molière* (Paris, 1964), ch. 7.

45 R. Morellus [Moreau], 'An pesti remedia αδοξα?', in Paris TMP, III in-fol., no. 574. At this date Moreau's scepticism was not always shared by the first generation of rationalists identified by Patin. See J. Duret, *Le général et souverain remède contre la maladie pestilentieuse* (Paris, 1623). Duret, doctor in 1584, died in 1629. A biographical notice on both Moreau and Duret can be found in Hazon, *Notice des hommes*.

46 Undated letter to Belin [*c.* 1631], in Triaire (ed.), *Lettres de Gui Patin*, p. 22. By 1649 Patin could claim that the *lapidus bezoardicus* was no longer heard of: letter to Spon, 18 June, in Patin, *Lettres*, ed. Réveillé-Parise, vol. I, p. 543.

47 See, for example, Fernel, *De abditis rerum causis*, pp. 157–69; Jean Lamperière, 'Estne in periaptis vis medica?' (1598); Guillaume Duval, 'An carbunculo sapphira?' (1611); Michel Duport, 'An curandis morbis amuleta?' (1643): Paris TMP, II in-fol., no. 276; III in-fol., no. 437; IV in-fol., no. 916.

48 Louis Robillart, 'An epilepsiae aetatis mutatio?' in Paris TMP, III in-fol., no. 519: 'amuleta, scripta, figura, characteres, ter insusuratta tria carmina'.

49 Admittedly, this is not how the rationalists perceived their achievement. Rather, they drew the distinction between Arabic and Greek medical practice. In their eyes they were cleansing the Graeco-Roman inheritance of its Arabic accretions.

50 For example, A. S. Curtaudus [Courtaud], 'Monspeliensis medicorum universitatis oratio' (21 October 1644), in BL, 1185 f 2(17).

51 *Lettres choisies de feu Monsieur Gui Patin ... dans lesquelles sont contenues plusieurs particularités historiques, sur la vie et la mort des savans de ce siècle, sur leurs écrits et sur plusieurs autres choses curieuses depuis l'an 1645 jusqu'en 1672,* 2nd edn (Paris, 1688), letter 3, pp. 8–10: a general defence of phlebotomy. Both Cousinots were identified by Patin as members of the rationalist coterie. Cousinot the younger was *premier médicin du roi 1643–6.*

52 Riolan the younger, *Curieuses recherches*, pp. 229–30.

53 *Ibid.*, p. 240. A short notice appears on Citoys in the *Dictionnaire de biographie française, sub nomine*.

54 Le Paulmier, *Lapis philosophicus*, pp. 118–22. There was a need, therefore, for stronger remedies which would be made safe by chemistry.

55 The physician and apothecary in *Le malade imaginaire* (1673).

56 Cf. Riolan the elder, 'Ad libros Fernelii de abditis rerum causis Commentarium', p. 166. Also, Lazare Rivière [Riverius], *Praxis medica cum Theoria*, 9th edn (Lyons, 1657), p. 355. Riverius, d. 1655, was a Montpellier professor with impeccable Fernelian credentials: see his description of the plague, *ibid.*, pp. 343–4. Riverius's *Praxis medica* was heartily disliked by Patin: comments in a letter to Belin, 10 May 1646 (Patin, *Lettres*, ed. Réveillé-Parise, vol. I, p. 122).

57 Cf. Patin's views on Gassendi. The philosopher was a great man who had ruined

his life by an excessive abstinence: letter to Spon, 23 August 1655, in Patin, *Lettres*, ed. Réveillé-Parise, vol. II, pp. 153–4.

58 *Schola salernitana, hoc est de valetudine tuenda* 'Animadversiones novae et copiosae Renati Moreau DMP' (Thomas Blasius: Paris, 1625). René Moreau was a leading influence among the second generation of rationalists. He was Patin's mentor and friend: see Hazon, *Notice des hommes, sub* Patin. On the history of this eleventh-century health guide, see the account by F. R. Packard in the reprint of Sir John Harington's 1607 English translation of the *Regimen sanitatis Salernitanum* (London, 1922), pp. 7–51.

59 N. Ellain, *Advis sur la peste* (Paris, 1604), pp. 31–44; biographical details in Hazon, *Notice des hommes, sub nomine*. On the growth of public health in France and Europe, see: J. Biraben, *Les hommes et la peste en France et dans les pays européens et méditerranéens*, 2 vols. (Paris, 1976), vol. II, pp. 85–101; C. Cipolla, *Cristofano and the Plague: A Study in the History of Public Health in the Age of Galileo* (London, 1973); C. Cipolla, *Public Health and the Medical Profession in the Renaissance* (London, 1976).

60 Hazon, *Notice des hommes, sub* Moreau. Little attention was paid to his request. Paris public health regulations really only began with Louis XIV: see J. Lévi-Valensi, *La médecine et les médecins français au XVIIe siècle* (Paris, 1933), pp. 70–80.

61 Hazon, *Notice des hommes, sub* Patin. The 1632 edition has not been seen. Patin's treatise was presumably his *Traité de la conservation de santé* published independently in the same year (n.p.). Guybert's work stressed the consultative role of the physician in its title: *Le medecin charitable enseignant la maniere de faire et preparer en la maison avec facilite et peu de frais les remedes propres à toutes maladies, selon l'advis du medecin ordinaire*, 1st edn (Lyons, 1623). Guybert was not specifically identified by Patin as one of the rationalist coterie but the value of his pharmacopoeia is vaunted in a number of letters: for example, to Belin, undated [*c.* 1631] and 18 January 1633, in Triaire (ed.), *Lettres de Gui Patin*, pp. 22 and 61–2. On the history of the self-help medical manual in the period under review, see A. Wear, 'Popularized ideas of health and illness in seventeenth-century France', *Seventeenth-Century French Studies*, 8 (1986), 229–42.

62 R. Pintard (ed.), *La Mothe le Vayer, Gassendi, Gui Patin: Etudes de bibliographie et de critique suivies de textes inédits de Gui Patin* (Paris, 1943), pp. 63–9.

63 Patin, *Lettres*, ed. Réveille-Parise, vol. I, p. 453, letter to Spon, 18 January 1649. Patin depicted all Fernelians as greedy. Cf. his picture of the *premier médecin du roi*, Vautier, in a letter to Spon of 29 May 1648: *ibid.*, vol. I, pp. 396–7.

64 The Jansenists aimed to restore strict adherence to the Ten Commandments in a moral universe dominated by Jesuit laxists. Their programme was promoted in a number of pamphlets in the 1640s and 1650s, notably in the *Lettres provinciales* (1655–6) of Pascal. Jansenism was particularly strong among the Paris lower clergy.

65 There is no evidence Patin belonged to the Jansenist movement but his correspondence continually refers sympathetically to its supporters: cf. his brief encomium to the movement's founding father in France, the Abbé Saint-Cyran: letter to Spon, 26 October 1643, in Patin, *Lettres*, ed. Réveillé-Parise, vol. I, p. 301.

66 The best recent account of the sect is A. Adam, *Du mysticisme à la révolte: les Jansénistes du XVIIe siècle* (Paris, 1968).

67 For a general introduction to this contemporary phenomenon, see H. Trevor-Roper, *The European Witchcraze of the Sixteenth and Seventeenth Centuries* (Harmondsworth, 1969).

68 Fernel, *De abditis rerum causis*, p. 159. 'Vidi execrationibus, precibus, verbis, sacrosanctis, votis et ieiuniis expederi i qui etiamnum saluberrime et integerimma mente degunt.'

69 George Scharpius, 'An solo contactu [,] visu, voce, afflatu, osculo, vel nudi lintei applicatione, vulnera et morbi naturaliter infligi et curari possint?', in Scharpius,

Quaestiones medicae (J. Gilet: Montpellier, 1617), pp. 21–2 (dissertations for a vacant chair: BN, T³¹ 265); Pierre Cognard, 'An a daemonibus, linguarum peregrinarum locutio, in maniacis et melancholicis?' (Montpellier, 1639): BL, 1185 f 2(15), pp. 8–10.

70 Riolan the elder, 'Ad libros Fernelii de abditis rerum causis Commentarium', pp. 134–5. 'Faverem peripateticis, nisi religioni christianae Platonicarum doctrina ex parte magis consentiret: malim errare cum ecclesia, quam cum philosophis bene sentire.'

71 [M. Marescot], *Discours véritable sur le faict de Marthe Brossier* (Paris, 1599). The examination took place only a year after the king had granted the Huguenots toleration through the Edict of Nantes. Marescot was identified as a first-generation rationalist by Patin. For an account of the Brossier case, see D. P. Walker, *Unclean Spirits: Possession and Exorcism in France and England in the Late Sixteenth and Early Seventeenth Centuries* (London, 1981), pp. 33–42; and R. Mandrou, *Magistrats et sorciers en France au XVIIᵉ siècle* (Paris, 1968), pp. 161–79.

72 Patin, *Lettres*, ed. Réveillé-Parise, vol. I, pp. 302–6, letter to Belin, 16 November 1643. The Brabantine physician Wier (1515–88) was author of *De praestigiis daemonum* (Basle, 1564), one of the first works to doubt the existence of witches. Del Rio (1551–1608) first published his book in 1599 at Louvain.

73 Patin, *Lettres*, ed. Réveillé-Parise, vol. III, pp. 211–12, letter to Falconet, 11 May 1660.

74 On the Loudun and Louviers cases, see Mandrou, *Magistrats et sorciers*, pp. 264–94; also, *ibid*, pp. 298–301 for Naudé's views on possession.

75 For a limited discussion, see Packard, *Patin*, pp. 259–65. Patin's correspondence is a good source for studying the mid-seventeenth century constitutionalist opposition to absolutism.

76 For example, G. Avenel (ed.), *Lettres, instructions diplomatiques et papiers d'état du Cardinal de Richelieu*, 8 vols. (Paris, 1853–77), vol. VII, pp. 911–14.

77 Patin and his correspondents seem to have kept their political opinions hidden. Patin from 1650 to 1672 held a medical chair at the Paris Collège Royal. This was an educational establishment, independent of the University, devoted to higher learning. As appointments were in the gift of the crown, Patin's elevation would have been impossible, had he been politically suspect. Evidently, his letters were never opened!

78 Patin's view of the court physician is discussed in Laurence Brockliss, 'The literary image of the *médecins du roi* in the literature of the Grand Siècle', in Vivian Nutton (ed.), *Medicine at the Courts of Europe 1500–1837* (London, 1990), pp. 124–9.

79 Patin, *Lettres*, ed. Réveillé-Parise, vol. I, p. 453; vol. II, p. 285; vol. II, p. 585: letter to Belin, 18 June 1649; to Spon, 13 March 1656; to Falconet, 15 August 1651.

80 'Taking the waters' was attacked in a number of faculty theses; for example; François Buonnier, 'An colico dolori narcotica cathartici miscenda?' (1618); Jean Pietre, 'An visceribus nutritis aestuantibus metallicarum aquarum potus salubris?' (1633): in Paris TMP, III in-fol., no. 578, and V in-fol., no. 790.

81 Patin, *Lettres*, ed. Réveillé-Parise, vol. II, p. 286n. Of the three fountains at Forges one became known as the Reinette and another, the Cardinale. For this and other popular seventeenth-century French spas, see L. W. B. Brockliss, 'The development of the spa in seventeenth-century France', in Roy Porter (ed.), *The Medical History of Waters and Spas*, suppl. 10, *Medical History* (London, 1990), pp. 23–47.

82 Louis XIV quite unfairly associated Jansenism with the Fronde. For the orthodoxy of Jansenist political thought, see R. Taveneaux (ed.), *Le Jansénisme et le politique* (Paris, 1965).

83 Details of Renaudot's tussle with the faculty are to be found in H. Soloman, *Public Welfare, Science and Propaganda in Seventeenth-Century France: The Innovations of Théophraste Renaudot* (Princeton, 1972), ch. 6. Renaudot was first denounced in 1640: see his *Factum du procez d'entre maistre Theophraste Renaudot, docteur*

en Medecine de la Faculté de Montpellier ... contre les Doyen et docteurs en medecine de la Faculté de Paris (n.p., n.d. [1640]). This is an interesting pamphlet because it points out that the faculty was divided over the use of metallic drugs. The faculty's case against Renaudot was defended in pamphlets by both Patin and Moreau; for example, René Moreau, *La Défence de la Faculté de Médecine contre son calomniateur ...* (n.p., 1641).

84 J. A. Hazon, *Eloge historique de la faculté de médecine, 16 octobre 1770* (Paris, 1773), pp. 50–1. The Parlement was the high court.

85 Brockliss, 'Medical teaching', pp. 231–5.

86 Riolan first published his *Anthropographia* in 1618. It had reached its fifth edition by 1628.

87 For Riolan's alternative theory of circulation, see his *Encheiridium anatomicum et pathologicum*, 4th edn (Paris, 1658), pp. 493–565; 1st edn 1648. Riolan's ideas are discussed in N. Mani, 'Jean Riolan II (1586–1657) and medical research', *Bulletin of the History of Medicine*, 42 (1968), 122–44.

88 C. Schmitt, 'Towards a reassessment of Renaissance Aristotelianism', *History of Science*, 11 (1973), 159–93.

89 It would be particularly interesting to know about the situation in Spain where an unacademic, empiricist and demonicist medical tradition survived among the Moriscos. Given the establishment hostility to Morisco culture, it seems probable that Spanish Galenists in the second half of the sixteenth and early seventeenth centuries would have found the Fernelian synthesis religiously suspect. Indeed, perhaps it is in Spain that rationalist Galenism first developed in this period. On Morisco medicine, see L. García-Ballester, 'Academicism versus empiricism in practical medicine in sixteenth-century Spain with regard to the Morisco practitioners', in A. Wear, P. K. French and I. M. Lonie (eds.), *The Medical Renaissance of the Sixteenth Century* (Cambridge, 1985), pp. 246–70.

90 Among French-educated Galenists in the first half of the century only one rationalist has been so far discovered who was not a Paris graduate. This was the Englishman James Primrose, M.D. Montpellier in 1617 (d. 1659). In his graduate theses he dismissed a belief in the efficacy of amulets as superstitious and claimed that they had only a psychosomatic value. See British Library, 1185 f 2(7), pp. 28–31.

6 'The mark of truth'

1 For interesting discussions of this thesis, see S. Y. Edgerton, Jnr, *Pictures and Punishment: Art and Criminal Prosecution during the Florentine Renaissance* (Ithaca, 1985), esp. pp. 157ff. and *The Heritage of Giotto's Geometry, Art and Science on the Eve of the Scientific Revolution* (Ithaca, 1991); J. Ackerman, 'Early Renaissance "Naturalism" and scientific illustration', in A. Ellenius (ed.), *Natural Sciences and the Arts*, Acta Universitatis Upsaliensis, 22 (Uppsala, 1985), pp. 1–17; and the essays by A. Crombie, Ackerman and Edgerton in J. Shirley and F. D. Hoeniger (eds.), *Science and the Arts in the Renaissance* (Cranbury, N.J., 1985).

2 W. Hunter, Lecture to the Royal Academy of Arts, 1770, in M. Kemp (ed.), *Dr William Hunter at the Royal Academy of Arts* (Glasgow, 1975), p. 40.

3 See M. Kemp, 'Taking it on trust: form and meaning in naturalistic representation', *Archives of Natural History*, 17 (1990), 127–88.

4 From Hunter's paper on the *Original* published in W. D. I. Rolfe, 'William Hunter (1718–1783) on Irish "Elk" and Stubbs' *Moose*', *Archives of Natural History*, 11 (1983), p. 270.

5 See. J. Edgerton, *George Stubbs 1724–1806* (London, 1984), pp. 118–19.

6 D. Knight, *Zoological Illustration* (Folkestone, 1977), p. 116.

7 The most substantial recent account of Leonardo's anatomical work is by C. Pedretti and K. Keele, *Leonardo da Vinci: Corpus of Anatomical Drawings in the*

Collection of Her Majesty the Queen, 3 vols. (New York, 1979–80). See also K. Keele, *Leonardo da Vinci's Elements of the Science of Man* (London, 1983).

8   Windsor, Royal Library, 19007v, see M. Kemp, 'Dissection and divinity in Leonardo's late anatomies', *Journal of the Warburg and Courtauld Institutes*, 35 (1972), p. 215, n. 85.

9   M. Kemp, 'A drawing for the *Fabrica* and some thoughts upon the Vesalius muscle men', *Medical History*, 14 (1970), p. 281.

10   M. Kemp, '"Il concetto dell'anima" in Lenardo's early skull studies', *Journal of the Warburg and Courtauld Institutes*, 34 (1971), 115–34.

11   Kemp, Dissection and divinity', p. 216. For a related issue, see M. Pardo, 'Memory, Imagination, figuration: Leonardo da Vinci and the painter's mind', in S. Küchler and W. Melion (eds.), *Images of memory* (Washington, D. C., 1991), pp. 47–73.

12   Windsor, Royal Library, 19013v.

13   For a good discussion of Verengario's principles, see R. French, 'Berengario da Carpi and the use of commentary in anatomical teaching', in A. Wear, R. French and I. Lonie (eds.), *The Medical Renaissance of the Sixteenth Century* (Cambridge, 1985), pp. 42–74.

14   Berengario da Carpi, *Isagogae breves* (Benedictum Hectoris: Bologna, 1522), fols. 63v–64r; and *A Short Introduction to Anatomy (Isagogae Breves)*, trans. L. Lind (Chicago, 1939), p. 160.

15   *Ibid.*, fol. 71r (trans., p. 172).

16   For these terms see French, 'Berengario', pp. 52–3.

17   J. B. de C. M. Saunders and C. D. O'Malley, *The Illustrations from the Works of Andreas Vesalius of Brussels* (Cleveland, 1952).

18   A. Vesalius, *De humani corporis fabrica libri septem* (J. Oporinus: Basle, 1543), notes to 59:1; and Saunders and O'Malley, *The Illustrations*, p. 168.

19   Kemp, 'A drawing for the *Fabrica*', pp. 281–4.

20   A. Vesalius, *Suorum de humani corporis fabrica librorum epitome* (Basle, 1543), introductory letter to the reader; and Saunders and O'Malley, *The Illustrations*, p. 204.

21   Saunders and O'Malley, *The Illustrations*, p. 46.

22   *Ibid.*, p. 47.

23   I have used the Italian edition: G. Valverde di Hamusco, *Anatomia del corpo humano* (Nicolò Bevilaqua; Rome 1560), notes for II, 1. The first edition, *Historia de la composicion del cuorpo humano*, was published in Spanish in Rome in 1556. See F. Guerra, 'Juan de Valverde de Amusco ...', *Clio Medica*, 2 (1962), 339–63. For the artistic sources of Gaspard Becerra's presentation of Valverde's muscleman, see amongst others Edgerton, *Pictures and Punishment*, pp. 216–19.

24   Valverde, *Anatomia*, introductory letter to the reader.

25   *Ibid.*, p. 26.

26   O. Brunfels, *Herbarum vivae eicones*, (I. Schott: Strasburg, 1530), and L. Fuchs, *De historia stirpium* (Carolus Guilard: Paris, 1543), which was much admired by Vesalius.

27   C. Estienne (Carolus Stephanus), *La dissection des parties du corps humain* (Simon de Colines, Paris, 1546); and facsimile edition with introduction by P. Huard and M. Grmek (Paris, 1965). The Latin edition, *De dissectione ...*, was published in Paris in 1545.

28   A. Monro (*primus*), 'The anatomy of the human bones and nerves' in A. Monro (*secundus*) (ed.), *The Works of Alexander Monro M.D.* (Edinburgh, 1781), pp. 46–7. The first edition, *The Anatomy of the Humane Bones*, was published in Edinburgh in 1726.

29   Monro, *Works*, pp. 29–30. Monro was referring to *Traité d'ostéologie, traduit de l'anglais de M. Monro* (Paris, 1759) illustrated by Suë for the French Academy of Arts.

30   W. Cheselden, *Osteographia or the Anatomy of the Bones* (London, 1733), preface. For Cheselden, see Z. Cope, *William Cheselden* (Edinburgh, 1953).

31 Cheselden, *Osteographia*, preface. For the study of anatomy at early British academies of art, including the involvement of Cheselden, see I. Bignamini in *The Artist's Model*, exhibition catalogue (with M. Postle) (Nottingham, 1991), pp. 8–15.

32 Cheselden, *Osteographia*, ch. VIII. See R. Ollerenshaw, 'The camera obscura in medical illustration: a belated reference', *British Journal of Photography* (1977), pp. 815–16.

33 Cheselden, *Osteographia*, preface; all subsequent quotations of Cheselden are also from this preface.

34 B. S. Albinus, *Tabulae sceleti et musculorum corporis humani* (Basle, 1747 and London, 1749); and *The Explanation of Albinus's Anatomical Figures of the Human Skeleton and Muscles* (London, 1754), p. xxii. See J. Elkins, 'Two conceptions of the human form: Bernard Siegfried Albinus and Andreas Vesalius', *Artibus et historiae*, 7 (1986), pp. 91–106.

35 Albinus, *Tabulae*, p. iv.

36 For such devices, see M. Kemp, *The Science of Art: Optical Themes in Western Art from Brunelleschi to Seurat* (London 1990), pp. 167–203. Elkins, 'Two conceptions', p. 93, misunderstands Albinus's grid technique.

37 Albinus, *Tabulae*, p. iv.

38 *Ibid.*, p. iii.

39 *Ibid.*, p. xxii.

40 *Ibid.*

41 For example, Albinus, *Dissertatio de arteriis et venis, intestinorum hominis adjecta icon coloribus distincta* (Leiden, 1736); *Dissertatio secunda de sede et caussa colores aethiopum et caeterorum hominum* (Leiden, 1737); *Icon durae matris in convexa superficie visae ...* (Amsterdam, 1738); and *Effiges penis humani injecta cera praeparati* (Leiden, 1741); all illustrated with colour prints by Jan Ladmiral.

42 Albinus, *Tabulae*, p. xv.

43 *Ibid.*, p. xix.

44 *Ibid.*, p. xxiv.

45 *Ibid.*, p. v.

46 P. Camper, *Epistola ad anatomicorum principem magnum albinum* (Gröningen, 1767).

47 W. Hunter, *Anatomia uteri humani gravidi (The Anatomy of the Human Gravid uterus)* (Birmingham, 1774), preface. The most important biographical material on Hunter is to be found in C. H. Brock (ed.), *William Hunter 1718–1783: A Memoir by Samuel Foart Simmons and John Hunter* (Glasgow, 1983). See also the essays in W. Bynum and R. Porter (eds.), *William Hunter and the Eighteenth-Century Medical World* (Cambridge, 1985).

48 Hunter, *Gravid Uterus*, notes to plate 10, fig. 1.

49 *Ibid.*, preface.

50 For Hunter as a collector of paintings, see A. McLaren Young, *Glasgow University's Pictures* (Glasgow, 1973).

51 J. Hunter, *The Natural History of the Human Teeth* (London, 1771).

52 J. Thornton, *Jacob van Rymsdyk* (Cambridge, 1982).

53 Hunter, *Gravid Uterus*, preface. For the lectures, see Kemp, (ed.), *Dr. William Hunter*.

54 Hunter, *Gravid Uterus*, preface.

55 *Ibid.*

56 W. Cumming, *The Proofs of Infanticide Considered Including Dr Hunter's Tract on Child Murder* (London, 1836). Hunter's paper was read to the members of the Medical Society on 14 July 1783.

57 *Gravid Uterus*, note to plate 1. See L. Jordanova, 'Gender, generation and science: William Hunter's obstetrical atlas', in Bynum and Porter (eds.), *William Hunter*, pp. 386–412.

58 C. N. Jenty, *Demonstratio uteri praegnantis mulieris* (Nuremberg, 1761); and his advertisement for his *Four Tables*.

59 Hunter, *Gravid Uterus*, preface.

7 The art and science of seeing in medicine

1 Judith Wechsler, *A Human Comedy: Physiognomy and Caricature in 19th Century Paris* (London, 1982); Janet Browne, 'Darwin and the face of madness', in W. F. Bynum *et al.* (eds.), *The Anatomy of Madness*, 3 vols. (London 1985), vol. I, pp. 151–65; Sander Gilman, *Seeing the Insane: A Cultural History of Madness and Art in the Western World* (New York, 1982); Sander Gilman, *Difference and Pathology: Stereotypes of Sexuality, Race and Madness* (Ithaca, 1985); Carlo Ginzburg, 'Morelli, Freud and Sherlock Holmes: clues and scientific method', *History Workship Journal*, 9 (1980), 5–36; Georges Didi-Huberman, *Invention de l'hystérie: Charcot et l'iconographie photographique de la Salpêtrière* (Paris, 1982); Mary Cowling, *The Artist as Anthropologist. The Representation of Type and Character in Victorian Art* (Cambridge, 1989).

2 Thomas Cooper, 'Observations respecting the history of physiognomy', *Memoirs of the Manchester Literary and Philosophical Society*, 3 (1790), 408–62.

3 Abraham Rees, *The Cyclopaedia: or, Universal Dictionary of Arts, Sciences, and Literature* (London, 1819), vol. XXVII (not paginated); *A New Royal and Universal Dictionary of Arts and Sciences* (London, 1771), vol. XI. Strictly speaking there is a special term to distinguish the study of static features (physiognomy) from that of the expression of the emotions (pathognomy). In practice, however, such a tidy distinction was rarely held to, not least because static features were understood as partly the product of habitual responses, themselves often the result of passion, emotion or the lack of it. Here I use physiognomy in the broadest sense compatible with contemporary accounts.

4 Other works that raise these questions include: J. Bourges, 'Esquisse d'un mémoire sur la physiognomonie', *Journal général de médecine, de chirugie, de pharmacie*, 18 (an 11), 129–43; James Parsons, *Human Physiognomy Explained* (London, 1747); and J. Pernetty, *Lettres philosophiques sur les physionomies*, 2nd edn (The Hague, 1758).

5 Richard Brown, *An Essay on the Truth of Physiognomy and its Application to Medicine* (Philadelphia, 1807). I have not been able to locate any biographical information on Brown. The British Library catalogue lists him as Richard Brown of Alexandria, U.S.A.

6 *Ibid.*, p. 9.

7 *Ibid.*, p. 11.

8 *Ibid.*, p. 19.

9 *Ibid.*, p. 23.

10 *Ibid.*, p. 38.

11 *Ibid.*, p. 41.

12 *Ibid.*, p. 65.

13 *Ibid.*, p. 66.

14 *Ibid.*, p. 78.

15 F. Cabuchet, *Essai sur l'expression de la face dans l'état de santé et de maladie* (Paris, an 10). All translations from this work are mine. I have not been able to locate any biographical information on Cabuchet.

16 *Ibid.*, p. 3.

17 P. Camper, *Dissertation physique de M. Pierre Camper, sur les différences réeles que présentent les traits du visage chez les hommes de différents pays* (Utrecht, 1791); P. Camper, *Discours prononcés par feu M. P. Camper sur le moyen de représenter d'une manière sure les diverses passions* (Utrecht, 1792); T. Cogan (ed.), *The Works of the Late Professor Camper* (London, 1821).

18 Cabuchet, *Essai*, p. 31.
19 On the idea of languages of nature, see L. Jordanova (ed.), *Languages of nature: Critical Essays on Science and Literature* (London, 1986).
20 I discuss the question of authors of nature, natural theology and physiognomy at greater length in 'Nature's powers: a reading of Lamarck's distinction between creation and production', in J. Moore (ed.), *The Humanity of Evolution* (Cambridge, 1989), pp. 71–98.
21 Cabuchet, *Essai*, p. 36.
22 On environmentalist approaches to medicine in this period, see J. Riley, *The Eighteenth Century Campaign to Avoid Disease* (Basingstoke, 1987).
23 C. Bell, *Essays on the Anatomy of Expression in Painting* (London, 1806), pp. vi–vii.
24 *Ibid.*, p. 13
25 *Ibid.*, p. 88.
26 J.-J. Suë, *Essai sur la physiognomonie des corps vivans* (Paris, 1797).
27 Bell, *Essays*, pp. vii–ix.
28 C. Bell, *The Hand, its Mechanism and Vital Endowments as Evincing Design* (London, 1837), p. 255.
29 *Ibid.*, p. 329.
30 *Ibid.*, p. 361.

8 The introduction of percussion and stethoscopy to Edinburgh

1 For descriptions of diagnostic practice in the eighteenth century, see C. Newman, 'Diagnostic investigation before Laënnec', *Medical History*, 4 (1960), 322–9; M. Nicolson, 'Giovanni Morgagni and physical examination in the eighteenth century', in C. Lawrence (ed.), *Medical Theory, Surgical Practice* (London, 1992); M. Nicolson, 'The art of diagnosis: medicine and the five senses' in W. F. Bynum and R. Porter (eds.), *Companion Encyclopaedia of the History of Medicine* (London, forthcoming).
2 The best account of the introduction of the new methods of diagnosis is S. J. Reiser, *Medicine and the Reign of Technology* (Cambridge, 1978). For the anatomico-clinical method in the early nineteenth century, see R. C. Maulitz, *Morbid Appearances: The Anatomy of Pathology in the Early Nineteenth Century* (Cambridge, 1987).
3 E. J. Bluth, 'James Hope and the acceptance of auscultation', *Journal of the History of Medicine*, 25 (1970), 202–10; S. J. Reiser, 'Aspects of the role of the stethoscope in the introduction of auscultation to Great Britain and the United States', in *Proceedings, Twenty-second International Congress for the History of Medicine, 1972* (London, 1974), pp. 832–40; also L. S. King, 'Auscultation in England, 1821–1837', *Bulletin of the History of Medicine*, 33 (1959), 446–53.
4 C. Newman, *Evolution of Medical Education in the Nineteenth Century* (Oxford, 1957), pp. 86–104; C. Newman, 'Physical signs in the London hospitals', *Medical History*, 2 (1958), 195–201.
5 P. J. Bishop, 'Reception of the stethoscope and Laënnec's book', *Thorax*, 36 (1981), 487–92; also P. J. Bishop, 'The evolution of the stethoscope', *Journal of the Royal Society of Medicine*, 73 (1980), 448–56.
6 For similar interpretations, see A. Sakula, 'Laënnec's influence on some British physicians in the nineteenth century', *Journal of the Royal Society of Medicine*, 74 (1981), 759–67; S. Jarcho, 'An early review of Laënnec's treatise', *American Journal of Cardiology*, 9 (1962), 962–9; S. Jarcho, 'An early mention of the stethoscope (Locock 1821)', *Bulletin of the New York Academy of Medicine*, 41 (1965), 374–7; S. Jarcho, 'Early impressions of mediate auscultation by James Clark', *American Journal of Cardiology*, 3 (1959), 254–6. But see also note 23 below.
7 What is missing is attention to the 'tacit', 'craft', or 'enculturational' elements of

medical knowledge; see M. Polanyi, *Personal Knowledge: Toward a Post-Critical Philosophy* (London, 1958); J. Ravetz, *Scientific Knowledge and its Social Problems* (Oxford, 1971); H. M. Collins, 'The TEA set: tacit knowledge and scientific networks', *Science Studies*, 4 (1974), 165–8. For medically relevant examples, see L. Fleck, *The Genesis and Development of a Scientific Fact* (Chicago, 1979) and the discussion of the work of Georges Canguilhem in M. Nicolson, 'The social and the cognitive: resources for the sociology of scientific knowledge', *Studies in the History and Philosophy of Science*, 22 (1991), 347–69.

8 Quoted in S. Jarcho, 'The introduction of percussion in the United States', *Journal of the History of Medicine*, 13 (1958), 259–60.

9 W. Cullen, *First Lines of the Practice of Physic*, 4 vols. (Edinburgh, 1789), vol. II, p. 314.

10 Anon., 'Review of Corvisart *Essai sur les maladies et les lésions organiques du coeur et des gros vaisseaux*', *Edinburgh Medical and Surgical Journal*, 7 (1811), 68–79. There is, however, a mention of a successful attempt to apply percussion in the lectures of Alexander Munro *secundus*, dating from *circa* 1772; see C. Lawrence, 'Ornate physicians and learned artisans: Edinburgh medical men, 1726–1776', in W. F. Bynum and R. Porter (eds.), *William Hunter and the Eighteenth-Century Medical World* (Cambridge, 1985), pp. 153–76.

11 For Corvisart and his advocacy of percussion, see E. Ackerknecht, *Medicine at the Paris Hospital 1794–1848*, (Baltimore, 1967), pp. 83–8.

12 For biographical details of Duncan, see J. D. Comrie, *History of Scottish Medicine*, 2 vols., (London, 1932), p. 507 *et passim*. The style and content of the Corvisart review are very suggestive of the writing of Andrew Duncan junior. Furthermore, the Duncans, father and son, ran the three journals with which they were associated as if they were a family business, doing most of the reviewing themselves. This was standard practice at the time. While other authors did work on preparing the 'Critical Analyses' for the *Edinburgh Medical and Surgical Journal*, they were mostly located outside Scotland. The author of the Corvisart review identifies himself as being Scots. Therefore it is most likely to have been Andrew Duncan junior, who was well known, moreover, for his close interest in Continental medicine.

13 Anon., 'Review of Corvisart *Essai*', p. 69.

14 A. Duncan, 'Three cases of inflammation of the heart, with appearances on dissection', *Edinburgh Medical and Surgical Journal*, 12 (1816), 43–71.

15 *Ibid.*, p. 59.

16 *Ibid.*, p. 64.

17 *Ibid.*, p. 66.

18 *Ibid.*, pp. 66–7.

19 *Ibid.*

20 A. Duncan, *Reports of the Practice in the Clinical Wards of the Edinburgh Royal Infirmary* (Edinburgh, 1819).

21 *Ibid.*, p. 83.

22 For example, *ibid.*, pp. 48–9.

23 The conclusion I offer here for Duncan's knowledge of percussion in 1818 is very similar to that suggested by Jarcho for James Clark's knowledge of the stethoscope in 1820: S. Jarcho, 'Auenbrugger, Laënnec and John Keats: some notes on the early history of percussion and auscultation', *Medical History*, 5 (1961), 167–72. See note 30 below.

24 A. Duncan (senior), *Observations on the Distinguishing Symptoms of the Three Different Species of Pulmonary Consumption, the Catarrhal, the Apostematous, and the Tuberculous*, 2nd edn (Edinburgh, 1816).

25 For an account of practice in the Royal Infirmary, see G. Risse, *Hospital Life in Enlightenment Scotland: Care and Teaching at the Royal Infirmary of Edinburgh* (Cambridge, 1985), pp. 240–66. For other examples of selective cultural transfer in this area see Maulitz, *Morbid Appearances*, pp. 134–57; S. Jacyna, 'Robert

Carswell and William Thomson at the Hôtel-Dieu of Lyons: Scottish views of French Medicine', in R. French and A. Wear (eds.), *British Medicine in an Age of Reform* (London, 1991), pp. 110–35.

26 R. T. H. Laënnec, *De l'auscultation médiate ou traité de diagnostic des maladies des poumons et du cœur fondé principalement sur ce nouveau moyen d'exploration*, 2 vols., (Paris, 1819); Bishop, 'Reception of the stethoscope'.

27 For example, A. B. Granville, 'On *Mediate Auscultation* by R. T. H. Laënnec', *London Medical and Physical Journal*, 43 (1820), 164–70.

28 For example, Reiser, *Medicine and the Reign of Technology*, pp. 22–32; Maulitz, *Morbid Appearances*.

29 J. Forbes, 'Translator's preface', in R. T. H. Laënnec, *A Treatise on the Diseases of the Chest* (London, 1821), pp. vii–xxviii, at p. ix.

30 Sir James Clark, like Forbes an Edinburgh M.D., was one of the first British physicians to see the stethoscope demonstrated in Paris: J. Clark, *Medical Notes on Climate, Diseases, Hospitals and Medical Schools in France, Italy, and Switzerland* (London, 1820).

31 Forbes, 'Translator's preface', pp. xxvi–xxvii. It will be noted that my interpretation of why Forbes reordered Laënnec's text is somewhat different from that recently advanced by Maulitz, *Morbid Appearances*, pp. 168–71.

32 For example, see Anon., 'De l'auscultation mediate par R. T. H. Laennec', *Quarterly Journal of Foreign Medicine and Surgery*, 2 (1819–20), 54–68.

33 C. Locock, *Dissertatio Medica Inauguralis de Cordis Palpitatione* (Edinburgh, 1821). This thesis has been discussed by S. Jarcho, 'An early mention of the stethoscope'.

34 Maulitz's remark that Locock's thesis was 'replete with the use of the stethoscope' cannot therefore be sustained: R. C. Maulitz, 'Metropolitan medicine and the man-midwife: the early life and letters of Charles Locock', *Medical History*, 26 (1982), 25–46, at p. 32.

35 W. Stokes, *An Introduction to the Use of the Stethoscope with its Application to the Diagnosis in Diseases of the Thoracic Viscera* (Edinburgh, 1825).

36 For example, *ibid.*, p. 45.

37 V. Collin, *De diverse méthodes d'éxploration de la poitrine* (Paris, 1824).

38 Stokes, *An Introduction*, p. ix; G. Andral, *Recherches sur l'expectoration dans les différentes maladies de poitrine* (Paris, 1821). I should perhaps make it clear that Stokes acknowledged the full extent of his debt to the French authors.

39 Stokes, *An Introduction*, pp. 217, 216 and 221.

40 Stokes's text has been cited as evidence for the assertion that 'by 1823, ausculation mediated by the stethoscope must have been something of a commonplace in Edinburgh': J. Coope, 'Mr Bampton's prize or the tale of an old stethoscope', *Lancet* (1952), II, 577–80. As we have seen this conclusion cannot be sustained on that basis. However it is also true that the fact that Stokes's *Introduction* does not mention his own use of the stethoscope does not prove that he had, at this time, no clinical experience with the instrument. Later, Stokes did publish an account of his own investigations with the stethoscope: W. Stokes, *Two Lectures on the Application of the Stethoscope* (Dublin, 1828).

41 J. Forbes, *Original Cases with Dissections and Observations Illustrating the Use of the Stethoscope and Percussion in the Diagnosis of Diseases of the Chest* (London, 1824), p. viii.

42 A. Duncan, 'Contributions to morbid anatomy – IV, Empyema and pneumothorax', *Edinburgh Medical and Surgical Journal*, 28 (1827), 302–32, at p. 307.

43 *Ibid.*, p. 311.

44 *Ibid.*

45 See *ibid.*, pp. 302–3. This was certainly how it was interpreted by his contemporaries, see Anon., 'Review of Duncan's "Empyema and pneumothorax"', *Medico-Chirurgical Review*, 8 (1828), 131–3.

46 Anon., 'Review of R. T. H. Laënnec *De L'Auscultation Médiate* and J. Forbes *A*

Treatise on the Diseases of the Chest', *Edinburgh Medical and Surgical Journal*, 18 (1822), 447–74.

47 The reviewer had experimented not only with the use of the stethoscope in the clinical situation (*ibid.*, p. 456), but also with modifications to the design of the instrument (*ibid.*, p. 451).

48 *Ibid.*, p. 457.

49 *Ibid.*, p. 456.

50 *Ibid.*, p. 457.

51 *Ibid.*, p. 456.

52 *Ibid.*

53 W. Cullen, *A Probationary Surgical Essay on Bronchotomy: Submitted to the Examination of the Royal College of Surgeons of Edinburgh* (Edinburgh, 1822). I am grateful to Mr John Symons of the Wellcome Institute Library for bringing the Library's recent acquisition of a number of these essays to my attention.

54 J. Russell, *A Probationary Essay on Emphysema: Submitted to the Examination of the Royal College of Surgeons of Edinburgh* (Edinburgh, 1823).

55 P. Huard and M. Grmek, 'Les élèves étrangers de Laënnec', *Revue d'histoire des sciences*, 26 (1973), 315–37, at p. 324.

56 J. Struthers, *Historical Sketch of the Edinburgh Anatomical School* (Edinburgh, 1867), p. 80.

57 J. P. Kay, 'Letter to the Editor', *Lancet* (1827–8), I, 757.

58 Huard and Grmekm, 'Les élèves étrangers de Laënnec', p. 327. Gregory and Cullen were not the only students to return to Edinburgh having studied in Paris. One might also mention Henry Harrington, Thomas Hodgkin and John Goldwyer. The last-named dedicated his M.D. thesis to Laënnec: J. Goldwyer, *Tentamen Medica Inaugurale de Pathologia Pulmonum* (Edinburgh, 1821).

59 Stokes's *Introduction to the Use of the Stethoscope* is dedicated to the younger Cullen. The dedication cites Cullen's 'unremitting attention to the light which mediate auscultation is now throwing on the obscurity of disease'.

60 J. Hope, *Dissertatio Medica Inauguralis de Aortae Aneurismate* (Edinburgh, 1825). Hope later published a translated and somewhat enlarged version of this work: J. Hope, 'On the diagnosis of aneurisms of the aorta by general and stethoscope signs', *London Medical Gazette*, 4 (1829), 353–8, 391–4, 417–24 and 449–53.

61 For biographical details of Hope, see Mrs J. Hope, *Memoir of the late James Hope M.D.* (London, 1842); N. Flaxman, 'The Hope of cardiology: James Hope (1801–1841)', *Bulletin of the Institute of the History of Medicine*, 6 (1938), 1–21.

62 I am grateful to Mrs J. M. Jeffrey, formerly Lothian Health Board Archivist, Medical Archive Centre, University of Edinburgh, for tracing the names in the patient register of the Royal Infirmary for me. The only discrepancies are that the register gives Lindsay Carstairs as having been 'relieved', and Agnes Downes as having been 'cured'. Hope records both of them as dying shortly after leaving the Infirmary.

63 Laënnec, *A Treatise*, pp. 274–7.

64 Hope, *De Aortae Aneurismate*, pp. 17–22.

65 Hope was not the first to disagree with Laënnec on the diagnosis of aortic aneurysm. The usefulness of the stethoscope in this regard had been defended, *contra* Laënnec, by R. J. H. Bertin, *Traité des Maladies du cœur et des Gros Vaisseaux* (Paris, 1824), pp. 138–50. However, Hope's account of the differential diagnostics is more detailed than, and distinctively different from, Bertin's.

66 R. Spittal, 'Case of aneurism of the abdominal aorta', *Edinburgh Medical and Surgical Journal*, 33 (1830), 303–7.

67 J. W. Turner, 'Observations on the cause of the sounds produced by the action of the heart', *Edinburgh Medico-Chirurgical Transactions*, 3 (1828), 205. For a full discussion of Laënnec's understanding of the heart sounds, see J. Duffin, 'The cardiology of R. T. H. Laennec', *Medical History*, 33 (1989), 42–71.

68 The work of Matthew Baillie Gairdner is discussed in G. W. Balfour, 'On the

evolution of cardiac diagnosis from Harvey's days till now', *Edinburgh Medical Journal*, 32 (1887), 1065–81; and W. P. Alison, *Outlines of Physiology*, 3rd edn (Edinburgh, 1839), p. 50.

69 There was a priority dispute between these two Edinburgh alumni on this issue, see R. T. O'Farrell, 'A famous cardiac controversy: Hope versus Williams', *Irish Journal of Medicine and Science*, 378, 6th series (1957), 278–85.

70 R. Spittall, *A Treatise on Auscultation Illustrated by Cases and Dissections* (Edinburgh, 1830), pp. 239–68.

71 N. P. Comins, 'New stethoscope', *London Medical Gazette*, 4 (1829), 427–30, at p. 427.

72 *Ibid.* I have retained Comins's description of his stethoscope as 'flexible'. Its design should not however be confused with that of the flexible rubber instruments of the late nineteenth and twentieth centuries. Comins's stethoscope consisted of two rigid tubes with a hinge between them which allowed the upper tube to be held at any angle relative to the lower one. The earpiece was also hinged.

73 *Ibid.*, p. 429.

74 *Ibid.*

75 *Ibid.*

76 *Ibid.*, p. 427.

77 Anon., ' "First lines of the practice of physic" by William Cullen, M.D.', *Edinburgh Medical and Surgical Journal*, 31 (1829), 191–6.

78 W. Cullen, *First Lines of the Practice of Physic*, new edn, 2 vols., W. Cullen and J. Crauford Gregory (eds.) (Edinburgh, 1829); see especially vol. I, p. 426, vol. II, pp. 348–68.

79 My point here is not so much that the evidence derived from stethoscopy was crucial to the making of the separation between pleurisy and peripneumony but that such evidence was central to the establishment of the new distinction within Edinburgh pedagogy.

80 W. P. Alison, 'Clinical lectures in medicine by Dr Alison, Edinburgh University', *Lancet* (1829–30), I, 732–7.

81 W. Stokes, 'A case of probable dislocation of the heart', *Edinburgh Medical and Surgical Journal*, 36 (1831), pp. 45–50.

82 Duncan, 'Contributions to morbid anatomy', p. 303.

83 G. Julius, 'Letter to Mrs Hope', in Mrs Hope, *Memoir*, pp. 325–32.

84 Edinburgh University Library, MS Gen 25, 'Copy of letter from John Nimmo to Dr William Stokes, 31/8/1825'. I am grateful to Dr Michael Barfoot, Lothian Health Board Archivist, Medical Archive Centre, University of Edinburgh, for bringing this manuscript to my attention.

85 Bluth, 'James Hope'; Kay, 'Letter to the Editor'; King, 'Auscultation in England'.

86 Duncan, 'Contributions to morbid anatomy', p. 303.

87 Anon., 'Review of Duncan's "Empyema and pneumothorax"', p. 131.

88 For example, Anon., 'Editorial', *Lancet* (1843–4), I, 267–8; H. Bennet, 'Remarks on the comparative value of auscultation practised with or without a stethoscope', *Lancet* (1843–4), I, 464; H. M. Hughes, *A Clinical Introduction to the Practice of Auscultation and other methods of Physical Diagnosis* (London, 1845).

89 See Maulitz, *Morbid Appearances*, pp. 143–7.

90 Andrew Duncan junior was one such exponent; see, for example, A. Duncan, 'Cases of diffuse inflammation of the cellular texture, with appearances on dissection and observations', *Transactions of the Medico-Chirurgical Society of Edinburgh*, 1 (1824), 470–650.

91 Maulitz, *Morbid Appearances*, p. 143.

92 Kay, 'Letter to the Editor'; C. Scudamore, *Observations on M. Laennec's Method of forming a Diagnosis of Diseases of the Chest by means of the Stethoscope and Percussion* (London, 1826), p. 51.

93 Forbes, 'Translator's preface', p. xix.

94 Forbes, *Original Cases*, pp. xxv–xxvi.
95 For the advocacy of the stethoscope by Scudamore, see Sakula, 'Laënnec's influence', and by Johnson, see Jarcho, 'An early review'.
96 S. Lawrence, 'Science and medicine at the London hospitals: the development of teaching and research, 1750–1815' (University of Toronto, Ph. D. thesis, 1985).
97 H. N. Segall, 'Introduction of the stethoscope and clinical auscultation in Canada', *Journal of the History of Medicine*, 22 (1967), 414–7.
98 For example, see Kay, 'Letter to the Editor', p. 757.
99 S. J. Reiser, 'The medical influence of the stethoscope', *Scientific American*, 240 (1979), 114–22; Newman, 'Physical signs'.
100 H. Bennet, 'Remarks on the comparative value'; A. T. Thomson, 'Lectures on medical jurisprudence. Lecture XXI: Corporeal disablement and simulation', *Lancet* (1836–7) I, 769–74.
101 C. J. B. Williams, *A Rational Exposition of the Diseases of the Lungs and Pleura* (London, 1828), p. 51; Stokes, *An Introduction*, pp. 11–12.

9 Educating the senses

1 See the essays in Andrew E. Benjamin, Geoffrey N. Cantor and John R. Christie (eds.), *The Figural and the Literal: Problems of Language in the History of Science and Philosophy, 1630–1800* (Manchester, 1987) for an introduction to the problems and questions in studying language and science.
2 At least 400 sets of manuscript lecture notes from 1700 to 1830 survive in various libraries and archives. The major repositories used for this essay are, in London: The Royal College of Surgeons of England (RCS); the Royal College of Physicians of London (RCP); The Wellcome Institute for the History of Medicine (WIHM); St Thomas's Hospital Medical School Library (StT); St George's Hospital Medical School Library (StG); the Willis Library in Guy's Hospital Medical School (Wills); in Bethesda, Maryland: the National Library of Medicine (NLM). Manuscript notes are also held by provincial record offices, such as that in Norwich (NRO), and probably in numerous other libraries and archives. The comprehensive register of English medical archives currently being compiled at the Wellcome Institute will undoubtedly reveal far more sources.
3 Owsei Temkin, 'The role of surgery in the rise of modern medical thought', *Bulletin of the History of Medicine*, 25 (1951), 248–59. Temkin reintroduced the idea that surgeons always had an orientation towards the body that centred on what could be learned through tacit experience, especially touch and anatomical localization. This inherent epistemological 'surgical point of view', he argues, when finally adopted by physicians, led to the modern perception of internally localized diseases.
4 N. D. Jewson, 'Medical knowledge and the patronage system in eighteenth-century England', *Sociology*, 8 (1974), 369–85; Malcolm Nicolson, 'The metastatic theory of pathogenesis and the professional interests of the eighteenth-century physician', *Medical History*, 32 (1988), 277–300; Malcolm Nicolson 'Giovanni Morgagni and eighteenth-century physical diagnosis', in Christopher Lawrence (ed.), *Medical Theory and Surgical Practice* (London, 1992).
5 Although explicit philosophical discussions are quite rare in the manuscript lecture notes, an analysis of how eighteenth-century London teachers approached the relationship between sensation, experience and reason could be based on their presentations of, for example, the nervous system, the mind, general physiology and madness. See Rom Harré, 'Knowledge', in G. S. Rousseau and Roy Porter (eds.), *The Ferment of Knowledge: Studies in the Historiography of Eighteenth-Century Science* (Cambridge, 1980), pp. 15–35 and G. S. Rousseau, 'Psychology', in *ibid.*, pp. 163–78.
6 WIHM MS 5976, William Saunders, *Elements of the Practice of Physic, for the Use*

of *Gentlemen who Attend the Lectures on that Subject. Read at Guy's Hospital*, [London], 1780), p. 6. See also, WIHM MS 858, Joseph Ager, 'Notes of lectures on the theory and practice of physic' (*c.* 1812–14), p. 16: Symptoms are 'the phenomena arising from the attend[ant] functions or action of a part either apparent to our senses or discoverable from the feelings of the patient'.

7 For an introduction to the importance of lay perspectives on medicine and their influence on medical knowledge and practice, see Roy Porter (ed.), *Patients and Practitioners: Lay Perceptions of Medicine in Pre-Industrial Society* (Cambridge, 1985); Irvine Loudon, *Medical Care and the General Practitioner, 1750–1850* (Oxford, 1986).

8 For descriptions of the surgeons' 'external' realm and the physicians' 'internal' one, see Loudon, *Medical Care*, pp. 19–20, 54–62 and 73–80; M. Jeanne Peterson, *The Medical Profession in Mid-Victorian London* (Berkeley, 1978), pp. 5–11.

9 Charles Newman, 'Diagnostic investigation before Laennec', *Medical History*, 4 (1960), 322–9.

10 Jewson, 'Medical knowledge.' Jewson's provocative model of client-dominated eighteenth-century medicine is too simplistic, as it concerns only the physician and his aristocratic patient, ignoring other practitioners and other classes. His insight, however, is useful for highlighting the vital role of patients' authority and expectations in the construction and application of medical knowledge. For an important extension of Jewson's work, see Nicolson, 'The metastatic theory of pathogenesis.'

11 Kenneth Keele, *The Evolution of Clinical Methods in Medicine* (London, 1963); Stanley Reiser, *Medicine and the Reign of Technology* (Cambridge, 1978), ch. 1. These scholars are extremely critical of the lack of separation between the 'subjective' (patient's) and 'objective' (practitioner's) data gained in clinical encounters, especially the eighteenth-century physicians' disinclination to perform physical examinations to obtain 'objective' knowledge. For a perceptive analysis of the peripheralization of the patient's account, see Mary Fissell, 'The disappearance of the patient's narrative and the invention of hospital medicine', in Roger French and Andrew Wear (eds.) *British Medicine in an Age of Reform* (London, 1991), pp. 92–109 and Kathryn Montgomery Hunter, *Doctors' Stories: The Narrative Structure of Medical Knowledge* (Princeton, 1991).

12 Michel Foucault, *The Birth of the Clinic* (New York, 1973); Toby Gelfand, *Professionalizing Modern Medicine: Paris Surgeons and Medical Science and Institutions in the Eighteenth Century* (Westport, Conn., 1980); Toby Gelfand, 'Gestation of the clinic', *Medical History*, 25 (1981), 169–80; Guenter Risse, *Hospital Life in Enlightenment Scotland: Care and Teaching at the Royal Infirmary of Edinburgh* (Cambridge, 1986).

13 Susan C. Lawrence, 'Entrepreneurs and private enterprise: the development of medical lecturing in London, 1775–1820', *Bulletin of the History of Medicine*, 62 (1988), 171–92; Susan C. Lawrence, 'Private enterprise and public interests: medical education and the Apothecaries' Act, 1780–1825', in French and Wear (eds.) *British Medicine*, pp. 45–73.

14 James Parkinson, *The Hospital Pupil; or an Essay Intended to Facilitate the Study of Medicine and Surgery in Four Letters* (London, 1800), pp. 42–52 and 75; James Lucas, *Candid Inquiry into the Education, Qualifications and Offices of a Surgeon Apothecary* (London, 1800), pp. 55–6. For student accounts, see Susan C. Lawrence, 'Science and medicine at the London hospitals: the development of teaching and research, 1750–1815' (University of Toronto, Ph.D. thesis, 1985), chs. 5 and 10. Several sets of manuscript lecture notes include records from several courses, demonstrating the students' broad educational programme. See, for example, RCS MS 42.d.12, 'Anatomical lectures delivered by Mr. Joseph Else, Surgeon, from October 1774 to April 1775 at his new Anatomical Theatre in St Thomas's Hospital'. These are followed in the same volume by notes of Hugh Smith's lectures on the 'Theory and practice of physic' (no location given), and by a few notes entitled

'Dr McKenzies [*sic*] maxims [on midwifery] to his pupils'. A few lectures also explicitly recognized that their audiences contained many men who would not be practising as 'pure' surgeons or physicians. See WIHM MS 3957, Percival Pott, 'Lectures on surgery' (*c.* 1770), p. 4.

15 Loudon, *Medical Care*, pp. 29–53; Lawrence, 'Science and medicine at the London hospitals', chs. 5 and 10; Joan Lane, 'The role of apprenticeship in eighteenth-century medical education in England', in W. F. Bynum and Roy Porter (eds.), *William Hunter and the Eighteenth-Century Medical World* (Cambridge, 1985), pp. 57–103.

16 William Hunter, *Two Introductory Lectures, Delivered by William Hunter to his Last Course of Anatomical Lectures at his Theatre in Windmill Street* (London, 1784), pp. 106–7. The utility of taking lecture notes for learning is repeated by Parkinson *Hospital Pupil*, pp. 44, 72–3 and 82.

17 As far as I know, no one has attempted to analyse medical lecture notes as a particular kind of 'literature' in eighteenth-century education. They clearly contain strategies for presenting a specific rhetorical approach to medical and scientific knowledge, but a detailed investigation is beyond the scope of this chapter. For important work on the role of audience and on strategies for establishing authority in science, see Benjamin *et al.* (eds.), *The Figural and the Literal*; Peter Burke and Roy Porter (eds.), *The Social History of Language* (Cambridge, 1987); J. V. Golinski, 'Utility and audience in eighteenth-century chemistry: case studies of William Cullen and Joseph Priestley', *British Journal for the History of Science*, 21 (1988), 1–31; J. V. Golinski, 'Language, method and theory in British chemical discourse, *c.* 1660–1770' (University of Leeds, Ph.D. thesis, 1984).

18 The large number of notes from William Hunter's and John Hunter's lectures highlight this bias. John Hunter became an especially heroic figure for nineteenth-century surgeons, and hence notes from his courses would far more likely have been kept by surgical families, and made their way back to hospital and other archives, than those from other lecturers. Stephen Jacyna, 'Images of John Hunter in the nineteenth century', *History of Science*, 21 (1983), 1–32. The popularity of John Hunter's theoretical approach to surgery, due not only to the content of his ideas but also to the boost he gave to the image of surgery as a science, is further demonstrated by the fact that, of all lecture notes examined so far, only those of John Hunter's courses were copied for years after his death. Clearly students transcribed notes taken by other pupils. See, for example, WIHM MS 2964, John Hunter, 'Lectures on surgery. A transcript of his original lectures, 1829'.

19 John Green Crosse, a London student in 1811–13, for example, kept his notes from John and Charles Clarkes' midwifery class, and Abernethy's surgical course. He also attended Dr George Pearson's lectures on the theory and practice of medicine, as well as Pearson's Saturday clinical lectures, but if Crosse took notes of these presentations, he did not value them enough to keep them with his other manuscripts. NRO MS 561/563, 'Clarkes' lectures on midwifery, 1812, taken down by John Green Crosse', 2 vols; NRO MS 468, John Green Crosse, 'Diary, 1811–1814', 20 January and 1 June 1812.

20 Joshua Brookes, Joseph Carpue, Dr Andrew Marshall and Dr George Tuthill are only a few who are known to have lectured for several years (Brookes and Carpue also having extensive anatomical collections), yet whose pupils, or the pupils' families, did not consider notes of their courses important. For one of the rare accounts of Brookes's course, see the recently catalogued WIHM 5602, 'Lectures on anatomy etc. by Joshua Brookes' (1811) taken down by Laurence Wrangle Brown. The scarcity of manuscripts about these less than famous men in itself probably reflects the ascendancy of the hospital schools in the mid-nineteenth century. Many of the private teachers did not, in retrospect, contribute to a long-term, 'respectable' institutional traditional and so their mementos had a marginal place in the construction of a professional heritage.

21 Published syllabi, or extended outlines, became popular for some courses. They were usually bound with blank interleaved pages for the students' own notes. See, for example, WIHM MS 5976, Saunders, *Elements*; Wills MS, William Babington and James Curry, *Outlines of a Course of Lectures on the Practice of Medicine, as Delivered in the Medical School of Guy's Hospital* (London, 1802–6), interleaved with notes by George Hickman (1806).

22 For manuscript notes by the lecturers themselves, see RCP MS 426–32, Thomas Lawrence, 'A course of lectures, 1751'. There is unfortunately no evidence that they were ever given as dictated – no student notes have yet appeared. The RCS holds manuscripts, 'Surgical lectures delivered 1796' and 'Notes for surgical lectures' (n.d.), apparently by Astley Cooper, but these have not yet been compared with any student notes, nor the identification confirmed; RCP MS 44, William Hamilton, 'Original MS of the first of a series of clinical lectures delivered at the London Hospital Medical College, 1787–90' (archivists' description).

23 On the business strategy that prevented popular teachers from publishing their lectures, see Roy Porter, 'William Hunter: a surgeon and a gentleman', in Bynum and Porter (eds.), *William Hunter*, p. 25; George Pearson, extramural lecturer and physician to St George's, published *Principles of Physic, to be Explained in a Course of Lectures* (London, 1805), but only one set of lecture notes has been discovered, and these have not yet been compared with the text. George Fordyce, physician to St Thomas's Hospital from 1770 to 1802, published various works, including the introductory *Elements of the Practice of Physic, in Two Parts*, 5th edn (London, 1784). Comparing this printed text with surviving manuscript notes quickly reveals that the printed version may have served as an extended outline of his course, but that his lectures were far richer, more detailed and certainly less formal that the stilted, almost aphoristic style of his publications.

24 Hunter, *Two Introductory Lectures*; see RCS MS 42.f.19–21, 'Lectures, anatomical and chirurgical, by William Hunter, 1779', taken down by Henry Gore Clough, 3 vols., vol. I, pp. 1–12. William Guy, who took notes of the course by Hunter and Cruikshank in 1780–1, omitted the introductory lectures entirely and began with the first substantive discussion, on the blood. WIHM MS 2961, 'Notes of a course of Dr Hunter's lectures' [1780–1].

25 The sample used to make this judgement is admittedly small, but none of the notes I have seen are duplicates. Compare, for example, WIHM MS 3956 (the first page of which is shown in fig. 49), WIHM MS 3957, RCS MS 42.d.39, and StG MS 15, four sets of lecture notes from Percival Pott's course on surgery at St Bartholomew's Hospital. The first three were compiled by anonymous students, dated *c.* 1770; the last, attributed to R. Edmunson, has an internal date placing the lectures in 1775–6. The texts are remarkably close in organization and style, but are certainly not identical. They reveal a complex interplay between verbatim reporting and student interpretation. This is most evident when the pupils used 'I', 'you' and, in some cases, 'Mr Pott' interchangeably, sometimes on the same page. In WIHM MS 3957, for example, the student wrote regarding a case of compound fracture: 'an instance of this kind you have seen in this house lately . . . I advised the man to submit to the operation [amputation] but he obstinately refus'd.' The 'I' here clearly referred to Pott and not the pupil. In WIHM MS 3956, the student, who regularly used 'I' for Pott, wrote: 'An instance of this kind I saw in the hospital lately . . . Mr Pott advised the man to Submit to the Operation but he obstinately refusing died at the end of four days.' In general, first person reporting reflects an account of what the student thought the lecturer said, not the pupil's personal experience. In a few instances, however, the student makes a clear distinction in order to show his own opinion. See WIHM MS 1672, 'Surgical operations by Henry Cline. Delivered 1788', p. 260; NLM MS B 5, Joseph Else, 'Lectures on anatomy' [*c.*1770], p. 270.

26 For illustrations of students' sometimes amusing errors and omissions, see WIHM

MS 2396–7. 'A new treatise on the practice of physic taken from Dr Fordyce's lectures', 2 vols. [c] 1775], vol. I, introduction; WIHM MS 2399, 'Notes from Dr Fordyce' [c. 1775], p. 134; One forthright and able student noted during John Abernethy's anatomy lectures: 'He spoke of 2 causes of distorted pelvis which I did not clearly hear or comprehend.' WIHM MS 817, 'Notes on Mr Abernethy's lectures on anatomy, 1813', 30 October 1813.

27 Joseph Ager's course on the Theory and Practice of Physic, (WIHM MS 858), for example, was an explicit exegesis of Cullen's nosology (pp. 21ff.). Most of the medical lectures (e.g. William Saunders and George Fordyce) for whom most manuscripts survive did not state their sources, or pupils did not record them. It is beyond the scope of this chapter to trace the intellectual roots of the ideas presented, although many obviously came from Edinburgh, Leiden and classical texts.

28 See Nicolson, 'Giovanni Morgagni'.

29 George Fordyce, for example, remarked that he would not discuss anatomy in any detail, 'for that you have elsewhere'. WIHM MS 2396–7. 'A new treatise on the practice of physic', vol. I, p. 70. William Saunder's lectures offer a telling example of the problem of 'rhetorical' versus 'real' practice. Saunders repeated the commonplace that the discovery of proximate causes required the observation of the course of the symptoms, the effects of remedies and 'the dissection of Dead Bodies'. (StT MS, c. 1788, p. 67). This advice closely follows Boerhaave's comments. See Robert James, *The Modern Practice of Physic, As Improved by the Celebrated Professors, H. Boerhaave and F. Hoffman*, 2 vols. (London, 1746), vol. I, p. 2. The important question then is whether Saunders offered any details to indicate that he substantiated the use of 'dead bodies' to his students. Certainly some pupils noted that he said dissection and/or post-mortems revealed useful knowledge, but Saunders did not put great weight on morbid anatomy. See, for example, RCP MS 96, 'Notes from Doctor Saunders' lectures on the theory and practice of physic, 1782', p. 154. When Saunders discussed the stages of inflammation, the pupil wrote: 'you will often see [adhesions] in dissecting the bowels from one another, Lungs from the Pleura, from some former slight inflammation'. Such passing comments provided only a limited paradigm for observing post-mortems.

30 D. D. Gibbs, 'Recommendations of Sir John Floyer on the education of a physician', *Proceedings of the XXIII International Congress on the History of Medicine* (London, 1974), p. 369; William Heberden, *An Introduction to the Study of Physic*, ed. LeRoy Crummer (London, 1929), pp. 119 and 122; Richard Davies, *The General State of Education in the Universities: With a Particular View to the Philosophical and Medical Education* (Bath, 1759), p. 4; Lucas, *Candid Inquiry*, pp. 55–6 and 79–81; Parkinson, *Hospital Pupil*, pp. 53–5 and 86–7.

31 See, for example, WIHM MS 2396–7, 'A new treatise on the practice of physic', vol. I, introduction; RCS MS 42.d.12, 'Anatomical lectures delivered by Mr Joseph Else, 1774', pp. 3–6; RCS MS 42.f.19–21. Hunter, 'Lectures, anatomical and chirurgical, 1779', vol. I, pp. 2–7; Hunter, *Two Introductory Lectures*, pp. 4–55; Matthew Baillie, 'Introductory lecture to the course of anatomy, Great Windmill Street' [1785], in *Lectures and Observations on Medicine* (London, 1825), pp. 3–40.

32 See, for example, WIHM MS 3957, Pott, 'Lectures on surgery', pp. 1–2. Pott criticized the surgeon who had only learned from books, the 'able Surgn [sic] in the Closet, apt in conversation', but who cannot operate. He equally disparaged those who had been trained by practice and a few texts only, for such men operated 'without knowing perhaps why it should be done'.

33 In addition to instruction in 'institutes', such as Boerhaave's or Cullen's, some lectures reminded their students that they needed to cultivate the polite manners that patients expected. William Saunders, to take an example from the 'utility' of science, stressed that students should learn chemistry for its social benefits: 'The Elegance of a prescription depends much on a good knowledge of Chymistry.'

WIHM MS 5976, Saunders, *Elements*, introduction, n.p.; see also Heberden, *Introduction to the Study of Physic*, pp. 90–2. For a general discussion of academic medicine and formal lectures, see Andrew R. Cunningham, 'Aspects of medical education in Britain in the seventeenth and early eighteenth centuries', (University of London, Ph.D. thesis, 1974), chs. 3–6; Nicolson, in 'The metastatic theory of pathogenesis', argues that physicians used a theoretical stance to promote their expertise over competitors, whether surgeons, apothecaries or 'quacks'. Here, I argue, surgeons and apothecaries hoped to appropriate inexpensively the physicians' language and behaviour to maintain their clientele.

34 William Graeme, *An Essay on the Method of Acquiring Knowledge in Physick* (London, 1729), pp. 9–10; Graeme went on to argue perceptively that, for example, the word 'bile' associated with a cause of jaundice presupposes an entire system of knowledge about bile and its place in physiology: 'for truly every Part is so connected with another, that it is impossible that any one Part can be thoroughly understood, without the knowledge of the rest, and that the Patient's Bed-side is not a convenient place for such a System to be taught' (p. 10).

35 RCP MS 44, Hamilton, 'Clinical lectures', pp. 3–4. Lester King, *The Medical World of the Eighteenth Century* (Huntington, N.Y., 1958).

36 Quoted in William Peachey, *A Memoir of William and John Hunter* (Plymouth, Devon, 1924), p. 18.

37 For Hunter's work, see Jacyna, 'Images of John Hunter'; Stephen Cross, 'John Hunter, the animal oeconomy and late-eighteenth century physiological discourse', *Studies in the History of Biology*, 5 (1981), 1–110. For an early example of a surgeon's attempts to build a theoretical superstructure on surgical cases see William Beckett, *Practical Surgery, Illustrated and Improved being Chirurgical Observations with Remarks upon the Most Extraordinary Cases, Cures and Dissections made at St Thomas's Hospital, Southwark* (London, 1740).

38 RCS MS 275.d.29–30, John Pearson, 'Lectures on surgery delivered in London in the years 1790 & 1791', 2 vols., vol. I, p. 78 and vol. II, pp. 79–80. Pearson was surgeon to the Lock Hospital and the Public Dispensary on Carey Street. He advertised lectures from at least 1783 to 1803 and appears to have given them at his home in Golden Square (*The Times*, 30 September 1794). A entire question yet to be studied is the development of formal nosological systems for surgical conditions. An excellent published example of this trend is Hugh Monro, *A Compendious System of the Theory and Practice of Modern Surgery, Arranged in a New Nosological and Systemic Method*, 2nd edn (London, 1800).

39 NLM MS B 47, Donald Monro, 'Lectures on the practice of physick, 1758', 2 vols., vol. II, p. 96; WIHM MS 5976, Saunders, *Elements*, pp. 83–99, 132 manuscript note; RCS MS 42.d.12, Smith, 'Theory and practice of physic' (n.d.), p. 299.

40 WIHM MS MSL 77, George Fordyce, 'Lectures on the practice of medicine [ascribed to John Coakely Lettsom], n.d.', pp. 42–3.

41 RCP MS 138, George Fordyce, 'Clinical lectures, 1785, taken down by Henry Rumsey', pp. 44–5. William Hunter noted that the hard pulse 'strikes the finger with great impetus', while the soft pulse, by definition, felt the opposite. Yet he went on to state that 'the Cellular Membrane lying betwixt the finger and the Artery makes it almost impossible to distinguish between them'. Even with this observational caution, he upheld the time-honoured view: 'The knowledge of the Pulse is a great improvement in Physick.' WIHM MS 2965, William Hunter, 'Lectures on anatomy' [c.1755], p. 17.

42 WIHM MS 5976, Saunders, *Elements*, manuscript note, p. 6.

43 RCP MS 140, George Fordyce, 'The substance of two courses of clinical lectures delivered by Dr Fordyce partly in 1785, 1786 & 1787, by Henry Rumsey', pp. 137–8. A different version of this remark appears in RCP MS 138, p. 49, along with a tirade against 'Systems of Medicine ... by Linnaeus, Sauvages & even Cullen'. Fordyce particularly objected to the idea of a single 'pathognomic

Symptom', since disorders in patients varied far too much for such a simplistic approach.

44 Joan Lane, '"The doctor scolds me": the diaries and correspondence of patients in eighteenth-century England', in Porter (ed.), *Patients and Practitioners*, pp. 205–48; Roy Porter, 'Laymen, doctors and medical knowledge in the eighteenth century: the evidence of the *Gentleman's Magazine*', in *ibid.*, pp. 283–314.

45 See, for example, the printed prospectus for the course on 'Therapeutics and materia medica' given at Guy's included in Saunders, *Elements* (WIHM MS 5976): 'Good specimens of each article will be produced and the various adulterations to which they are subject, pointed out.' John Burgess, physician to St George's Hospital 1774–87, whose materia medica collection was eventually donated to the RCP, probably used his material in the private courses he offered outside the hospital. RCP MS 182, 'Synopsis of a course of lectures on materia medica' (n.d.); RCP MS 183, 'Lectures on Materia Medica' (n.d.).

46 StG MS 2, Colin Mackenzie, 'Midwifery' (1770), p. 11 and lecture 10.

47 William Hunter's work has been covered by numerous authors. See, in particular, Peachey, *William and John Hunter*; Toby Gelfand, 'The "Paris manner" of dissection: student anatomical dissection in early-eighteenth century Paris', *Bulletin of the History of Medicine* 46 (1972), 99–130; C. J. Lawrence, 'Alexander Monro *Primus* and the Edinburgh manner of anatomy,' *Bulletin of the History of Medicine*, 62 (1988), 193–214, discusses Monro's demonstration method of anatomical teaching within the traditions and expectations of natural philosophy. London teachers clearly separated the anatomical lectures *per se*, with their carefully orchestrated demonstrations, from the dissection courses. During the latter, it appears that demonstrators, usually assistants to the lecturers, aided the students in their work.

48 Hunter, *Two Introductory Lectures*, p. 108; Heberden, *Introduction to the Study of Physic*, pp. 93–7.

49 StT MS, [Henry Watson], 'Notebook: midwifery and anatomy notes by John Turner, 1763', p. ... 154; WIHM MS 1678–80, Henry Cline, 'Anatomical lectures at St Thomas's Hospital, 1793', 3 vols.; WIHM MS 2965, Hunter, 'Lectures on anatomy', pp. 11 and 195; RCS MS 42.d.12, 'Anatomical lectures delivered by Mr Joseph Else, 1774', p. 8; WIHM MS 817, 'Notes of Mr Abernethy's lectures on anatomy, 1813', 2 November 1813 (see fig. 48).

50 Hunter, *Two Introductory Lectures*, p. 87. For Hunter's method using preserved preparations and fresh specimens, see pp. 87–93. Hunter's students did not record the epistemological advice given in Hunter's published introduction. It was, nevertheless, an obvious theme in his lectures. See WIHM MS 2966, William Hunter, 'Lectures anatomical and chirurgical, 1775', lecture 2. The student noted Hunter's emphasis on demonstration material, 'for they are the objects of the senses'.

51 Hunter, *Two Introductory Lectures*, pp. 103–5 and 108–10. Hunter described how he presented material to the class on pp. 111–13. Large specimens were shown at the front of the theatre; smaller ones 'shewn at two or three places successively that everyone present may get a distinct view' and the smallest 'sent 'round the company'. That pupils were not encouraged to stray from the specific point at hand when observing the preparation is clear from Hunter's injunction to pay attention to 'that part only' being discussed. He also strictly asked that the students not touch the preparations: 'No experiment is to be made, by pressing or bending, to try their strength or texture.' (p. 112). See also Baillie, 'Introductory lecture', pp. 87–9.

52 See, for example, RCP MS 138, Fordyce, 'Clinical lectures, 1785', pp. 9–10.

53 Parkinson, *Hospital Pupil*, p. 87.

54 RCP MS 44, Hamilton, 'Clinical lectures', p. 15.

55 Several authors who advised on medical education emphasized training the senses during the pupil's preliminary education. William Heberden, for example, urged

that 'it is absolutely necessary to make a collection of the materia medica, for without seeing the drug itself, it will be difficult to conceive & almost impossible to remember what is said about it'. *Introduction to the Study of Physic*, p. 89; see also pp. 82–5. *Introduction to the Study of Physic*, p. 89; see also pp. 82–5. Richard Lovell Edgeworth, an educationalist, wanted parents to choose their sons' professions as early as possible, in order to rear them correctly. For the nascent physician: 'the first thing to be attended to, even from the pupil's infancy, is the cultivation of his senses; acuteness, and accuracy, of smell, of taste, of feeling are peculiarly necessary to a physician, both in the practice of his art, and the pursuit of sciences by which medicine can be improved'. *Essays on Professional Notes Education*, (London, 1809), p. 203.

56 D. W. Hamlyn, *Sensation and Perception: A History of the Philosophy of Perceptions* (London, 1961), p. 93–148; Sergio Moravia, 'The Enlightenment and the sciences of man', *History of Science*, 18 (1980), 247–52; Karl Figlio, 'Theories of perception and the physiology of the mind in the late eighteenth century', *History of Science*, 13 (1975), 177–212.

57 For an extended discussion of William Hunter's approach to knowledge and the assumed priority of vision, see L. J. Jordanova, 'Gender, generation and science: William Hunter's obstetrical atlas', in Bynum and Porter (eds.), *William Hunter*, pp. 385–412.

58 WIHM MS 2663, 'Physiology by Dr Haighton, 1801', pp. 49–57 and 235; Wills MS, John Haighton, 'Lectures on the physiology of the human body, delivered at Guy's Hospital, 1796, written down by Martin Tupper', pp. 75–7. StG MS 8–9, 'Notes of lectures delivered by John Hunter' (n.d.). For discussions of the rhetorical role of reporting on experiments as a means of structuring legitimate knowledge, see the references in note 17 above.

59 NLM MS B 47, Monro, 'Practice of physick, 1758', vol. I, p. 87. Donald Monro, son of Alexander Monro *primus* received his Edinburgh M.D. in 1753. He was elected physician to St George's Hospital in 1758, resigning in 1786 probably due to his commitments as a physician in the army. How long he lectured in London is unknown.

60 WIHM MS 2401, George Fordyce, 'Lectures on the theory and practice of physic, 1787, taken down by William Lambe', p. 3.

61 WIHM MS 2396–7, Fordyce, 'A new treatise on the practice of physick', vol. II, p. 370.

62 RCS MS 42 f.19–21, Hunter, 'Lectures, anatomical and chirurgical, 1779', vol. II, p. 68.

63 StT MS, Astley Cooper, 'Lectures on surgery, 1808, taken down by William Davies', p. 13.

64 RCP MS 254, 'Notes on surgery, taken from the lectures read by Henry Thompson at the London Hospital, by Gilchrist Stirling, 1759', lecture 6.

65 WIHM MS 1672, Cline, 'Surgical operations, 1788', p. 54.

66 NLM MS B 47, Monro, 'Practice of physick, 1758', vol. II, pp. 66 and 217.

67 WIHM MS 2396–7, Fordyce, 'A new treatise on the practice of physick', vol. II, p. 535.

68 WIHM MS 1678–80, Cline, 'Anatomical lectures, 1793', vol. I, p. 36, original emphasis; NLM MS B 5, Else, 'Lectures on anatomy', pp. 309–10; WIHM MS 2396–7, Fordyce, 'A new treatise on the practice of physic', p. 557. vol. II, p. 557. Here Fordyce discussed diagnosing inflammation of the uterus: 'a Swelling and heat may be felt by introducing a finger into the vagina'.

69 WIHM MS 2966, Hunter, 'Lectures anatomical and chirurgical, 1775', n.p.

70 Part of the difficulty in interpreting how practitioners gained knowledge of internal diseases, such as dropsy or enlargements of the abdominal viscera, stems from the mode of expression commonly used. When, for example, Boerhaave wrote that an external liver abscess would be 'evident to the sight and touch' (James, *Modern*

Practice of Physic, vol. II, p. 9), these sensations could have been what the patient experienced and reported, not the practitioner's direct perceptions. Similarly, Fordyce's comment about liver inflammation, that 'we have often another Symptom, which is perceiving a fluctuation, which is sometimes to be felt, in any part of the liver, immediately under the Integuments' (WIHM MS 2396–7, Fordyce, 'A new treatise on the practice of physick', vol. II, p. 523) does not directly specify who does the perceiving. Such passive descriptions have generally been taken to suggest that physicians did not touch the patient (Charles Newman, 'Diagnostic investigation before Laënnac', *Medical History*, 4 (1960), 322–9). Yet many physicians wrote entirely in the passive voice as a matter of course. They rarely, if ever, used the first person in their narratives, which suggests stylistic convention as much as an actual distancing from the patient. Equally significant, moreover, is a preliminary observation that surgeons also used the passive voice in describing certain clinical experiences. John Abernethy, for example, when discussing the diagnosis of lumbar abscess, chronicled the general symptoms such as 'severe pain in the loins with fever'. He went on: 'If he [the patient] coughs an impulse may be felt upon the fascia of the thigh'. (WIHM MS 814, John Abernethy, 'The principles and practice of surgery, 1808', p. 95). Just because Abernethy was a surgeon should not cause us to assume that in this case he would do the feeling as opposed to asking the patient about his sensations. A consistent sensitivity to style in eighteenth-century medical and surgical prose would help, I suggest, the unravelling of conventions and contexts of medical language.

71 WIHM MS 1672, Cline, 'Surgical operations, 1788', pp. 163 and 165.
72 NLM MS B 47, Monro, 'Practice of physick, 1758', vol. II, p. 222.
73 WIHM MS 3957, Pott, 'Lectures on surgery', p. 67; RCS MS 42.d.39, Percival Pott, 'Lectures on the practice of surgery' (n.d.), pp. 135–9.
74 Reiser, *Reign of Technology*, pp. 4–7; Keele, *Clinical Methods*, p. 18, notes Galen's use of pain near the clavicle to diagnose disease of the liver. This is but one example of a well-known sensation often used to determine the 'seat' of a disorder. For its repetition in eighteenth-century lectures, see, for example, WIHM MS 1678–80, Cline, 'Anatomical lectures, 1793', vol. II, p. 42. David B. Morris offers an extensive analysis of patients, pain and medical culture in his *The Culture of Pain* (Berkeley, 1991).
75 WIHM MS 2396–7, Fordyce, 'A new treatise on the practice of physick', vol. II, p. 526.
76 RCP MS 96, 'Notes from Doctor Saunders' lectures . . . , 1782',
77 RCS MS 42.f.19–21, Hunter, 'Lectures, anatomical and chirurgical, 1779', vol. II, p. 22; RCP MS 139, George Fordyce, 'Clinical lectures, 1787', pp. 71–2.
78 WIHM MS 1672, Cline, 'Surgical operations, 1788', p. 175.
79 RCP MS 138, Fordyce, 'Clinical lectures, 1785', pp. 14–38.
80 WIHM MS 4371, William Saunders, 'Clinical and physical lectures, 1782', p. 2; WIHM MS 2966, Hunter, 'Lectures anatomical and chirurgical, 1775', n.p.
81 See, for example, WIHM MS 1675, Henry Cline, 'Surgical lectures, *c.* 1790', pp. 103–4. In strangulated hernia, the practitioner knows that gangrene has begun when the tumour, 'hard & tense with a great deal of pain', becomes 'soft, flaccid & easy having an emphysematous feel'. Then 'the patient flatters himself better but in fact these are symptoms of mortification'.
82 WIHM MS 814, Abernethy, 'Principles and practice of surgery, 1808', pp. 23–6 and 43: 'I could prove that if a man had no Constitutional, he would have no local disease . . .' This theme is apparent in most of Abernethy's published works. See, for example, his *On the Constitutional Origin and Treatment of Local Diseases*, 1st edn (London, 1809); reprinted in his *The Surgical and Physiological Works*, 2 vols., (London, 1825), vol. I, pp. 1–144.
83 WIHM MS 814, Abernethy, 'Principles and practice of surgery, 1808', p. 389.

10 The rise of physical examination

1 See R. L. Engle and B. J. Davis, 'Medical diagnosis: present, past and future', *Archives of Internal Medicine* 112 (1963), 512–43; I. Galdston, 'Diagnosis in historical perspective', *Bulletin of the History of Medicine* 9 (1941), 367–84. S. Reiser comments in *Medicine and the Reign of Technology* (Cambridge, 1978), p. 7: 'The failure of doctors to examine the body in the presence of internal disease, and the reluctance of patients to allow it, were common in the early nineteenth century'. E. Shorter, *Bedside Manners: The Troubled History of Doctors and Patients* (New York, 1986).

2 P. Strong, *The Ceremonial Order of the Clinic* (London, 1979).

3 See D. Armstrong, *Political Anatomy of the Body: Medical Knowledge in Britain in the Twentieth Century* (Cambridge, 1983).

4 M. Nicolson, 'The introduction of percussion and stethoscopy to early nineteenth-century Edinburgh', in this volume.

5 Michaela Reid, *Ask Sir James* (London, 1987), p. 201. Queen Caroline, wife of George II, had earlier resisted physical examination, not wishing it to be widely known that she had a rupture: Lord Hervey, *Some Materials Towards Memoirs of the Reign of King George II*, ed. R. Sedgwick, 3 vols. (London, 1931), vol. III, pp. 879ff.

6 S. Lawrence, 'Educating the senses: students, teachers and medical rhetoric in eighteenth-century London', in this volume; S. Lawrence, 'Science and medicine at the London hospitals: the development of teaching and research 1750–1815' (University of Toronto, Ph.D. thesis, 1985).

7 J. Y. T. Grieg (ed.), *The Letters of David Hume*, 2 vols. (Oxford, 1969), vol. II, pp. 311–20.

8 *Ibid.*

9 *Ibid.*

10 *Ibid.*

11 *Ibid.*, pp. 324–5.

12 *Ibid.*, pp. 310–20.

13 *Ibid.*, p. 325.

14 H. Brody, *Stories of Sickness* (New Haven, 1987); A. Kleinman, *Illness Narratives: Suffering, Healing, and the Human Condition* (New York, 1988).

15 D. Porter and R. Porter, *Patient's Progress: The Dialectics of Doctoring in Eighteenth-Century England* (Cambridge, 1989), ch. 5.

16 J. M. Adair, *Essays on Fashionable Diseases . . .* (London, 1790).

17 J. Mulhallen and D. J. M. Wright, 'Samuel Johnson: amateur physician', *Journal of the Royal Society of Medicine*, 76 (1983), 217–22.

18 R. W. Chapman (ed.), *The Letters of Samuel Johnson*, 3 vols. (Oxford, 1984), vol. III, p. 850. See also vol. II, p. 476; Mulhallen and Wright, 'Samuel Johnson'.

19 W. Buchan, *Observations on the Prevention and Cure of Venereal Disease* (London, 1796), p. xv.

20 B. Mandeville, *A Treatise of the Hypochondriack and Hysterick Diseases*, 2nd edn (London, 1730; reprinted Hildesheim, 1981).

21 Francis McKee, 'The earlier works of Bernard Mandeville, 1685–1715' (University of Glasgow, Ph.D. thesis, 1991).

22 J. Lane, 'The doctor scolds me: the diaries and correspondence of patients in eighteenth-century England', in R. Porter, (ed.), *Patients and Practitioners* (Cambridge, 1985), pp. 207–47, at p. 217.

23 For postal diagnosis see Porter and Porter, *Patient's Progress*, ch. 5, and G. Risse, 'Doctor William Cullen, physician, Edinburgh: a consultation practice in the eighteenth century', *Bulletin of the History of Medicine* 48 (1974), 338–51.

24 C. Lawrence, 'Incommunicable knowledge: science, technology and the clinical art in Britain, 1850–1914', *Journal of Contemporary History* 20 (1985), 503–20.

25 Nicolson, 'Introduction of percussion and stethoscopy'.

26 Ernest Heberden, *William Heberden 1710–1801: Physician of the Age of Reason* (London, 1989).

27 M. MacNeil, *Under the Banner of Science: Erasmus Darwin and his Age* (Manchester, 1987).

28 A. Seward, *Memoirs of the Life of Darwin* (London, 1804), p. 3.

29 *Ibid.*

30 The Earl of Ilchester (ed.), *Lady Holland's Journal*, 2 vols. (London, 1908), vol. II, p. 173.

31 C. C. Hankin (ed.), *The Life of Mary Anne Schimmelpenninck*, 2 vols. (London, 1858), vol. I, p. 152.

32 T. Trotter, *A View of the Nervous Temperament* (London, 1807), pp. 289–90.

33 Quoted in R. Hunter and I. Macalpine, *Three Hundred Years of Psychiatry* (Oxford, 1963), p. 463.

34 On the pioneering role of surgery *because* of willingness to touch, see Owsei Temkin, 'The role of surgery in the rise of modern medical thought', *Bulletin of the History of Medicine*, 26 (1951), 248–59. Generally M. Foucault, *The Birth of the Clinic* (London, 1972); Reiser, *Medicine and the Reign of Technology* and C. Lawrence, 'Incommunicable knowledge'.

35 R. Porter, 'The exotic as erotic', in G. S. Rousseau and R. Porter (eds.), *Exoticism in the Enlightenment* (Manchester, 1989), pp. 117–44.

36 M. Pelling, 'Appearance and reality: barber-surgeons, the body and disease', in A. L. Beier and R. Finlay (eds.), *London 1500–1700: The Making of the Metropolis*, pp. 82–112; W. F. Bynum, 'Treating the wages of sin: venereal disease and specialism in eighteenth-century Britain', in W. F. Bynum and R. Porter (eds.), *Medical Fringe and Medical Orthodoxy, 1750–1850* (London, 1987), pp. 5–28.

37 See I. R. Cutter and H. R. Viets, *A Short History of Midwifery* (Philadelphia, 1964); J. H. Aveling, *English Midwives: Their History and Prospects* (London, 1872; reprinted London, 1967); H. R. Spencer, *The History of British Midwifery 1650 to 1800* (London, 1927; reprinted New York, 1978); J. Donnison, *Midwives and Medical Men* (New York, 1977); and E. Shorter, *A History of Women's Bodies* (Harmondsworth, 1980).

38 S. Gilman, 'Touch, Sexuality and Disease', in this volume. See also F. Bottomley, *Attitudes to the Body in Western Christendom* (London, 1979); B. S. Turner, 'The body and religion: towards an alliance of medical sociology and sociology of religion', *Annual Review of the Social Sciences*, 4 (1980), 247–86; B. S. Turner, *The Body and Society: Explorations in Social Theory* (Oxford, 1984).

39 M. Bakhtin, *Rabelais and His World* (Cambridge, Mass., 1968); P. Camporesi, *La carne impassabile* (Milan, 1983), translated as *The Incorruptible Flesh: Bodily Mutation and Mortification in Religion and Folklore* (Cambridge, 1988); cf. R. Porter, 'Bodies of thought: thoughts about the body in eighteenth-century England', in J. Pittock and A. Wear (eds.), *Interpretations and Cultural History* (London, 1991), pp. 82–108.

40 F. Barker, *The Tremulous Private Body* (London, 1984); cf. R. Porter, 'History of the body', in Peter Burke (ed.), *New Perspectives on Historical Writing* (Cambridge, 1991), pp. 206–32.

41 R. Latham and W. Matthews (eds.), *The Diary of Samuel Pepys*, 11 vols. (London, 1970–83), vol. VIII, p. 422.

42 H. Whitbread (ed.), *I Know My Own Heart: The Diary of Anne Lister (1740–1840)* (London, 1987), p. 228.

43 N. Elias, *The Civilising Process* (Oxford, 1983); R. Sennett, *The Fall of Public Man* (Cambridge, 1976); and, more generally, E. Goffman, *The Presentation of Self in Everyday Life* (Harmondsworth, 1969). See also F. Childs, 'Prescriptions for manners in eighteenth-century courtesy literature' (University of Oxford, D. Phil. thesis, 1984).

44 E. Hall (ed.), *Miss Weeton: Journal of a Governess 1807–11*, 2 vols. (Oxford, 1936), vol. II, p. 384.

45 *Ibid.*

46 W. Bray (ed.), *Diary of John Evelyn* (London, 1966), p. 191 (4 October, 1683).

47 E. Bristow, *Vice and Vigilance: Purity Movements in Britain since 1700* (Dublin, 1977).

48 For prudery, see P. Fryer, *Mrs Grundy: Studies in English Prudery* (London, 1963); M. Jaeger, *Before Victoria* (London, 1956); and E. Trudgill, *Madonnas and Magdalens* (London, 1966).

49 G. A. Bonnard (ed.), *Edward Gibbon: Memoirs of my Life* (London, 1966).

50 See R. Porter, 'A touch of danger: the man-midwife as sexual predator', in G. S. Rousseau and R. Porter (eds.), *Sexual Underworlds of the Enlightenment* (Manchester, 1987), pp. 206–32; and R. Porter, 'Barely touching: a social perspective on mind and body', in G. S. Rousseau (ed.), *The Languages of Psyche: Mind and Body in Enlightenment Thought* (Berkeley, 1990), pp. 45–80.

51 P. Thicknesse, *Man Midwifery Analysed* (London, 1764), p. 8. For Thicknesse, see P. Gosse, *Dr Viper* (London, 1952). See also *The Danger and Immodesty of the Present Too General Custom of Unnecessarily Employing Men-Midwives* (London, 1772); and John Blunt [pseud.], *Man-Midwifery Dissected, or the Obstetric Family Operator* (London, 1793).

52 Quoted in A. Maclaren, *Reproductive Rituals* (London, 1986), p. 100.

53 P. Wagner, *Eros Revived: Erotica of the Enlightenment in England and America* (London, 1988); W. G. Smith (introd.), *The Amorous Illustrations of Thomas Rowlandson* (London, 1983); P. Pinkus, *Grub Street* (London, 1968); R. Straus, *The Unspeakable Curll* (New York, 1970); D. Foxon, *Libertine Literature in England, 1660–1745* (New York, 1965).

54 Latham and Matthews (eds.), *Diary of Samuel Pepys*, vol. II, p. 43.

55 See J. Levine, *Dr Woodward's Shield* (Berkeley, 1977), pp. 9 and 17; R. Porter, 'John Woodward, "a Droll Sort of Philosopher"', *Geological Magazine*, 126 (1979), 395–417; Richard Mead, *The Life and Adventures of Don Bilioso de L'Estomac* (London, 1719).

56 J. Percival, *Medical Ethics* (Manchester, 1803), p. 84. The other side was that it was acknowledged that doctors could perform procedures on poor and charity patients, especially in hospital, which private patients would never tolerate; above all, experimentation with new therapies. See Erasmus Darwin, *Zoonomia*, 6 vols. (London, 1801), vol. IV, pp. 463–7.

57 Bristow, *Vice and Vigilance*.

58 See P. Burke, *Popular Culture in Early Modern Europe* (London, 1978); R. Paulson, *Popular and Polite Culture in the Age of Hogarth and Fielding* (Notre Dame, Ind., 1979); R. Darnton, 'In search of the Enlightenment: recent attempts to create a social history of ideas', *Journal of Modern History*, 43 (1971), 113–32; R. Darnton, 'The High Enlightenment and the low life of literature in pre-Revolutionary France', *Past and Present*, 51 (1971), 81–115; R. Darnton, *Mesmerism and the End of the Enlightenment in France* (Cambridge, Mass., 1968); H. C. Payne, 'Elite versus popular mentality in the eighteenth century', *Studies in Eighteenth-Century Culture*, 8 (1979), 201–37.

59 [S. J. Rolleston], *A Philosophical Dialogue Concerning Decency* (London, 1751), p. 9.

60 *Ibid.*, p. 10.

61 *Ibid.*, p. 10.

62 B. Mandeville, *The Virgin Unmask'd* (London, 1709), esp. pp. 1–4. 'A discourse upon nakedness and dress'; and L. G. Crocker, *An Age of Crisis: Man and World in Eighteenth-Century Thought* (Baltimore, 1963). See also McKee, 'Works of Mandeville'.

63 See discussion in Roy Porter, 'Libertinism and promiscuity', in J. Miller (ed.), *The*

Don Giovanni Book: Myths of Seduction and Betrayal (London, 1990), pp. 1–19, esp. p. 17. Female modesty, of course, preoccupied Boswell, for he wanted women to be sexy and modest at the same time. Boswell apparently believed the good wife should be modest 'to all but husband', with others she should be 'as a young girl before new married'.

64 P. Quennell (ed.), *The Private Letters of Princess Lieven to Prince Metternich, 1820–1826* (London, 1937), p. 91.

65 R. H. Fox, *Dr John Fothergill and his Friends* (London, 1919), p. 32; A. Barbeau (ed.), *Life and Letters at Bath in the Eighteenth Century*, preface by A. Dobson (London, 1904).

66 Porter and Porter, *Patient's Progress*, ch. 5.

67 Buchan, *Observations*, p. 136.

68 M. Bloch, *The Royal Touch* (London, 1973); and R. Crawford, *The Kings' Evil* (Oxford, 1911).

69 M. Ramsey, *Professional and Popular Medicine in France, 1770–1830: The Social World of Medical Practice* (Cambridge, 1988). J. Devlin, *The Superstitious Mind* (New Haven, 1987). For mesmerism, see R. Darnton, *Mesmerism*; and V. Buranelli, *The Wizard from Vienna: Franz Mesmer and the Origins of Hypnotism* (London, 1976). For Charcot see J. Goldstein, *Console and Classify: The French Psychiatric Profession in the Nineteenth Century* (Cambridge, 1987).

70 B. B. Kaplan, 'Greatrakes the Stroker: the interpretations of his contemporaries', *Isis*, 73 (1982), 178–85. The early history of English mesmerism awaits study. For contemporary accounts and attacks see J. Martin, *Animal Magnetism Examined* (London, 1790), and [anon.], *The Mysteries of Animal Magnetism Displayed* (n.p., 1789). See also R. Porter, '"Under the influence": mesmerism in 18th century England', *History Today* 35 (1985), pp. 22–9; J. Miller, 'Mesmerism', *The Listener* (22 November 1973), pp. 685–90.

71 R. Cooter, 'Bones of contention? Orthodox medicine and the mystery of the bone-setter's craft', in Bynum and Porter (eds.), *Medical Fringe and Medical Orthodoxy, 1750–1850* pp. 158–73.

72 See N. Steneck, 'Greatrakes the Stroker: the interpretations of historians', *Isis*, 73 (1982), 161–77; and A. Brian Laver, 'Miracles no wonder! The mesmeric phenomenon and organic cures of Valentine Greatrakes', *Journal of the History of Medicine*, 33 (1978), pp. 35–44.

73 Porter, '"Under the Influence"'.

74 J. W. Tibble and A. Tibble (eds.), *The Prose of John Clare* (London, 1951), p. 74.

75 Porter and Porter, *Patient's Progress*, ch. 10.

76 Whitbread (ed.), *I Know My Own Heart*, p. 160. While suffering from the infection, Miss Lister slept with another girlfriend, Tib, and passed it on to her. When Tib complained of an infection, Miss Lister played the innocent.

77 *Ibid.*

78 *Ibid.*

79 *Ibid.*, p. 161.

80 *Ibid.*, p. 163.

81 *Ibid.*, p. 229

82 *Ibid.*, p. 287.

83 A. Freemantle (ed.), *The Wynne Diaries*, 3 vols. (Oxford, 1935–40), vol. III, entry for 3 December 1803.

84 A. E. Rodin and J. D. Key, *Medical Casebook of Doctor Arthur Conan Doyle: From Practitioner to Sherlock Holmes and Beyond* (Malabar, Fl., 1984), p. 25.

85 Lathan and Matthews (eds.), *Diary of Samuel Pepys*, 17/11/1663, vol. IV, p. 385; J. Broadhurst, 'Peeps with Pepys at hygiene and medicine', *Annals of Medical History*, 1st series, 10 (1928), pp. 165–72.

86 D. Vaisey (ed.), *The Diary of Thomas Turner* (Oxford, 1984), p. 230.

87 *Ibid.*

88 *Ibid.*

89 R. Porter, *Health for Sale: Quack Medicine in Eighteenth-Century England* (Manchester, 1989), ch. 4.

90 J. Haslam, *Considerations on the Moral Management of Insane Persons* (London, 1817), p. 4.

91 For background see R. Rolls, *The Hospital of the Nation: The Story of Spa Medicine and the Mineral Water Hospital at Bath* (Bath, 1988); and M. R. Neve, 'Natural philosophy, medicine and the culture of science in provincial England', (University College, London, Ph.D. thesis, 1984), pp. 92f.

92 A. Cleland, *An Appeal to the Publick or a Plain Narrative of Facts Relating to the Proceedings of a Party of the Governors of the New General Hospital at Bath against Mr Archibald Cleland (One of the Surgeons of the Said Hospital)* (London, 1743).

93 *Ibid.*, p. 19.

94 *Ibid.*

95 *Ibid.*, p. 21.

96 *Ibid.*

97 *Ibid.*, p. 23.

98 *Ibid.*, p. 24.

99 *A Short Vindication of the Proceedings of the Governors of the Hospital at Bath in Relation to Archibald Cleland, Late Surgeon ot the Said Hospital* (Bath, 1744).

100 Cleland, *Appeal*, p. 24.

101 *A Short Vindication*, p. 17.

102 *Ibid.*, pp. 28–9.

103 *Remarks on an Appeal to the Publick by Mr Cleland and on a Letter to Him . . .* (London, 1743), p. 7.

104 Cleland, *Appeal*, p. 24.

105 A. Scull and D. Favreau, 'The clitoridectomy craze', *Social Research*, 53 (1986), 243–60.

11 Touch, sexuality and disease

1 Ashley Montague, *Touching: The Human Significance of the Skin* (New York, 1971).

2 Michel Serres, *Les cinq sens* (Paris, 1985); Desmond Morris, *Intimate Behavior* (New York, 1971); Marielene Putscher (ed.), *Die fünf Sinne: Beiträge zu einer medizinischen Psychologie* (Munich, 1978). See also R. E. Siegel, *Galen on Sense Perception: His Doctrines, Observations and Experiments on Vision, Hearing, Smell, Taste, Touch and Pain, and their Historical Sources* (Basle, 1970); M. J. Morgan, *Molyneux's Question: Vision, Touch and the Philosophy of Perception* (Cambridge, 1977); M. L. Bloch, *The Royal Touch: Sacred Monarchy and Scrofula in England and France* (London, 1973).

3 On the nature of touch, see the discussion in Vernon B. Mountcastle (ed.), *Medical Physiology*, 2 vols. (St Louis, 1968), vol. II, pp. 1345–675. On the cognitive approach to touch, see William Schiff and Emerson Foulke (eds.), *Tactual Perception: A Source Book* (Cambridge, 1982).

4 See Leo Steinberg, *The Sexuality of Christ in Renaissance Art and in Modern Oblivion* (New York, 1983).

5 On the history of pain, see R. Janzen, *et al.* (eds.), *Schmerz: Grundlagen, Pharmakologie, Therapie* (Stuttgart, 1972).

6 A. Kent Hieatt, 'Eve as Reason in a tradition of allegorical interpretation of the Fall', *Journal of the Warburg and Courtauld Institutes*, 43 (1980), 221–6.

7 See Carl Nordenfalk, 'Les cinq sens dans l'art du Moyen Age', *Revue de l'Art*, 34 (1976), 17–28. As early as the Cluny unicorn tapestries, the female comes to personify the senses, especially the sense of touch. This is true even in the earlier

manuscript illustrations to Alain de Lille which Nordenfalk brings, in which it is clear that, while all of the other senses are represented by a gender-neutral figure (and the appropriate horse representing the sense), the figure representing touch is female.

8 Plato, *Phaedo*, 60b–c.

9 *The Life of St Teresa of Jesus*, trans. David Lewis (London, 1888), p. 233.

10 Adapted from Lucretius, *Of the Nature of Things*, trans. W. E. Leonard (London, 1921), p. 61. See Ursula Schoenheim, 'The place of touch in Epicurus and Lucretius' (Cornell University, M.A. thesis, 1956).

11 Alani de Insulis, *Opera omnia* (Patrologia Latina) (Paris, 1855), cols. 522–3.

12 See Lactantius, *Divinae institutiones*, VI, in his *Opera omnia*, vol. I (Patrologia Latina) (Paris, 1844), col. 705.

13 *Marsilio Ficino's Commentary on Plato's Symposium*, trans. Sears Reynolds Jayne. University of Missouri Studies, 19, no. 1 (Columbia, Mo., 1944), p. 130.

14 I am indebted to the presentation by Marielene Putscher, 'Das Gefühl: Sinnengebrauch und Geschichte', in Putscher (ed.), *Die fünf Sinne*, pp. 147–59.

15 See J. F. Conway, 'Syphilis and Bronzino's London allegory', *Journal of the Warburg and Courtauld Institutes*, 49 (1986), 250–5.

16 On the later history of this image, see Neil Hertz, 'Medusa's Head: male hysteria under political pressure', *Representations* 4 (1983), 27–54.

17 Francisco Lopez de Villalobos, *Somario de la medicina con un tratado sobre las pestiferas bubas* (Madrid, 1498), fol. 27r.

18 Charles Hope, 'Problems of interpretation in Titian's erotic paintings', *Tiziano e Venezia* (Venice, 1980), 111–24.

19 See Otto Brendel, 'The interpretation of the Holkham *Venus*', *Art Bulletin*, 28 (1946), 65–75. On the general question of the relationship between the senses and sexuality, see A. P. de Mirimonde, 'La musique dans les allégories de l'amour', *Gazette des Beaux-Arts*, 68 (1966), 265–90 and 69 (1967), 319–46.

20 See the tabulation in Anton Pigler, *Barockthemen*, 2 vols. (Budapest, 1956), vol. I, pp. 462–5.

21 On the background, see W. von Leyden, *Seventeenth Century Metaphysics* (London, 1968).

22 Caravaggio's work stands in contrast to the traditional image of the senses as a woman. The young boy who is represented recoiling from the bite of the lizard could easily be read as a homoerotic counter-image to this tradition, especially with regard to the clear sexual implications of the animal represented. On Caravaggio's use of the lizard, see J. Slatkes, 'Caravaggio's "Boy Bitten by a Lizard"', *Print Review*, 5 (1974), 148–53 and Jane Costello, 'Caravaggio, lizard, and fruit', in Moshe Barasch and Lucy Freeman Sandler (eds.), *The Ape of Nature: Studies in Honor of H. W. Janson* (New York, 1981), 375–85. One could argue that the erotic is merely subsumed by the painful in Caravaggio's painting; see Donald Posner, 'Caravaggio's homo-erotic early works', *The Art Quarterly*, 34 (1971), 301–24.

23 See the two essays on this topic: Herbert Rudolph, '"Vanitas": Die Bedeutung mitteralterlicher und humanistischer Bildinhalte in der niederländischen Malerei des 17. Jahrhunderts', in the *Festschrift Wilhelm Pinder zum sechzigsten Geburtstage überreicht …* (Leipzig, 1938), pp. 419–45 and Hans Kaufmann, 'Die Fünfsinne in der niederländischen Malerei des 17. Jahrhunderts', in Hans Tintelnot (ed.), *Kunstgeschichtliche Studien* [Festschrift for Dagobert Frey] (Breslau, 1943), pp. 133–57.

24 Svetlana Alpers, *The Art of Describing: Dutch Art in the Seventeenth Century* (Chicago, 1983).

25 Herbert Friedmann, *A Bestiary for Saint Jerome: Animal Symbolism in European Religious Art* (Washington, D.C., 1980), p. 269.

26 Lorenz Oken, *Elements of Physiophilosophy* (London, 1847), p. 651.

27 See the discussion by Stephen Jay Gould, *The Flamingo's Smile: Reflections in Natural History* (New York, 1985), pp. 200–9.

28 Havelock Ellis, *Studies in the Psychology of Sex: Sexual Selection in Man* (Philadelphia, 1926), p. 6.
29 *Basic Writings of Nietzsche*, edited and translated by Walter Kaufmann (New York, 1968), p. 504.
30 Sander L. Gilman, 'Black sexuality and modern consciousness', in Reinhold Grimm and Jost Hermand (eds.), *Blacks and German Culture* (Madison, 1986), pp. 35–53.
31 Dorothy Nelkin and Stephen Hilgartner, 'Disputed dimensions of risk: a public school controversy over AIDS', *Milbank Memorial Fund Quarterly* 64, supplement 1 (1986), 118–42.
32 Sander L. Gilman, *Difference and Pathology: Stereotypes of Sexuality, Race, and Madness* (Ithaca, 1985), pp. 131–49.
33 James H. Jones, *Bad Blood: The Tuskegee Syphilis Experiment – A Tragedy of Race and Medicine* (New York, 1981).
34 S. Piomelli, 'Chronic transfusions in patients with sickle cell disease: indications and problems', *American Journal of Pediatric Hematology and Oncology* 7 (1985), 51–5.
35 Gilman, *Difference and Pathology*, pp. 76–108.
36 A good overview of this material is to be found in Charles Michael Helmken, *AIDS: Images for Survival* (Washington, D.C., 1989). See also the discussion of images of AIDS in my *Disease and Representation: Images of Illness from Madness to AIDS* (Ithaca, 1988), pp. 245–312.

12 Sense and sensibility

1 Samuel D. Gross, *A System of Surgery*, 2 vols. (Philadelphia, 1882), vol. I, p. vii.
2 J. Warren Collins, *To Work in the Vineyard of Surgery*, ed. E. D. Churchill (Cambridge, 1958), p. 4.
3 Stephen Smith, *The Principles and Practice of Operative Surgery*, 2nd edn (Philadelphia, 1887), p. 111.
4 For discussion of heroism in surgery, see Martin S. Pernick, *A Calculus of Suffering* (New York, 1985).
5 Henry J. Bigelow, *Introductory Lecture*, Massachusetts Medical College (Boston, 1850), p. 20.
6 *Ibid.*, p. 21.
7 John Brown, 'Rab and his friends', in *Horae Subsecivae*, 3 vols. (Edinburgh, 1882), vol. II, p. 366.
8 Elizabeth Johns, *Thomas Eakins: The Heroism of Modern Life* (Princeton, 1983), p. 56.
9 Samuel D. Gross, *Autobiography*, 2 vols. (Philadelphia, 1887), vol. I, p. 171.
10 *Ibid.*, p. 162.
11 Gross, *A System of Surgery*, vol. I, p. 482.
12 Samuel D. Gross, 'A century of American medicine: surgery', *American Journal of the Medical Sciences*, 71 (1876), 431–84.
13 Reginald Fitz, 'Perforating inflammation of the vermiform appendix; with special reference to its early diagnosis and treatment', *Transactions of the Association of American Physicians* 1 (1886), 107–36; and Charles McBurney, 'Experience with early operative interference in cases of disease of the vermiform appendix', *New York Medical Journal*, 50 (1889), 676–84.
14 Gert H. Brieger, 'American surgery and the germ theory of disease', *Bulletin of the History of Medicine*, 40 (1966), 135–45.
15 E. H. Gombrich, 'The visual image', *Scientific American* 227 (1972), 82–96.
16 The literature on Eakins is growing. Of most help were the standard biography by Lloyd Goodrich, *Thomas Eakins*, 2 vols. (Cambridge, 1982); Johns, *Thomas Eakins*; Gordon Hendricks, *The Life and Work of Thomas Eakins* (New York, 1974); Darrel Sewell, *Thomas Eakins, Artist of Philadelphia* (Philadelphia, 1982).

17 William Schupbach, *The Paradox of Rembrandt's 'Anatomy of Dr. Tulp'* (London, 1982), Supl. 2, *Medical History*.

18 For the Paris period, see especially Gerald M. Ackerman, 'Thomas Eakins and his Parisian masters Gerome and Bonnat', *Gazette des beaux-arts*, 73 (1969), 235–56. For any biographical point about Eakins, whether it be his life or his work, the two-volume study by Goodrich, *Thomas Eakins*, is indispensable.

19 Phyllis Rosenzwieg, *The Thomas Eakins Collection of the Hirshhorn Museum and Sculpture Garden* (Washington, D.C., 1977), p. 30.

20 Quoted by Lois Dinnerstein, 'Thomas Eakins' *Crucifixion* as perceived by Mariana Griswold van Rensselaer', *Arts Magazine*, 53 (1979), 140–5.

21 William C. Brownell, 'The art schools of Philadelphia', *Scribner's Magazine*, 18 (1879), 737–50, at p. 745.

22 *Ibid.*, p. 744.

23 Charles Bregler, 'Thomas Eakins as a teacher', *The Arts*, 17 (1931), 379–86; 18 (1931), 29–42; Elizabeth Johns, 'Thomas Eakins and "Pure Art" Education', *Archives of American Art*, 23 (1983), 2–5; Louise Lippincott, 'Thomas Eakins and the Academy', in *In This Academy: The Pennsylvania Academy of Fine Arts, 1805–1876* (Philadelphia, 1976), pp. 162–87.

24 Linda Nochlin, *Realism* (New York, 1971), pp. 127 and 192; see also Lloyd Goodrich, 'Realism and Romanticism in Homer, Eakins and Ryder', *Art Quarterly*, 12 (1949), 17–29.

25 Goodrich, *Thomas Eakins*, vol. I, p. 31, and Hendricks, *Life and Work*, p. 47. Hendricks has added commas for easier reading.

26 Goodrich, *Thomas Eakins*, vol. I, p. 31.

27 Clarence Darrow, 'Realism in literature and art', *Arena*, IX (1893), 98–113; reprinted in Neil Harris (ed.), *The Land of Contrasts, 1880–1901* (New York, 1970), pp. 179–88, at p. 186.

28 Especially useful articles about *The Gross Clinic*, in addition to chapters in the four major books on Eakins cited above, are Michael Fried, 'Realism, writing, and disfiguration in Thomas Eakins's *Gross Clinic*', *Representations*, 9 (1985), 33–104; Elwood C. Parry, '*The Gross Clinic* as anatomy lesson and memorial portrait', *Art Quarterly* 32 (1969), 373–91; Gordon Hendricks, 'Thomas Eakins's *Gross Clinic*', *Art Bulletin*, 51 (1969), 57–64.

29 Austin Flint, 'Memoir of Samuel D. Gross', in Gross, *Autobiography*, vol. I, pp. xii–xxxi.

30 Quoted in Hendricks, 'Eakins's *Gross Clinic*', p. 61.

31 *Ibid.*, p. 63.

32 *Ibid.*

33 *Ibid.*, p. 62.

34 *Ibid.*

35 *Ibid.*

36 Theodor Billroth, *Lectures on Surgical Pathology and Therapeutics*, trans. from 8th edn. 2 vols. (London, 1878), vol. II, p. 210.

37 For cogent analyses of *The Agnew Clinic*, see especially Margaret S. Smith, '*The Agnew Clinic*: "Not cheerful to look at"', *Prospects*, 11 (1987), 161–83; Diana E. Long, 'The medical world of *The Agnew Clinic*: a world we have lost?', *Prospects*, 11 (1987), 185–98; Patricia Hills, 'Thomas Eakins' *Agnew Clinic* and John S. Sargent's *Four Doctors*: sublimity, decorum, and professionalism', *Prospects*, 11 (1987), 217–30.

38 Goodrich, *Thomas Eakins*, vol. II, p. 46.

39 For Agnew's biography, see especially J. Howe Adams, *History of the Life of D. Hayes Agnew, M.D., LL.D.* (Philadelphia, 1892); J. William White, 'Memoir of D. Hayes Agnew, M.D., LL.D.', *Transactions of the College of Physicians of Philadelphia* 15 (1893), xxix–lxv.

40 For Agnew as a teacher and the history of the Barton chair, see Gert Brieger,

'Surgery', in Ronald Numbers (ed.), *Education of American Physicians* (Berkeley, 1980), pp. 180–2.

41 Adams, *Life of Agnew*, pp. 220–49.

42 Abraham Flexner, *Medical Education in the United States and Canada* (New York, 1910), p. 116.

43 Quoted by Rudolph M. Matas, 'William Stewart Halsted 1852–1922: an appreciation', in William S. Halsted, *Surgical Papers*, 2 vols. (Baltimore, 1924), vol. I, p. xxiv.

44 Allen O. Whipple, *The Evolution of Surgery in the United States* (Springfield, Ill., 1963), p. vii.

45 Matas, 'William Stewart Halsted', vol. I, p. xxxvi.

46 *Ibid.*

13 Training the senses, training the mind

1 Merriley Borell, 'Extending the senses: the graphic method', *Medical Heritage*, 2 (1986), 114–21.

2 Stella V. F. Butler, 'Science and the education of doctors in the nineteenth century: a study of British medical schools with particular reference to the development and uses of physiology' (University of Manchester, Ph.D. thesis, 1981).

3 See especially Arleen M. Tuchman, 'From the lecture to the laboratory: the institutionalization of scientific medicine at the University of Heidelberg' and Timothy Lenoir, 'Science for the clinic: science policy and the formation of Carl Ludwig's institute in Leipzig', in William Coleman and Frederic L. Holmes (eds.), *The Investigative Enterprise: Experimental Physiology in Nineteenth-Century Medicine* (Berkeley, 1988), pp. 65–99 and 139–78.

4 Stanley Joel Reiser, *Medicine and the Reign of Technology* (Cambridge, 1978); Audrey B. Davis, *Medicine and its Technology: An Introduction to the History of Medical Instrumentation* (Westport, Conn. 1981); Christopher Lawrence, 'Moderns and ancients: the "new cardiology" in Britain 1880–1930', *Medical History*, supplement 5 (1985), 1–33; Joel D. Howell, 'Early perceptions of the electrocardiogram: from arrhythmia to infarction', *Bulletin of the History of Medicine*, 58 (1984), 83–98; Robert G. Frank, Jr, 'The telltale heart: physiological instruments, graphic methods, and clinical hopes, 1854–1914', in Coleman and Holmes (eds.), *The Investigative Enterprise*, pp. 211–90.

5 Merriley Borell, 'Instrumentation and the rise of modern physiology', *Science and Technology Studies*, 5 (1987), 53–62, and Merriley Borell, *The Biological Sciences in the Twentieth Century*, Album of Science (I. Bernard Cohen, gen. ed.), vol. IV (New York, 1989).

6 Lawrence, 'Moderns and ancients'; Howell, 'Early perceptions'; Frank, 'The telltale heart'.

7 C. Ludwig, 'Beiträge zur Kenntniss des Einflusses der Respirationsbewegungen auf den Blutlauf im Aortensysteme', *Müller's Archiv für Anatomie und Physiologie und wissenschaftliche Medicin* (1847), 242–302.

8 E.-J. Marey, *La méthode graphique dans les sciences expérimentales et principalement en physiologie et en médecine* (Paris, 1878).

9 J. Burdon-Sanderson (ed.), *Handbook for the Physiological Laboratory*, 2 vols. (London, 1873), vol. I, p. 218.

10 *Ibid.*

11 'The Thompson-Yates Laboratories' and 'The School of Physiology', *The Sphinx: University College Students Magazine*, 6 (1898), 3–8 and 9–12, at p. 11. I am extremely grateful to Stella Butler for providing me with copies of these interesting essays attributed to Sherrington by John Eccles. See Sir John Eccles, 'Two hitherto unrecognized publications by Sir Charles Sherrington', *Notes and Records of the Royal Society of London*, 23 (1968), 86–100. Sherrington was then Holt Professor of Physiology.

12 For details, see Merriley Borell, 'Instruments and an independent physiology: the Harvard Physiological Laboratory, 1871–1906', in Gerald L. Geison (ed.), *Physiology in the American Context, 1850–1940* (Bethesda, 1987), pp. 293–321.

13 'The School of Physiology', p. 11.

14 *Ibid.*

15 Gerald L. Geison, *Michael Foster and the Cambridge School of Physiology: The Scientific Enterprise in Late Victorian Society* (Princeton, 1978), p. 56.

16 M. S. Pembrey, *Practical Physiology*, 3rd edn (London, 1910), p. v.

17 *Ibid.*

18 Edward T. Reichert, 'Some forms of apparatus used in the course of practical instruction in physiology in the University of Pennsylvania', reprint from *The University of Pennsylvania Medical Bulletin* (June 1901), 31pp., quoted from pp. 1–2. From Cambridge University, Whipple Museum of the History of Science, Cambridge Scientific Instrument Company collection, bound 'Pamphlets No. 7', item 5. I am grateful to Susan Ray, Librarian, for assistance in locating this material, and to Margaret E. A. Pamplin, Manuscripts Room, Cambridge University Library, for drawing my attention to its existence.

19 *Ibid.*, pp. 2–3.

20 Cambridge Scientific Instrument Company, List No. 9 (July 1885), p. 6. Cambridge University Library, Cambridge Scientific Instrument Company collection; 'Distribution of driving power in laboratories', *Nature*, 33 (14 January 1886), 248–50.

21 William Stirling, *Outlines of Practical Physiology, being a Manual for the Physiological Laboratory, including Chemical and Experimental Physiology, with Reference to Practical Medicine*, 3rd edn (London, 1895), pp. 383–7 and pp. 194–5.

22 Borell, 'Instruments and an independent physiology', p. 317, n. 29, and Merriley Borell, 'Marey and d'Arsonval: The exact sciences in late nineteenth-century French medicine', in J. L. Berggren and B. R. Goldstein (eds.), *From Ancient Omens to Statistical Mechanics: Essays on the Exact Sciences Presented to Asger Aaboe* (Copenhagen, 1987), pp. 225–37, at p. 231.

23 Baird & Tatlock (London) Ltd, 'Price list of chemical apparatus, chemicals, and reagents' (London, 1910), and 'Price list of chemical & scientific apparatus and pure chemicals' (London, October 1891). A history of the company is found in the centenary insert in Baird & Tatlock (London) Ltd, 'Laboratory apparatus & scientific instruments' (London, 1981). I have been unable to locate a copy of the separate physiological list described in the 1910 catalogue. The medical science and physical science collections of the Science Museum, London, as well as the Science Museum Library, hold selected Baird & Tatlock catalogues. I am very grateful to Ghislaine Lawrence, Keith Parker, Stephanie Watt and Ian Carter for assistance in locating and using these materials.

24 University of Cambridge, 'Presentation of the School of Physiology by the Worshipful Company of Drapers and its opening by H.R.H. Prince Arthur of Connaught on Tuesday 9 June 1914' (Cambridge, 1914), 15pp. I am grateful to Tilli Tansey for providing me with a copy of this document.

25 See especially Frank, 'The telltale heart'.

26 Merriley Borell, Deborah J. Coon, H. Hughes Evans and Gail A. Hornstein, 'Selective importation of the "exact method": experimental physiology and psychology in the United States, 1860–1910', in British Society for the History of Science and the History of Science Society, 'Program, Papers, and Abstracts for the Joint Conference, Manchester, England, 11–15 July 1988' (Madison, Wis., 1988), pp. 189–96. On William James, see Deborah J. Coon, 'Courtship with anarchy: the socio-political foundation of William James' pragmatism' (Harvard University, Ph.D. dissertation, 1988).

27 Lisa Rosner, 'The professional context of electrotherapeutics', *Journal of the History of Medicine and Allied Sciences*, 43 (1988), 64–82; Joel Howell, 'Early use

of X-ray machines and electrocardiographs at the Pennsylvania Hospital', *Journal of the American Medical Association*, 255 (1986), 2320–3.

28 Borell, 'Instruments and an independent physiology'.

29 Richard C. Cabot, 'The historical development and relative value of laboratory and clinical methods of diagnosis', *Boston Medical and Surgical Journal*, 157 (1907), 150–3, at p. 151. I am grateful to Hughes Evans for drawing my attention to this article.

30 Joel Howell, 'Machines' meanings: British and American uses of technology 1880–1930' (University of Pennsylvania, Ph.D. thesis, 1987).

31 Leslie Cromwell, Fred J. Weibell, Erich A. Pfeiffer and Leo B. Usselman, *Biomedical Instrumentation and Measurements* (Englewood Cliffs, N.J., 1973), p. 4.

32 Christopher Lawrence, 'Incommunicable knowledge: science, technology and the clinical art in Britain 1850–1914', *Journal of Contemporary History*, 20 (1985), 503–20.

33 Paul R. Torrens, 'Historical evolution of health services in the United States', in S. J. Williams and Paul R. Torrens (eds.), *Introduction to Health Services*, 2nd edn (New York, 1984).

34 Cabot, 'Historical development', pp. 150, 152 and 153.

35 See Borell, 'Instruments and an independent physiology', p. 319, notes 62, 64, 65 and 68 for a list of such texts.

36 Russell Burton-Opitz, *Advanced Lessons in Practical Physiology for Students of Medicine* (Philadelphia, 1920), p. 17.

37 Richard C. Cabot, *Case Teaching in Medicine: A Series of Graduated Exercises in the Differential Diagnosis, Prognosis and Treatment of Actual Cases of Disease* (Boston, 1908), p. vii.

14   Technology and the senses in twentieth-century medicine

1 James Sawyer, 'Clinical thermometry', *Birmingham Medical Review*, 4 (1875), 109–17, at p. 116.

2 Henry Catell, 'Roentgen's discovery, its application in medicine', *Medical News*, 68 (1896), 170.

3 C. A. Wunderlich, *On the Temperature in Diseases: A Manual of Medical Thermometry* (London, 1871), p. 75.

4 National Commission on Allied Health Education, *The Future of Allied Health Education* (San Francisco, 1980).

5 *Ibid.*

6 J. Burdon-Sanderson, 'The Characteristics of the arterial pulse...', *British Medical Journal*, (1867, 2), 19–22, 39–40 and 57–8, at p. 39.

7 Alvan R. Feinstein, *Clinical Judgment* (Baltimore, 1967), pp. 4–8, 29, 285–6 and 324–34.

8 Julius Herisson, *The Sphygmometer, an Instrument which Renders the Action of Arteries Apparent to the Eye* ..., trans. E. W. Blundell (London, 1835), p. 14.

9 Willem Einthoven, 'The different forms of the human electrocardiogram and their signification', *Lancet* (1912, 1), 853–61, at p. 854.

10 Walter C. Alvarez, *Nervousness, Indigestion, and Pain* (New York, 1943), p. 111.

11 Walter C. Alvarez, 'Diagnostic time savers for overworked physicians', *Journal of the American Medical Association*, 122 (1943), 933–7, at p. 933.

12 Denise Grady, 'Going overboard on medical tests', *Time* (25 April 1988), p. 80.

13 John D. Stoeckle (ed.), *Encounters Between Patients and Doctors: An Anthology* (Cambridge, Mass., 1987), p. 49.

14 Fred E. Masarie, Jr., Randolph A. Miller and Jack D. Myers, 'INTERNIST-I properties: representing common sense and good medical practice in computerized medical knowledge base', *Computers and Biomedical Research*, 18 (1985), 458–79.

See also R. A. Miller, 'INTERNIST-I/CADUCEUS: problems facing expert consultant programs', *Methods of Information in Medicine*, 23 (1984), 9–14.

15 James B. Herrick, 'The importance of the history and physical examination to diagnosis', *Journal of the Indiana State Medical Association*, 24 (1931), 69–72, at p. 71.

16 George L. Engel, 'Are medical schools neglecting clinical skills', *Journal of the American Medical Association*, 236 (1976), 852–5. See also Stanley J. Reiser, *Medicine and the Reign of Technology* (Cambridge, 1978), pp. 165–70.

Index